The Deaf Way II Reader

The Deaf Way II Reader

Perspectives from the Second International Conference on Deaf Culture

Harvey Goodstein
Editor

Gallaudet University Press ❖ **Washington, DC**

Gallaudet University Press
Washington, DC 20002
http://gupress.gallaudet.edu

© 2006 by Gallaudet University Press
All rights reserved. Published 2006
Printed in the United States of America

Library of Congress Cataloging-in-Publication Data

International Conference on Deaf Culture (2002 : Washington, D.C.)
   The Deaf way II reader : perspectives from the second international conference on deaf culture / Harvey Goodstein, editor.
     p. cm.
   Includes bibliographical references and index.
   ISBN-13: 978-1-56368-294-0 (alk. paper)
   ISBN-10: 1-56368-294-X (alk. paper)
   1. Deaf—Social conditions—Congresses. I. Goodstein, Harvey. II. Title.
III. Title: Deaf way 2 reader. IV. Title: Deaf way two reader.
HV2359.I487 2006
362.4′2—dc22   2006030661

∞ The paper used in this publication meets the minimum requirements of American National Standard for Information Sciences—Permanence of Paper for Printed Library Materials, ANSI Z39.48-1984.

Contents

Foreword ❖ I. King Jordan   xi

Preface   xiii

PART ONE: Advocacy and Community Development

Changing the World—Together ❖ Benjamin Soukup   3

Our Inalienable Rights: Global Realization of the Human Rights of Deaf People ❖ Liisa Kauppinen   10

Are Deaf People in Developing Countries Advocating on a Political Level? A South African Perspective ❖ Wilma Newhoudt-Druchen   17

World Deaf Leadership Project Enhances Deaf Empowerment in Thailand ❖ Peoungpaka Janyawong   21

Communication, Sign Language, Culture, and Education as Human Rights ❖ Yukata Osugi   26

Hands across the Pacific: Partnerships for Progress ❖ Jan Fried, Nancy Bridenbaugh, and Linda Lambrecht   32

Partnership in the Irish Deaf Community ❖ Kevin Stanley   38

Deaf Empowerment in Greece ❖ Vassili Kourbetis and Kostas Gargalis   42

A Model in Accessing the Community for Deaf-Blind Adults ❖ Maricar Marquez and Ilissa Rubinberg   48

Improving Development Assistance from American Organizations to Deaf Communities in Developing Countries ❖ Amy Wilson   52

PART TWO: Economics

How We Can Better the Lives of Deaf People in Developing Countries through Business Investment ❖ Adebowale Ogunjirin   61

Successful Entrepreneurship in Third World Countries ❖ Alok Kumar Kejriwal   64

Successful Strategies for Deaf Business Professionals ❖ Emilia Chukwuma, Ronald Sutcliffe, Jim Macfadden, Yuri Maximenko, David Barber, and Bernard Brown   66

A Comparative Investigation of Entrepreneurship among Deaf Populations in Developed and Developing Countries ❖ Isaac O. Agboola   73

PART THREE: Education

Deaf Education: Whose "Way" Is It? ❖ Laurene Simms   81

Signs of Literacy: Naturalistic Inquiry into ASL/English Bilingualism at Home and at School ❖ Carol J. Erting, Cynthia Neese Bailes, Lynne C. Erting, Carlene Thumann-Prezioso and Marlon Kuntze   87

Deafness and the Pedagogy of Difference ❖ Gladis Perlin   96

American Sign Language Curriculum for First-Language ASL Students ❖ Heather Gibson   100

Asian Deaf Perspectives on Deaf Education ❖ Cynthia J. Plue   107

Academic Writing of Deaf Students in Higher Education: Processing and Improving ❖ Krister Schönström   114

PART FOUR: Family

Deaf Couples and Adoption ❖ Rune Anda   121

The Psychological Support Offered to "New Parents" of Deaf and Hard of Hearing Children in Cyprus ❖ Kika Hadjikakou   127

The Missing Link in Literacy Development—A Parent's Perspective ❖ Nayantra Kanaye   134

The Silent Garden: Reaching Out to Your Deaf Children ❖ Paul W. Ogden   141

Deaf Parents with Teenage Children ❖ Paul Preston   145

Deaf Parents with Hearing Children: A CODA Symposium ❖ Thomas H. Bull, Elizabeth Beldon, and Bert Pickell   152

PART FIVE: Health and Mental Health

Mental Health and Deafness Go Global ❖ Barbara Brauer   163

Mental Health Services in the Philippines: A Deaf Perspective ❖ Maria Tanya L. de Guzman   166

Cancer Awareness Project: Deaf Cancer Wise ❖ Carly Munro   172

AIDS and Deaf People: Health Service Delivery and Prevention for Deaf People by Deaf People ❖ Julie Elaine Roy and Michel Turgeon   178

Reconstructing Deafness: A Solution-Focused Approach to Mental Health ❖ Sue E. Ouellette   181

PART SIX: History

Russian Deaf Towns ❖ Elena Silianova   189

Iranian Deaf Culture ❖ Abbas Ali Behmanesh   193

Our Civil Rights Movements: A Guide for All ❖ Kelby Brick   199

Houses out of Sand: Building a Deaf Community in Israel ❖ Meir Etedgi   205

The Status of Deaf People in Developing Countries ❖ Raphael Domingo   213

PART SEVEN: Language and Culture

The Domino Effect: Changing Values = Changing Language = New Styles of Training ❖ Clark Denmark and Frances Elton   219

How Is Asian Deaf Culture Different from American Deaf Culture? ❖ Steven Chough and Kristina Dobyns   227

Sign Language Use among Indigenous Populations ❖ Jeffrey E. Davis   233

Onomatopoeia in British Sign Language? or, The Visuality/Sensation of Sound ❖ David Fowler and Mark Heaton   241

What Is Deafhood and Why Is It Important? ❖ Paddy Ladd   245

Deaf View Image Art: A Manifesto Revisited ❖ Betty Miller, Deborah Sonnenstrahl, Alex Wilhite, and Paul Johnston   251

PART EIGHT: Literature

Crossing the Divide: Helen Keller and Yvonne Pitrois Dialogue about Vaudeville ❖ Rachel M. Hartig   267

The Poetics and Politics of Deaf American Literature ❖ Cynthia Peters   272

ASL Literacy in Early Childhood: ASL Poetry ❖ Robyn Sandford   278

Conceptual "Rhymes" in Sign Language Poetry ❖ Sarah Taub   284

PART NINE: Recreation, Leisure, and Sport

The Role of Deaf Sport in Developing and Maintaining Deaf Identity in Great Britain ❖ Jordan Eickman   293

Deaf Women and Sports in Nigeria: Problems and Prospects ❖ Anthonia Ngozika Euzouwa   301

The D/deaf Community, Leisure, and Public Recreation ❖ Gina A. Oliva   305

PART TEN: Sign Language and Interpreting

How to Be All Things to All People: ASK! ❖ Carole Lazorisak and Lynne Eighinger   315

Variation in Sign Languages: Methodological Issues and Research Findings ❖ Ceil Lucas, Robert Bayley, Ruth Reed, Rob Hoopes, Steven Collins, and Karen Petronio   322

Linguistic Development and Deaf Identity in Rural Rio Grande do Sul, Brazil ❖ Ricardo Vianna Martins   336

The Role of the U.S. Court Interpreter in the New Millennium ❖ Carla M. Mathers   340

Narratives in Tactile Sign Language ❖ Johanna Mesch   344

PART ELEVEN: Technology

Genetics: A Future Peril Facing the Global Deaf Community ❖ Joseph J. Murray   351

Making Ourselves Heard: The Promise of No-Barriers Communication ❖ Raymond J. Oglethorpe   357

The Dilemma of Pediatric Cochlear Implants ❖ John B. Christiansen and Irene W. Leigh   363

The Impact of Genetics Research on the Deaf Community ❖ Jane Dillehay and Kathleen Arnos   370

WISDOM: Wireless Information Services for Deaf People on the Move ❖ Gunnar Hellström   376

Telecommunications Access: An American Civil Right ❖ Karen Peltz Strauss and Gregory Hlibok   380

Accessible Educational Media: Research, Development, and Standards ❖ Larry Goldberg, Madeleine Rothberg, and Mary Watkins   386

PART TWELVE: Youth

Climbing the Seven Summits: A Deaf Woman's Dream ❖ Heidi Zimmer   393

What Makes a Good Deaf Leadership Camp in Germany, Thailand, and the United States? ❖ Dan Brubaker, Beverly Buchanan, Stefan Goldschmidt, and Simeon Hart   398

A National Organization of Deaf-Blind Youths ❖ Linda Eriksson, Eva Jansson, and Emil Beijersten   405

The Past, Present, and Future of Deaf Youth in Russia ❖ Vladimir V. Kotenev   410

Vital Self-Determination of Deaf Youth in Russia in Conditions of Social
    Instability ❖ DMITRY REBROV   414

Contributors   417

Index   419

Foreword

About seventeen years ago, a small group of individuals at Gallaudet University began to discuss the idea of a Deaf Way international conference. We agreed that in the past, every time people came together to talk about deafness, people talked about problems such as the difficulty of educating deaf children, for example. The focus always seemed to be on how to help deaf people. Our group at Gallaudet knew that was wrong. We knew deaf people have a lot to brag about and that deaf people have a lot to be proud of. We wanted people to come together and celebrate the Deaf way. Many people, even people at Gallaudet, were skeptical about our idea of a conference like this and told us that this kind of conference would not attract many people. They said a few researchers, a few interested students, and perhaps some local deaf and hard of hearing people would come, but other than that, we would not be able to attract people to come together to celebrate deafness. Those skeptics were really, really wrong. Some of you today were among the five thousand people who came to the first Deaf Way in 1989. At that time the five thousand people who attended the conference made that the largest international gathering of deaf people ever. Of course it is not the largest anymore: today we see the largest international gathering of deaf people ever, with ten thousand people here.

During the first Deaf Way, we celebrated deaf cultures from around the world. We listened, we learned, and we had many discussions and debates. It was a rich and rewarding experience. More important than that week itself were the long-term results. Because of Deaf Way, many, many people have many wonderful stories about what happened afterward and how their lives changed as a result of Deaf Way. For me, I think the most significant long-term result was what I call personal to-do lists. Many of us left Deaf Way with lists of what we would do in the future to help change the world for deaf people. We made lists of actions we promised ourselves we would do. Our lists were each unique, of course. Some things on our lists were like going back home and convincing the government to provide better access to education and job opportunities. Our lists included the notion of returning to school to earn a degree, or even an advanced degree, sometimes in fields where before deaf people did not frequently study. Others knew they could change jobs or enter the business world and become deaf entrepreneurs. However, all of our lists had things in common also. We all agreed to stay active today and tomorrow and to continue to celebrate and honor the diversity of the deaf community throughout the world. Each of us in our own way has helped keep the spirit of Deaf Way alive.

This week we will talk about what we have accomplished during the thirteen years since the first Deaf Way. This week we come together again but in even larger numbers. This week we have an opportunity to share our knowledge, our hearts, and our community. I know that we will learn a great deal this week. We will enjoy ourselves also. More important, I hope that Deaf Way II will reinforce our commitment to work together toward positive change. I hope that we will leave with new to-do lists filled with ideas of how we can work together. Start your list this morning. Start now. Take out paper and a pen, or if you have a high-tech notebook, take that out. Start your list. Carry your pen with you every day to all of the meetings. Help make the world a better place for deaf people.

I. King Jordan

Preface

By all indications, the Deaf Way II international conference and arts festival (DWII) hosted by Gallaudet University in Washington, D.C., on July 8–13, 2002, was an outstanding success. The exciting and unique event, patterned after the first successful Deaf Way (also hosted by Gallaudet University on July 9–14, 1989), exceeded all expectations as described in the vision statement adopted by the Deaf Way II Organizing Committee (DWOC):

> Deaf Way II, an international gathering to be held in Washington, D.C., USA, July 8–13, 2002, will be an opportunity to reflect on the past and imagine the future of the world's Deaf community. Bringing together thousands of participants to share and celebrate the experiences of deaf people, the conference and cultural arts festival will enlighten, enrich, and expand society's concept of deaf life.
>
> Deaf Way II will:
>
> 1. Encourage cross-cultural and cross-continent exchanges through an international conference on language, culture, history, and art of deaf and hard of hearing people.
> 2. Examine technology use by, for, and on deaf people, and consider the interconnectedness of deaf, hard of hearing, and hearing people in an increasingly technologically sophisticated world.
> 3. Celebrate the visual, performing, and literary arts of deaf and hard of hearing people through a Cultural Arts Festival.
> 4. Foster greater tolerance and understanding among deaf, hard of hearing, and hearing people through scholarly discussions and experiential cultural events for participants, and extensive outreach to the general public.
> 5. Heighten opportunities for deaf and hard of hearing people by bringing to light our artistic, leadership, and professional capabilities and diverse contributions to societies around the world.

There were 9,675 participants from 121 countries officially registered for DWII by the end of the DWII week. Nearly all of them registered for the entire conference rather than for a day or two. Of that number, 3,108 registrants (32 percent) were from international countries, including 1,642 people from developing nations or economies. The opening celebration, conference program, and on-campus theatrical performances were open only to registrants (closed to the general public). However, it has been estimated that a total of 12,000 people attended the DWII events open to the public at the two primary convening areas at the Washington Convention Center (WCC) and Gallaudet University during the DWII week.

In addition, an estimated total of 400,000 people attended the DWII-related events, art exhibits, and theatrical performances at approximately ten public venues in the Washington, D.C., metropolitan area, over a period of several months, from May to September 2002. Two venues were related to the Smithsonian. A Smithsonian official expressed pleasure at a significant surge of at least 100,000 attendees at the Arts and Industries Building, which housed the History through Deaf Eyes exhibit. Also, the Smithsonian conducts its annual Folk Life Festival on the National Mall around the first week of July every year, which is open to the public and has hundreds of thousands of attendees. For July 2002, its Asian-oriented theme was the Silk Road. On Saturday, July 6, it featured DWII artists, namely the Hong Kong Theatre of the Deaf, My Dream (Chinese classical dance), Karthika and Astad Deboo (contemporary Indian dance), and the Japanese Theatre of the Deaf. One observer remarked that lots of people carrying and using DWII's orange bulletin as "fans" all over the National Mall that day created a wonderful sight.

We have reached many more people nationally and worldwide using direct mail, articles in newspapers (including the *Washington Post*, the *New York Times*, and newspapers and newsletters in other countries), the Internet (www.deafway.org, washingtonpost.com, and others), and the National Public Radio.

The two primary programs during the DWII week were 1) the conference program, including exhibition booths, which was held at the WCC and Grand Hyatt Hotel in the mornings and afternoons, and 2) the arts festival program, which was held at Gallaudet University and many local public venues around the Washington, D.C., area, mostly in the afternoons and evenings. In addition to these two programs, DWII events and activities included the opening celebration, DWII youth programs, the international Deaf club/kids' fun center, tours of Gallaudet University, and the closing banquet.

The purpose of the opening celebration was first to enable Gallaudet University President I. King Jordan to officially welcome the participants to the DWII international conference and arts festival and to state the importance of the six-day gathering. The opening celebration was also an opportunity for host Gallaudet University to create an academic and festive atmosphere by giving the participants in the audience a sampling of the speakers, presenters, and artists involved in the conference and festival. This program, which took place on Monday night, July 8, in the tightly packed 7,000-seat Hall A of the WCC, was so spectacular that it set a highly enthusiastic and festive mood for the week.

The international conference component included 301 presenters in 198 time slots of forty-five minutes each from Tuesday, July 9, through Saturday, July 13. Some presentations were made individually or jointly, and others were in symposium or panel formats, some of which extended over two time slots. Also included were seventeen plenary and keynote presentations and about twenty poster sessions on various topics. There were twelve different strands or topics of interest within the conference program: advocacy and community development; economics; education; family;

health and mental health; history; language and culture; literature; recreation, leisure, and sports; sign language and interpretation; technology; and youth. The names of all presenters and titles and brief descriptions of presentations could be found in the 186-page *Deaf Way II Program Book*, which was distributed to all of the registrants.

It is of interest to note that technology was not a major topic for discussion during the first Deaf Way in 1989. During the 1990s, federal laws were enacted enhancing telecommunications (telephone relay services) and media (captioning) access for deaf and hard of hearing people. Also, over the past decade a number of significant technological innovations and enhancements (including Web cam, video relay interpreting, and wireless two-way pagers) were developed in the areas of communications useful to deaf and hard of hearing people. Another topic of increasing interest was the adoption of children by deaf parents and other family issues.

The conference also included exhibition booths, which were open to the public at the WCC for three days, Tuesday, July 9, through Thursday, July 11, instead of the entire week. However, attendees made it clear that the booths had so much to offer that they needed at least one additional day. Altogether, there were more than 150 booths for the attendees to browse and experiment with new products. The "international alley," featuring arts, crafts, and many other small-shop operators, took up roughly one-half of the total booths. The corporate booths, occupied mostly by the various telecommunications companies exhibiting latest technological advances, comprised about one-third of the total booths. Various Gallaudet University units clustered at a "Gallaudet island," including the Office of Admissions, Graduate School, Laurent Clerc National Deaf Education Center, Gallaudet University Press, and the bookstore, occupied the remaining booths. In addition, in a lounge area situated in the middle of the exhibit area, the attendees were able to watch a replica of the 1965 Shelby Cobra Roadster being assembled from a kit by some ten deaf high school students attending Gallaudet University's Summer 2002 Youth Scholars Program.

Although the conference presentations were open to only the registrants, the arts festival program was open to the public, primarily at Gallaudet and at off-campus venues in the Washington, D.C., metropolitan area. The orange festival program was widely distributed at the public venues to heighten public awareness about DWII and Gallaudet University.

The arts festival included thirty-two deaf theater and dance companies selected to perform, which involved a total of 369 individual performers and 125 crew and staff. There also were 15 storytellers (solo performers), 15 writers, 15 filmmakers, 68 featured visual artists, and 6 emerging visual artists.

Three featured deaf artists were invited to work on campus as artists-in-residence prior to the start of DWII and to do commissioned work. Chuck Baird (USA) was here for more than a year from early summer 2001 through end of summer 2002. He served as a consultant for the DWII Visual Arts Committee, created a number of paintings for Gallaudet University, and served as a curator for DWII visual arts. He also worked with a number of student interns and co-taught, along with Peggy Reichard, a course titled "Internship: Art Exhibit Planning and Installation" to sixteen students in spring 2002. Abelardo Jimenez (Columbia) arrived in June 2002 to complete a large stone sculpture called "Universal Knowledge," which was installed on campus about fifty yards from the southwestern corner of College Hall. Sander Blondeel (Belgium) arrived in June 2002 but was unable to complete a large oval glass piece due to the late arrival of glass ordered from a New York shop. He returned to Gallaudet in fall 2002 to complete his commissioned work, which is now hung by a large window on the second floor of College Hall. In addition, a local Emmy award–winning puppet maker, Ingrid Crepeau, was on campus for the spring 2002 semester and taught a unique course in giant puppet making. Each student designed and completed a large bird puppet, which was used in DWII's opening celebration.

One of the challenges was to secure sufficient performance spaces for use during the DWII week to accommodate the more than 9,500 registrants and thousands of other ticket buyers. At Gallaudet, we were able to use Elstad Auditorium, Elstad Black Box, and Ely Center Auditorium. Also at Gallaudet, one large tent was set up on Olmsted Green holding two theaters, each theater seating 300, aptly named Bernard Bragg Theatre on the Green and Phyllis Frelich Theatre on the Green in honor of the two nationally acclaimed deaf performing artists. Additional performance spaces were obtained at off-campus public venues through partners such as the Kennedy Center (Millennium Stage), Smithsonian (Discovery Theater), Maryland-National Capital Park and Planning Commission (Publick Playhouse/Harmony Hall), and the Smith Center at the University of Maryland (Kay, Kogod, and Gildenhorn Theatres).

The art exhibits were open to the public for a period much longer than the six-day DWII event, and the History through Deaf Eyes exhibit had the longest opening period, from May 9 to September 10, 2002. At Gallaudet, the exhibits were at Chapel Hall (sculpture), the Edward Miner Gallaudet (EMG) building (photography), the Gallaudet University Kendall Conference Center (GUKCC; glass, silver, and ceramics), and Washburn Arts Center (the "main course," i.e., a sampling of art from most of the sixty-eight artists). Art exhibits were also shown at the following off-campus venues: the Kennedy Center, the Arthur M. Sackler Gallery of Art, the Swedish Embassy, the National Zoo, the Mexican Cultural Institute, the National Arboretum Administration Building, the Millennium Arts Center, and the Smithsonian Arts and Industries Building.

The film and video festival component was open to the public and held at the GUKCC. Approximately twenty films and videos of varying lengths were shown. Deaf and hearing filmmakers came together in person to present films and videos that include deaf individuals.

The Deaf Way II Anthology, a 196-page book published by Gallaudet University Press prior to DWII, included literary contributions made by sixteen deaf and hard of hearing writers. This collection included poetry, essays, short stories, and one play that bear witness to the Deaf experience. Copies of the book, funded in part by the National Endowment for the Arts, were distributed to the DWII registrants during the DWII week. In addition, there were symposiums and workshops during the week for the attendees to exchange their writing experiences, concerns, and ideas.

Children and teenagers were able to register for any one of the four DWII youth educational programs conducted on campus during the week. Shuttle buses were provided so that children could be picked up at and brought back to the WCC daily. Because of space limitations, we had to regretfully turn down additional applications for those programs. The programs were (1) young children's world (for those two to five years old), with twenty-one children registered; (2) child education program (six to eight years old), with thirty-two registered; (3) pre-teen educational program (nine to twelve years old), with fifty-six registered; and (4) teen programs (thirteen to seventeen years old), with fifty registered in either the culture enrichment camp or the sports camp. The activities included cooking, arts and crafts, team-building activities, computer literacy activities, leadership program, and culture exchange, to name a few. There also were hands-on workshops led by DWII featured artists. The children and teenagers loved the programs so much that every morning they could hardly wait to get on the shuttle buses for Gallaudet for additional activities. Parents also were very pleased with the contents of the programs.

The International Deaf Club (IDC), set up at the WCC, was a place where the participants could relax, socialize, and dance each night from 8 p.m. to 2 a.m. Some claim that the IDC was the largest walled deaf club in the world! It measured 300 feet by 300 feet, with six large video screens and music amplifiers so powerful that the volume had to be turned down to one-fourth of its full power. There were a number of stage shows and movies. There were many more talented artists than the available number of invitations we could allow within our scheduled arts festival. The IDC provided opportunities for those artists to display their talents by performing mime, magic, storytelling, and so forth on stage. Adjacent to the IDC was the kid's fun center, which provided different sports and arcade games as well as several air-blown plastic and rubber mats for the kids (and adults!) to explore and jump on. The IDC also included food booths where people could order meals or snacks and many round tables at which people could sit, eat, and chat.

Gallaudet University has been universally regarded as a flagship institution promoting education, training, and empowerment of deaf and hard of hearing students. Shuttle buses were provided for transportation to Gallaudet University, where tours were arranged by our Visitors Center during the week. Visitors could appreciate its historic significance and learn more about its current academic programs at the undergraduate and graduate levels, including services and programs for international students who need to learn English or wish to participate in exchange programs. There was a strong demand for visits to Gallaudet all week long; indeed, even on the last day of the week, when there was a significant reduction of on-campus planned activities, we had to secure additional buses to transport an unanticipated large congregation of registrants. Evidently, they wanted to learn as much about Gallaudet as they could. Although the new Student Academic Center and the Student Union Building were not quite completed at that time, the visitors were able to walk through the buildings and have a look at several prototype high-tech classrooms and laboratories designed for use by deaf and hard of hearing students. Fortunately, the Gallaudet bookstore opened just in time for the registrants and other guests. The volume of sales of DWII and Gallaudet items was high.

The closing banquet was held from 7 p.m. until midnight on Saturday, June 13, at the elegant Great Hall of the National Building Museum, which was the site of the inaugural ball for Gallaudet University President I. King Jordan in 1988. The registrants needed to buy tickets at an additional charge for this sold-out event, which was limited to 1,650 people. The attendees had an opportunity to wear their best formal clothes representative of their countries. The event included a showing of video clips of DWII highlights of the week, music, a short program, and dancing. A toast was made as the evening came to a close. Everyone was recognized for attendance, participation, and support, which made Deaf Way II a successful international celebration of deaf and hard of hearing people's capabilities and accomplishments and created anticipation for many positive things to come.

Communication access has always been a challenge at any international conference or gathering because of differences in written, sign, and spoken languages. At the World Federation of the Deaf conferences, which occur every four years, three official languages are used for discourse, namely: the host country's sign language, International Sign (standardized signs and grammar derived mostly from European countries), and written/spoken English. The presenters, interpreters, and captions were projected on large screens to enhance visibility and readability. Most international conferences follow a similar model and setup; in the case of DWII, the official languages used were American Sign Language, International Sign, and written/spoken English.

DWII Interpreting Committee coordinated the interpreting, and every presentation at the DWII conference had output in the three official languages, including spoken English and real-time captioning (written English) projected on large screens. The international groups that were not fluent in any of the three official languages brought their own interpreters, who could translate spoken English into their native sign language. Conversely, international presenters who brought their interpreters could make presentations in their own native languages for the interpreters to translate into spoken English, so that successive interpreting could be done in the official languages and real-time captioning in English could be projected onto the large screens. The DWII Interpreting Committee also worked out the logistics with foreign sign language interpreters to make sure that they could stand on a riser close to their international groups throughout the assembly.

Another committee, known as the Developing Nations Support Service (DNSS) Committee, was expanded to provide support and assistance to all international registrants. The DNSS coordinated the insertion of twelve different icons representing the twelve conference topics, three icons representing the three arts festival major areas, and three keywords describing each presentation or activity in the program book to facilitate its navigation by international participants. In addition, the DNSS developed a video and used a large room in the Washington Convention Center for walk-in sessions to orient and assist the international participants in the selection of presentations relevant to their needs.

A total of thirty-four Deaf-Blind/tactile and fifty-one Deaf-Blind/close vision individuals constituted about 1 percent of all the DWII registrants. On the basis of requests made by Deaf-Blind individuals at least two months in advance, the DWII Interpreting Committee coordinated the provision of Deaf-Blind tactile or close vision interpreters during the week. Support service providers (SSP) were also provided to work with Deaf-Blind participants during breaks, meals, travel between events, and so forth. Alternate versions of the program book were also provided in Braille and large print for them to read.

Many international constituents who know written English eagerly volunteered to become the regional or country contact people and spread the word about DWII in their own languages by giving translated presentations or materials and providing assistance in filling out registration forms in written English. Some of them went even further and asked for permission to do partial translation of the DWII Web site into native languages on their Web sites. We gladly gave them permission to do so and created links from the DWII Web site to theirs. There were thirteen links altogether.

A total of ninety-two registrants identified themselves as individuals with "other access needs" on the application form. About 10 percent of them contacted the DWII office in advance about their disabilities and desired accommodations, and we made plans accordingly; we even made contingency plans for a few additional registrants who asked for assistance after they got here. A DWII staff member with a focus on disability access consulted with a staff member from the Office for Students with Disabilities and made the necessary arrangements by providing personal care assistants (PCAs), vehicles with hydraulic lifts, and other transportation, including taxis, as requested.

By all indications, the DWII international conference and arts festival was a well-run and enormously successful event that allowed for exchange of academic, professional, artistic, and cultural content. To be sure, Gallaudet University has invested a lot in the unique event by providing large amounts of financial, human, and physical resources. Was it a worthwhile investment on Gallaudet University's part? My answer definitely is a resounding yes! The world certainly looks up to Gallaudet as a flagship institution in the education, training, and empowerment of deaf and hard of hearing people. It would be most appropriate for Gallaudet University to continue to host a significant event such as Deaf Way at least once every eight to ten years to keep instilling hope for great achievements in all the disciplines and attainment of a high quality of life for deaf people.

The positive impact of DWII on Gallaudet University is briefly highlighted next. Also, the positive impact of DWII on international participants is described with a number of examples.

During the four years of planning, student involvement increased incrementally and then exponentially as the DWII week approached. We had pre-college students at the Clerc Center who observed and did some artwork with a DWII artist in residence. Internship opportunities were provided to students, such as making tall bird puppets for the opening celebration. Other opportunities enabled students to become curators of DWII artwork and hang them at a number of art exhibits in the Washington metropolitan area. Students could sign up for classes about conducting research in disciplines including English and history. Some students worked in the DWII office as assistants to committee leaders and gained hands-on experience in the managing of a large international conference, most notably in the areas of registration and application processes for conference presenters and festival artists. We had at least three hundred student volunteers who provided remarkable leadership support to various committees. There were at least one hundred alumni volunteers who worked with us with dedication and pride during the week. Numerous partnerships were created between Gallaudet University and a number of institutions, including the Smithsonian, the Kennedy Center, and the University of Maryland. We also fostered a working relationship with the U.S. Department of State regarding visa matters and with other federal agencies on grants. Contacts were made with our current and new individual and corporate supporters to make donations and contributions to DWII and

Gallaudet University. Public awareness about deaf and hard of hearing individuals' capabilities and accomplishments in the professional, corporate, and artistic worlds was enhanced.

During the thirteen years since the first Deaf Way in 1989, there were significant new developments that needed to be shared and discussed at a large international gathering. Indeed, new bodies of research on history, culture, arts, and literature concerning deaf and hard of hearing people were collected during those years. Federal laws were enacted promoting human rights and accessibility for deaf and hard of hearing individuals including the Americans with Disabilities Act of 1990, the TV Decoder Circuitry Act, the Individuals with Disabilities Education Act, and the Telecommunications Act of 1996. Another phenomenon was the emergence of Internet, wireless communications, broadband access, and digital video technologies with useful applications for deaf and hard of hearing people. During those years, we saw a large growth of deaf and hard of hearing professionals, business owners, artists, and advocates of human rights and equal access who have done well and serve as excellent role models for many individuals from all over the world. DWII provided a forum for such information sharing, showcasing individual skills and new technologies and increasing our appreciation for art and culture. Many international participants left the conference feeling empowered, with increased hope and determination to improve education, services, and the quality of life for deaf and hard of hearing people at home.

The special fall 2002 issue of *Gallaudet Today* about DWII contains some excellent examples of the positive impact on international participants, some of which are extracted here.

- ❖ "The many Canadian participants were proud of [Max] Fomitchev, who at Deaf Way II performed a one-man show and served as the Opening Celebration's master of ceremonies. 'It feels good to be a free man, and to represent a free country,' he said. 'I want to show the world what deaf people can do,' he continued. 'I want other deaf people to achieve their dreams and have big goals. That's what Deaf Way I [in 1989] did for me, and I want to return the favor'" (p. 17).
- ❖ "Takeo Sato from Japan said his most lasting impression were formed by the services for deaf people he saw that week, giving him hope for the way life can someday be at home. The easy access to interpreters was one of the things that astounded him. 'There are so many interpreters here!' he exclaimed. 'There are not enough in Japan, and we need to get more.'" (p. 17).
- ❖ "Dar and Aditi Patel, visiting from India, said that Deaf Way II made them see that the time has come for progress at home. 'In India, deaf women are very suppressed; they must live at home until they get married,' said Dar Patel. 'Now, I realize that many deaf women from around the world live on their own'" (pp. 17–18).
- ❖ "Kehinde Akewusola and Odutola Odusanya from Nigeria said they, too, want to see changes to improve life for deaf people in their country. They came to learn how to make it happen, and to ask for help. . . . Odusanya, who is a university teacher, said things have gotten a little better since he started teaching 20 years ago, but it is not enough. . . . 'First and foremost,

we need good role models. We need people to come and volunteer to help improve the deaf curriculum'" (p. 19).

❖ "While staying at the Renaissance Hotel in Washington, D.C., a group of 56 Deaf Way II participants from Switzerland got together to discuss how to improve services for deaf people in their country. 'Right now the Swiss parliament is formulating and rewriting the Equity Act—similar to the Americans with Disabilities Act . . .' said Roland Hermann, president of the Swiss-German Deaf Association. . . . So the group wisely decided that Deaf Way II would be a great opportunity to expose the powerbrokers in Switzerland to what deaf people around the world have accomplished. En masse, the group went to the Swiss Embassy and invited the Swiss ambassador to attend Deaf Way II. Their efforts paid off. The following morning, Susanne Blickenstorfer, the wife of the Ambassador of Switzerland agreed to come."

That same issue of *Gallaudet Today* contains 48 pages of excellent articles and pictures about DWII. There also is an exciting pictorial book, about 200 pages long, titled *Deaf Way II: An International Celebration*, published by the Gallaudet University Press in 2004. The pictorial book brings the wonderful programs and activities of DWII to life through pictures and brief narratives. In addition, videos in DVD and VHS formats were published by the Gallaudet University Press in 2004 covering the opening celebration, the highlights of the week, and an interview with King and Linda Jordan.

It has been a challenge getting the presenters to submit a final version of their presentations for follow-up publication and archiving. That may be attributable in part to differences in languages and difficulties expressing thoughts and concepts in written English as requested. Video recording and captioning transcripts were done at each presentation, but a few videos and transcripts are missing at this time. Nonetheless, we are fortunate to have most of the presentations covered by using a combination of the outlines, final papers, videos, and captioning transcripts, which are now in the archives here at Gallaudet and are available for use by students, faculty, and researchers.

This book includes about seventy-five selected papers that were presented during the DWII conference. We made an attempt to include every keynote and plenary presentation in their proper section. For the sections based on the twelve conference strands, several papers were selected so that the authors came from different countries and the papers covered varying subtopics, as far as possible. We hope that from these representative papers in the book the reader will appreciate the wide range of topics covered and exchanged during the conference.

The tremendously successful DWII would be impossible without the strong, unwavering support from Gallaudet University, particularly president I. King Jordan and his office, the administration, faculty, staff, students, and volunteers during the planning and operational stages. It is impossible to thank every individual involved because there are too many of them. Nevertheless, the members of the Deaf Way Organizing Committee (DWOC) are to be commended for their steadfast dedication and commitment to make DWII a memorable event that all of us here at Gallaudet will cherish with great pride for many years to come.

The DWOC members include chair, Harvey Goodstein; vice chair—Operations Committee, Dwight Benedict; program assistant, Laura Brown; special assistant to chair and Development Office liaison, Cathy Sweet-Windham; international coordinator, Rosanne Bangura; coordinator of international affairs, John Lewis; coordinator—Conference Program Committee, Mike Kemp; coordinator—Cultural Arts Committee, Jay Innes; Performing Arts Subcommittee producers, Tim McCarty and Paul Harrelson; Visual Arts Subcommittee coordinator, Peggy Reichard; coordinator—Volunteers Program Committee, Mary Anne Pugin; coordinators—Interpreting Committee, Diana Markel and Juniper Sussman; consultant, Jan DeLap; coordinator—Marketing Committee, Roz Prickett; coordinators—Technology Committee, Jeff Murray and Lloyd Ballinger; coordinator—Merchandise Committee, Astrid Goodstein; coordinator—Advertising Committee, Vladimir Kotenev; liaison—Office of Public Relations, Mercy Coogan; liaisons—Office of Sponsored Programs, Stan Matelski and Audrey Wineglass; liaisons—Business and Auxiliary Services Division, Fred Kendrick and Mike Lockhart; liaison—Finance Office, Billy Hughes; photo editor/Web designer, Ralph Fernandez; and art/layout designer, Zhou Fang.

Gallaudet University as the host institution was the largest sponsor of the DWII conference. We were fortunate to also receive support from many sponsors that enabled us to make DWII a truly worthwhile and memorable international conference and festival. Some of the major sponsors need to be mentioned here with thanks, and they are Communication Service for the Deaf, Inc. (CSD); Sprint; America Online; MCI; NBC4; Freiss Foundation; Macfadden and Associates, Inc. (MAI); Washington Metropolitan Area Transit Authority (Metro); and washingtonpost.com.

For this book, thanks go to Laura Brown, who contacted the authors and collated the papers. I am most thankful to receive significant editorial assistance and support from Ivey Wallace and Deirdre Mullervy of the Gallaudet University Press.

Finally, many thanks go to Astrid and our family for their steadfast support throughout all these years since 1998, from the first day of planning for the DWII conference and beyond to the publication of this book.

Harvey Goodstein, Editor

PART ONE

Advocacy and Community Development

Changing the World—Together

BENJAMIN SOUKUP

I know a story about an eight-year-old child, a little boy, who had an experience with his parents, his father in particular. He had a deaf mother and a deaf father, and a brother and sister who were also deaf. This eight-year-old boy loved his father very much and hoped some day he would be able to be just like his father and be a farmer. His father worked hard in the fields every day, and the son was thrilled at the thought that someday he would follow in his father's footsteps and run the family farm. The eight-year-old boy watched one day as a storm passed through and destroyed the crops and some of the buildings. The insurance did not cover the damages, and so the father took the young son with him to the bank to see what could be done. The father wrote back and forth to the banker explaining what had happened to this farm and his crops and the need for additional funding so they could continue operating the farm. The little boy watched all of this as they communicated back and forth via paper and pen. The banker said, "I don't know if we can loan you any money; we don't feel that a deaf person has the ability to run a farm. I suggest that you look at other options." But there were no other financial options or sources, and so they were forced to auction off their possessions.

The day of the auction was probably one of the saddest days of the boy's life. He saw piece by piece—the cultivator, the tractor, the livestock—being sold until nothing was left. This little eight-year-old boy saw the family lose the farm. They had to relocate to town, and the father became a carpenter, but he was not happy. His father passed away when the boy was twelve, and this boy never forgot what his father went through, how his deafness was looked down upon, and how his mother had to take care of the family. He graduated from the South Dakota School for the Deaf, and as he was growing up he wondered if he would ever have his own farm. He would have been proud to be a farmer, but that was not meant to be.

This boy later went to Gallaudet University, and when he came back to his home, he worked at a meatpacking plant. He remembered the passion that his father had; he saw the things that his father tried to accomplish and the frustration that resulted because of stereotypes, attitudes, discrimination, and oppression. This led the boy to work with the deaf community to change that from happening to others. He saw so many other deaf individuals who went through life experiencing frustrations because of barriers and limited opportunities. They were not given the chance as others often are. That little eight-year-old boy was me. I learned at a young age the realities of deafness and was instilled with the passion to change things for the better. That passion in that eight-year-old old boy is still burning today. It has never gone out.

When I became the president of South Dakota Association of the Deaf (SDAD), I studied the organization's history, the organization's structure, and everything that it stood for. They have fought for individuals' rights since it began in 1902. It was located in a very rural area, and many people would travel one hundred miles on horse and buggy just to gather and attend conferences. My father was involved with the organization, and again, I wanted to follow in his footsteps. When I was able to become the president of this group, we helped establish Communication Service for the Deaf, Inc. (CSD). As a result, I was asked to become the CEO, and John Buckmaster took my place as president of SDAD. He was a tremendous influence on me, a wonderful advocate fighting for the rights of deaf individuals who always listened to their needs and was always willing to stand by the deaf community, willing to testify. He was very heavily involved with the American Athletic Association of the Deaf (AAAD). A lot of people consider him to be the father of the AAAD softball and baseball tournaments. And he was just a simple potato farmer. When he was the president of SDAD and I was the CEO of our organization, we started a very close journey together that would last for many years, and we worked with many fine individuals. Many of these individuals are in the audience today. They are the people who established a very strong foundation for CSD, and that is why CSD is where it is today.

Another thing I would like to tell you about is the value of the community. After I came back from Gallaudet University, I returned to the South Dakota deaf community. They had a softball team, social events, and a very small core of probably forty or fifty deaf people living in the local town. Most of these deaf people worked at John Morrell & Company, a meatpacking plant that was one of the largest and highest-paying employers in the area. I became employed there myself because I wanted to be with the rest of the group, and it was a wonderful experience. During our break times, we would get together and chat about deaf issues and plan deaf events and sport activities. When we were not doing this at work, we were doing this on the weekends at a deaf club located on the third floor of a downtown building.

One day, we were informed that we were no longer able to hold our deaf club meetings there because the building was no longer safe for use. We decided to relocate the club, and that is where the community found a beginning. Until that point, we took it for granted that we would have a place to congregate, but now there was an issue placed before us. We were challenged with meeting an immediate need for the greater good of the group. What were we going to do? We had to find a solution, and we did just that. We worked quickly and efficiently. We found an old army barracks that was in disrepair, and that is where it started. We were challenged, we had a vision, we knew what this deaf club would look like, and we worked very, very hard to create what we thought was one of the most beautiful deaf clubs around. This seemingly insignificant event encouraged us. We realized what we could do if we worked together. We began to seriously discuss other issues facing the deaf community: the lack of interpreting services or community support services and meeting the needs that many individuals had. We went to the SDAD convention at that time and discussed how we could better our lives. We then pursued funding avenues with the state and with other organizations and started a snowball affect. My main point is the value of community.

I went to a National Association of the Deaf (NAD) conference in my younger years, and I fell in love with the NAD goals and mission, their objectives. Later, when the NAD was experiencing a very difficult time in their history, dealing with finances, staffing, programs, and a myriad of other issues, I was given a chance to join their board. We worked hard and long to address the issues, and it was a wonderful growing and developing experience for me. We continued our efforts to find solutions and address the issues, including the education of deaf children, cochlear implants, and a wide variety of other important national issues. We worked on finding new sources of funding and reorganizing the structure of the NAD organization. I believed that we could make a difference in the lives of deaf and hard of hearing people on a greater, national level. We still faced many, many barriers and discrimination, and I knew that the NAD alone could not do the job itself. It required a lot of people—people from the local level to the national level working together. We established the State Association Presidents Conference (SAPC) to encourage this. We thought that this would be a way of improving communication and involvement. The SAPC was very successful, it still is today, and we have seen improvements in communication among the national, state, and local levels. A lot of communication is taking place through the Internet.

We also established the NAD tour. We felt there was a need to bring the organization to the people and to provide information to the membership about the organization, its purpose, its structure, and its strengths. The NAD cannot be a strong organization without the involvement of its membership, so we had the national tour. In our travels across Deaf America, we saw a lot of people with passion and dreams—people who felt that they could achieve a better place in life. I saw people with desire, people wanting opportunities, and people needing direction and guidance. The NAD tour increased the membership of the organization, and I think many of our agenda items that we established were due to the forums that we created at the NAD. This provided the membership with an opportunity to express their views and what they would like to see the NAD prioritize as far as projects. It is not possible for the NAD to do everything. The NAD has a very small staff; they are achieving a lot of miracles every day for all of us.

The only way we can really make a substantial difference is by working together with them. If you work alone, you will only continue to be isolated, and that is a challenge. We often isolate ourselves, we divide ourselves, and we limit our potential as a result. We may not always have all the answers, but I and many other people in Deaf America—throughout the world even—believe that we can find solutions and that the best way of doing that is by working with each other. The NAD will always have a special place in my heart, and I will always be there for the NAD, because it is one organization that truly advocates for the rights for deaf and hard of hearing people. They have for more than one hundred years.

The SDAD gave me their full support. They believed that we should move in a certain direction, so I started working closely with a wonderful partner, Sprint. We bid for contracts together, and we were involved with them because we were a deaf-consumer-driven organization. By working together, we believed we could provide high-quality services in the area for the deaf and hard of hearing people. CSD would provide the facilities, management, and support, and Sprint would provide the technology and the engineering. It has been a truly wonderful and successful partnership that has led directly and indirectly to many other things. In fact, not very long ago we celebrated our ten-year partnership together. Today, CSD is now involved with video relay, which was partially developed by CSD, and Sprint is helping us market this service. You will be able to see that product here at Deaf Way. You will see a lot of activities taking place with our deaf relay services and our video relay services; we are trying to branch out on a global basis with these new products. I think this has taught all of us a valuable lesson—the value of working with other businesses, those in the community, state government, and others.

In the past, service organizations have relied on federal and state grants and funding sources to support human services. This social service concept was and is widespread. At CSD, we changed our philosophy about how we provide businesses and human service models. The many political changes that take place affect and drive funding sources. Any time you see a change in political leadership, priorities change. The economy may change, and that greatly impacts services and funding sources. In addition, we cannot expect to rely solely on the government to meet all of our needs. We have the responsibility to find businesses that are willing to share the same mission, a philanthropic mission of supporting the community. This leads to partnerships whereby businesses and human service models can work together. By using the philosophy of working with businesses to address social responsibilities, we are able to establish our own direction. We are still a nonprofit organization, but we work with other for-profit organizations to provide certain services and products. We then utilize funds that we generate from certain products to help subsidize our human services. This way, if there is a human service we want to provide, we can find a way to do it. For example, we have a variety of senior citizen programs; we have transportation, apartments, and housing programs for deaf people; we have a recreational program and activities within our deaf community center. Where is it that you can find funding to support all of these venues? For us to have our own destiny, for us to create our own destiny, we must take the responsibility to find the funding for services. I do not think that there is really another way of accomplishing this.

Today CSD has well more than two thousand employees. There is a mixture of deaf and hearing people alike working together. Our hearing employees believe very strongly in what we are trying to accomplish. In the same light, our deaf employees have opportunities that they may not otherwise have had in other companies. We strongly believe that working together, we will find solutions and will address many of the issues that face deaf and hard of hearing people. It is up to us to take the responsibility of establishing our own destiny rather than depending on someone else to create that destiny for us, and I think that is a great value.

CSD has been involved with many partnerships and national organizations. One in particular is the USADSF—the USA Deaf Sports Federation—led by Dr. Bobbie Beth Scoggins, who is the president of this organization. We met some time ago and had the chance to sit down and look at the possibilities of a partnership between CSD and USADSF, and we felt that both organizations could contribute and complement each other. We recently announced our partnership and will be working very closely together, sharing resources, and supporting each other. One of the exciting new developments is the establishment of a museum for USADSF. There is a rich history of many, many activities, national sporting events, and tournaments. Some of these athletes have participated in the World Games for the Deaf. This is a wonderful thing for the future of our children, who are able to come in and see the museum and their role models. If you have the opportunity to come and visit us, feel free to stop by our campus and see our new center. We feel that this will be ready for the public in the fall of 2002.

I also want to share our involvement with the WFD—the World Federation of the Deaf. When I was the president of the NAD, Nancy Bloch and I represented the NAD at the WFD conference in Vienna, Austria. It was a very long flight, and I suppose many of you experienced the same thing flying here to Washington, D.C. My travel there was one of the highlights of my life. It really opened my eyes about how much we share worldwide. We had the chance to meet many different leaders throughout the world who used different languages and signs—we tried to learn as many international signs as we could. It was a wonderful opportunity to share common experiences, some funny, some very sad, and it was a rich learning experience for all of us. Yerker Andersson, who was president of the WFD at that time, shared many of his experiences in his travels, including some very difficult experiences in very dangerous areas. That is something Yerker was always willing to do—help individuals try to establish schools and programs, deal with governments and politicians, and educate them about how they can improve the lives of deaf people. There are not very many people in the world who are able to dedicate as much time and commitment as Yerker. He is definitely one of my role models, and I look forward to the new president, Liisa Kauppinen. I also admire her, an outstanding woman who has worked very diligently. She was the secretary for the WFD under Yerker before she became president. I had an opportunity to visit with her when she came to South Dakota. We recently had a symposium on deaf education, and Liisa was able to join us. I had a chance to really get to know her, her work, what she is trying to achieve, and the funding support she is hoping to acquire for her organization. CSD is committed to supporting the WFD. We believe in their work and encourage more people to be more involved and to be more supportive of the WFD. Some of us are very fortunate to live in America or in European countries. We have many conveniences, but there are many other deaf and hard of hearing brothers and sisters in other parts of the world who are experiencing needs, and it is our obligation to assist them. When we talk about change, we need to work together with them for everyone's benefit. I think we can do it, but it requires our collaboration worldwide.

There is value in supporting the community and also the value of our employees. I really admire the employees at CSD, their energy, their dedication, and their passion. They come to work every day in hopes of making improvements in the lives of deaf and hard of hearing people. What drives them? I have found that all of them have passion. Not long ago, we had an executive from a large corporation who came to visit us and said, "One of the things that impresses me the most about CSD is that you allow every individual in your organization to dream. Don't ever lose that. This is a place where everyone feels they are part and parcel of the organization. They have ownership. They have ownership of the future." I am very proud of that. It is a place where anyone can contribute. We have employees, both deaf and hearing, who have technical expertise, and they focus on finding technical enhancements to improve the lives of deaf people. There are human service employees trying to improve lives, making sure that daily needs are being met, and making sure that people have equal opportunities to participate and receive services that they need. There are administrative and support employees who provide services that make all of the programs possible, the kind of internal services that help a company run. From the groundskeepers to the CEO's office, we have a wonderful mixture of deaf, hard of hearing, and hearing people all working hand in hand toward the same goals and mission. Our employees are not only involved and committed to CSD but other organizations as well, providing support to them. Some are involved with the NAD. Some of them are involved on a local level, working with youth groups. Some volunteer their time in working in communities. They truly are role models for others, and it is a very beautiful thing to see. About forty of our employees are here with us at Deaf Way II. All of them have been very motivated about attending this event. You might see them here, proudly displaying their CSD shirts. They want to share their stories and knowledge with you, so take the time to visit with them and ask them to share their dreams and their experiences with you. I am sure they will be happy to do so.

There is no greater investment than in our youth. When I was on tour as the NAD president or in my travels on behalf of CSD and different communities, I truly enjoyed meeting many outstanding young deaf people, who were very articulate, intelligent, and destined to be our future leaders. Unfortunately, I believe we are not investing as much as we should in youth programs. CSD established a youth camp for leadership and literacy training. Joe Murray, who will be giving a presentation this week, has been involved with the WFD youth programs and with youth around the world, and I think this is a great investment for our youth today. How can we invest in these people in creative ways? We have found that our experiences with interns from Gallaudet, the National Technical Institute for the Deaf (NTID), and California State University (CSUN) has been very inspirational. Many of these students have realized their potential, and they find a passion in life, not necessarily continuing their work with CSD, but continuing elsewhere in their lives in many different ways and areas. We need to continue those kinds of opportunities for youth. Gallaudet University, the world's only liberal arts college for deaf and hard of hearing students, has been doing many wonderful things. We do appreciate Gallaudet University's efforts to empower and encourage deaf and hard of hearing people, not only here in America but also throughout the entire world. Also, Rochester Institute of Technology (RIT) is a wonderful technical college for deaf students, where the NTID is one of seven colleges at RIT allowing deaf and hard of hearing students to learn more about technology and many other majors. CSUN is yet another fine university for deaf and hard of hearing students. All over the world, there are many other fine universities, which could provide an education to deaf and hard of hearing students. We just need to have a chance to have everyone work together to allow those investments in youth to take place. If there is not enough funding, we should find other creative ways to get the needed funding for youth programs. We need to explore ways that do not limit the opportunities for children to go to camp or to get an appropriate education, so that they may fully realize their potential.

As you can see, we have a rich history of accomplishment through the years. We have been involved in civil rights, trying to implement programs, establish goals, create opportunities, and improve many things. We have been trying to change the world by working together. CSD's new slogan is actually "Changing the World Together." We want to continue to work with new technology, address new challenges, and create new dreams. I often tell my staff that we are here today, not to benefit ourselves but to benefit others and to ensure that the future is better than what we have today. We have the responsibility and the obligation to establish a new direction for future generations by planning appropriately and by working together.

Our Inalienable Rights: Global Realization of the Human Rights of Deaf People

LIISA KAUPPINEN

The topic of my presentation is "Human rights are our inalienable rights." We need to discuss how to realize human rights for each and every Deaf person in the world. I have listed three themes in my presentation: (1) human rights belong to everyone; (2) human rights documents can ensure Deaf people's equal entitlement to all human rights; and (3) governments are responsible for the practical implementation of human rights for all. These three themes provide different approaches to achieving a good life.

We Deaf people see good life anchored to the use of sign language. It is our right to use our language and our right to be ourselves as Deaf people. But very often, other people cannot see life as a Deaf person as a positive thing. Additionally, there is an ongoing discussion on bioethics and what a "normal" human being should be. That view of a human being is narrow and should be condemned. Deaf people struggle to attain our right to live as Deaf people in today's societies and to lead happy lives. Deaf people are remarkable in our capacity for creativeness. If we sense a deficiency in an environment where we live, we find our own solution to correct that deficiency. We have developed visual languages and are ingenious in our ways of creating lifestyles based on visual solutions. However, that's something that is underestimated and held in low esteem by the uninitiated public. Very often, however, we as individuals and as a community do not have the political power to make decisions for ourselves. All these issues are human rights issues. I want to focus on that and on the global situation in regard to education.

It is really important for all of us to bear in mind that human rights are our rights—rights that belong to each and every one of us. All the different human rights instruments exist for the sole purpose to ensure that governments allow us to exercise our human rights. Deaf people realize that even though some sign languages are becoming more widespread, they are not being completely recognized by governments and society nor are our points of views listened to and respected enough.

The right to life is automatically a human right as indicated in the first three articles of the Universal Declaration of Human Rights adopted by the United Nations in 1948. Everybody has the right to life, freedom and security of person. We have discussed these rights insufficiently. We need to discuss education, we need to discuss sign language, but we need also to intensify discussions about the right to life and related issues. Joe Murray mentioned the case of the two Deaf women who wanted to have a Deaf baby that resulted in lots of discussion in the global press and on the Internet. The mothers were accused of giving birth to a baby that was condemned to lead an unhappy life. I have been pondering where this kind of thinking stems from.

I would like to discuss the doctoral dissertation by Simo Vehmas (2002) that was just recently published, "Deviance, Difference, and Human Variety: The Moral Significance of Disability in Modern Bioethics." His work focuses on the right to life, the right to exist. The latest advancements in biotechnology have greatly influenced bioethical discussion from the medical view on the pathological aspects and undesirableness of Deafness. When many bioethicists discuss the quality of life and the criteria for a good life, their emphasis invariably shifts to scientifically improving the physical qualities of human beings who are perceived to be disabled.

Deaf people often assert that we are not disabled people, but rather that we are a culturally linguistic minority. But our situation in the hearing world is actually the same as those of physically disabled people. The larger world does not appreciate our views, our knowledge, nor our experience and they label us as disabled people who need to be cured. This narrow point of view devalues us as human beings. The medical professionals involved in these discussions share the mistaken philosophy that disability always causes suffering to individuals and to their families, and incurs tremendous expense to the government. This kind of thinking encourages the development of biotechnology to prevent disability. There are, however, researchers who don't feel this perception is right. They believe that disabled people are unhappy when society does not treat them as valid human beings, but instead defines them as defective according to medical criteria. Disabled people suffer as a result of that pathological attitude. The same goes for Deaf people. If our language is not accepted, if our ways of living are not accepted, then we suffer. When we can use our language and when we can use our solutions as our way of life, then we can lead very satisfying lives.

A Scandinavian survey about mental health issues investigated what sorts of results medical help produced in treating psychiatric issues. The survey showed that neither medical help nor intensive psychological therapy were the most effective in treating mental health issues. In fact, social interaction with friends and within different networks and domains were the most effective therapy. That's exactly the situation for Deaf people.

The larger society's belief that it is overwhelmingly expensive to support people with disabilities is simply not right. In fact, not one government has gone bankrupt because of its support for people with disabilities. Governments' complaints about the excessive cost of disability support reflects their questionable and warped values. Governments spend a tremendous amount of money on the military and big sports stadiums; there's always enough money budgeted for that. So it's not a question of whether something is really expensive or not; it's a question of values and priorities.

Deaf people are not involved enough in bioethical discussions. We need to first engage in these discussions within our own community, and then we need to expand the circle to include our friends who work with us and the politicians who make policy and fiscal decisions in order to be ready to discuss these issues with bioethicists and consultants. We must participate in these discussions to help the "experts" broaden their views. In his dissertation, Vehmas also criticizes parents' authority to decide whether or not to abort a fetus if they learn it is disabled. He argues that because doctors often give narrow one-sided information to these parents, their decisions cannot be fully informed. Whether or not they have made the right decision then becomes really questionable.

Parents have the responsibility for the well being of their future child, taking care of the child, and giving the child a good life. But nowadays our values seem to be based on a the business world model. Education seems more about quality criteria, standards, and outcome expectations than learning. Now we seem to be setting the same sorts of criteria for fetuses, criteria that children need to fulfill in order to be allowed to be born. If they don't meet those criteria, then is it justifiable to get rid of them by aborting them? If so, our ethics have really taken a wrong turn; it's a dangerous situation. We should do something to help future children to have the right to life, regardless of the differences and variations in human characteristics.

Deaf people have faced difficulties in explaining what a good life is for us. Cultural anthropologists, sociologists, linguists, and other researchers have conducted studies demonstrating what deaf people need for a positive quality of life but their research has had surprisingly little effect. What more do we need to do to convince people that we do know what a good life for us is? For centuries, generation after generation of the larger society has sought ways to "correct" Deaf people in order to make us more like hearing people. And their attempts have always attracted appreciation and support. It is only when Deaf people manage to learn to talk or behave like hearing people that they get respect from society. Yet, when we ourselves create different solutions, achieve access and communication, lead rich lives, and contribute to society, society seems to dismiss our accomplishments.

When parents learn that their child is deaf, they usually are not given a full spectrum of information. They are not aware about the realities, possibilities and successes for Deaf people nor are they aware that anything is possible for us. Parents of Deaf children never receive this information; consequently, they can't understand why they shouldn't grieve and are unable to accept our solutions. They may fear losing their children to a foreign language or a cultural group. They want to keep their children; they see us in an opposite camp. It is really unfortunate this is the current situation, which leads to many misconceptions and hardships in the lives of Deaf children, including being deprived of their natural language.

The current situation results in many needlessly illiterate Deaf people who lack social interaction, have linguistic, social, and information inadequacies, cannot find work, have difficulties in coping and managing their own lives, and experience mental health problems. These situations exist simply because the Deaf points of view are not heard by the larger society. Our experiences and solutions are simply dismissed.

Being oppressed because we are Deaf is a human rights issue and we must work hard to overcome and attain all of our human rights. The right to integrity is also a human right. I have met with people who work with children's rights; they conduct surveys and research on children's rights. The Convention of the Rights of the Child, which the United Nations General Assembly ratified in 1989, states that the child's right comes first and is paramount. The parents' rights are secondary to the well being of the child—including the right to be born, the right to exist as is, and the right to integrity and security. These people I know in the field of children's rights say that it's like Deaf adults have abandoned Deaf children. The larger society views Deaf children as needing medical interventions. Who decides whether these children have the right to live as Deaf people? Who advocates for them as Deaf children? This is a question of human rights. Is it right to live as a Deaf person? Who is the one who can define our human rights? It's us, and we must do that for ourselves. We must define what our rights are. The bioethical experts can't do that. The outsider views and documents on human rights have defined overarching human rights that pertain to everybody, but we must define, clarify, and interpret to society the human rights for Deaf people.

According to Phillipson and Skutnabb-Kangas, "people who are deprived of linguistic human rights may thereby be prevented from enjoying other human rights, including fair political representation, a fair trial, access to education, access to information and freedom of speech, and maintenance of their cultural heritage" (2001). So if we want to promote our human rights, we must bear these issues in mind.

It's really crucial that we study human rights tools as developed by the United Nations. There are certain things that we have to learn in life. In school we learn multiplication tables until we know them by heart. We have learned our national anthems, and we know those by heart as well. I believe we also should learn human rights issues by heart as part of our educational curriculum. We need to master these tools to help us gain equality in life. We must also know the national and international processes, practices of appeal, and the ways of influencing the development of legislation. These will enable us to attain our freedom of speech and the right to promote our language and our culture. You receive education so that you can better participate in life of the society. Knowledge and application of human rights secure possibilities and opportunities for us.

The United Nations has enacted human rights acts and declarations that define the rights and freedoms all humans are entitled to. The most important human rights include the right to exist, the right to our language, and the right to our culture. The first and most important covenant within the U.N. system is the Universal Declaration of Human Rights (1948). The other important covenants of significance to Deaf people are the International Covenant on Civil and Political Rights, the International Covenant on Economic, Social and Cultural Rights, the Convention on the Rights of the Child, the Convention on the Elimination of All Forms of Discrimination against Women, and others like the Standard Rules on the Equalization of Opportunities for Persons with Disabilities, ILO's Agreements 159 and 169, and the UNESCO's Salamanca Statement and Framework for Action on Special Needs Education.

National governments have ratified those instruments and cooperate with the different U.N. agencies that are responsible for monitoring the implementation of these declarations. But very often nothing is said in the reports about Deaf people's human rights. Hence it is our responsibility to gather and provide information about the status of Deaf people's lives to our governments and the U.N. agencies so that they can monitor the implementation of Deaf people's human rights. The Standard Rules on the Equalization of Opportunities for Persons with Disabilities includes the right to sign language, interpreting services, and related issues.

There is a strong tendency to modify an individual rather than to modify the environment. But the Standard Rules emphasize a developmental process by which society and various environmental systems (i.e., services, activities, information, and documents) are placed within everyone's research and in particular, within disabled people's reach. These excellent support documents can be used when you go to your own governments and advocate for your rights as a linguistic and cultural minority group.

All our rights are derived from the basic rights to our own language and culture. The solution and principle of human rights is not to change the Deaf individual but to modify the environment so that it will be good for everyone. The World Federation of the Deaf (WFD) views being Deaf as a sociocultural issue where language and culture serve as a basis for equality. Sign language deprivation at an early age leads to obstacles and serious disability, whereas the use of sign language minimizes barriers and restrictions in the environment. We must have a clear vision of Deaf people as members of a linguistic and cultural group, as well as part of the disability movement.

I have seen Deaf people throughout the world. Eighty percent of Deaf people, most of whom live in developing countries, do not receive an education. There are developing countries where school enrollment for all approaches 95 percent but only 5 percent of Deaf children receive an education. This results in much discrimination in regard to their further education, employment, and receipt of community services. Discrimination and abuse of Deaf children are highly common everywhere in the world. Educational rights, linguistic rights, freedom of expression, the right to be heard, self determination, and the right to integrity remain elusive goals.

For Deaf people in developing countries, many different factors impact their lives. Poverty is an obvious factor. There are countries in Asia, Africa, and Latin America where the majority of people have to live with an income of less than one dollar per day. There are countries where there are no service structures, no telecommunication devices, and even no electricity so it's not easy for Deaf people to make progress in these countries given these limitations. We must bear in mind that people from the developing countries are not any less intelligent or capable than us; they just don't have the same basic possibilities that we have for solutions. Nonetheless, they do have their own ways of helping each other. For instance, in Zambia there is a group of Deaf women who weren't able to find employment. All of them had children, and had problems finding food for their families. So they decided to buy some chicks, raise them, and sell the eggs. They shared clothes with one another and passed children's clothes on to younger children. They created and sold some handcrafts. They created their own solutions, and their own ways of coping.

Much progress has been made in the past twenty years with the increasing availability of bilingual education and the recognition of sign language in more than thirty countries. Yet tens of millions of Deaf people are still without the most rudimentary conditions for life; many live in areas that often suffer natural catastrophes, pollution, drought, and a lack of clean water and food. War is the worst obstacle to progress, with women and children suffering the most. So although much new development has occurred, with much success, there still remains so much to do in so many countries. And therefore, we need cooperation.

Access to education should be rapidly increased. Literacy and trained interpreters are needed so that Deaf people can assert for themselves the provision of education and services with officials and politicians. Joint development cooperation projects with Deaf people and their organizations in third-world countries can be arranged. These help Deaf people to upgrade their know-how in the fields of management, planning, and economics.

Deaf people need cooperation, ideas, and training because that gives confidence in ourselves—confidence that we can do whatever we want to. We are capable. We can influence our living environment. In lots of countries, however, Deaf people are still unaware of how to use their government's political process to achieve legislation that would allow them to mandate change in their favor.

Several countries in Asia, Africa, and Latin America have achieved good results through involvement and cooperation. Prominent Deaf leaders from one country have then helped Deaf leaders in other countries to develop and gain skills. We need this type of cooperation to enable us to be aware of our lives, our culture, and ourselves—and what constitutes a good life for us, from our point of view. We must define that for ourselves, by ourselves. With the current global situation and ongoing bioethical discussions throughout the world, we must be active and proactive in that determination. We need a strategy, and a plan, at the national and international levels in order for us to promote our human rights and our agenda.

Strategies you can use for the future to improve the lives of Deaf people include becoming aware of the significance of sign language, Deaf culture and the history of Deaf people; becoming aware of Deaf people's rights, the U.N. Human Rights mandates, the U.N. Standard Rules, the Salamanca Statement; learning about political and economic power, legislation, and services provided in your own country; and being aware of the changes, development, and planning that involve Deaf issues.

The Statutes (Article 2) of the WFD prioritize the implementation and promotion of human rights as a duty of our organization. WFD has adopted a strategy plan for the next five years titled "Facing the New Millennium: Equality is Quality of Life." We are heavily engaged in all U.N. Human Rights work that promotes the rights of Deaf people and also taking part in preparing the emerging Convention on Human Rights for Persons with Disabilities, but it is the U.N. member states and governments who have the power to decide their outcome. Therefore it is very important that the members of WFD must try to influence the representatives of the member states! Your involvement is needed to influence your government's representatives who make decisions for and recommendations to the United Nations. At the moment, because of groundbreaking developments in the field of human rights with already existing mandates, cooperation needs to continue at both national and international levels.

As an interesting aside, when the General Assembly of the United Nations approved the drafting of a new Convention on Human Rights of Persons with Disabilities, the WFD was not sure whether we should join that process or not. We consider Deaf people to be a linguistic and cultural group rather than a disabled group. However, there isn't that much networking in the field of linguistic minorities and there are no conventions in the rights of linguistic minorities. Moreover, the other linguistic minorities still aren't ready to accept us as one of them. Thus we decided to join the disability movement instead. I do appreciate the efforts of the disability movement, and at the international level we have received so much support from disability organizations. At a meeting on persons with disabilities in Mexico just a couple of weeks ago, we received much support for a linguistic rights clause within the Convention on Human Rights for Persons with Disabilities. But the drafting work is still going on. We do submit suggestions and propose text, but it's the government who ultimately decides. My Finnish government delegate who had attended U.N. meetings came back to Finland, looked me up, and asked me point blank, "Why don't the other Deaf associations in other countries contact and collaborate with their respective governments? Every time I attend a U.N. meeting, I noticed that the other government representatives don't know anything about Deaf people. They don't have a clue about sign language, so I have to teach them!"

So we all have the responsibility to contact our governments and teach them about our issues. Please make sure that you contact and keep in contact with your U.N. delegates on issues important to us. That's the way we can advance our issues. And I really hope that in the future U.N. meetings, the ones who make the decisions on different instruments and conventions will be aware of Deaf issues. The only way they can learn those things are with your help and with the help of your organizations. Your cooperation is essential. If we don't do that, then there's no point in hoping that we will attain our human rights. Please remember that WFD is not a government, we don't have a decisive voting power within the United Nations—we are just there as consultants. And lastly, please remember that human rights are your rights. With these different documents, conventions, and covenants, it is the government's responsibility to implement them, but Deaf people must advance our agenda and assist our government representatives. Let's all sign and sing this together:

> *Get up, stand up*
> *stand up for your rights*
> *Get up, stand up*
> *don't give up the fight*
> *Get up, stand up*
> *life is your right*
>   Bob Marley

Are Deaf People in Developing Countries Advocating on a Political Level? A South African Perspective

WILMA NEWHOUDT-DRUCHEN

For many years, our history in South Africa was *dominated* by apartheid, a social and political policy of racial segregation and discrimination enforced by white minority governments in our country from 1948 to 1994. The laws and policies of apartheid had a tremendous negative affect on our country and how people viewed disabled people in our country. South Africa has had a very strong welfare system, but it remained just that: a welfare system that did not encourage people on welfare to think about their human rights and to become independent.

Disabled People of South Africa (DPSA) was started during apartheid in 1984. The DPSA's goal is to promote the human rights of people with disabilities. The DPSA has monitored the human rights of deaf people and advocated for their human rights. From the beginning, the DPSA has had a very good relationship with the African National Congress (ANC), which is now the ruling and majority party in South Africa. The DPSA has also worked with Scandinavian countries in joint projects in South Africa to monitor the human rights of deaf people and disabled people. The DPSA is a nongovernmental organization; it is not a political organization. There was a disabled member of parliament back in 1994; she was a woman in a wheelchair and also a member of the DPSA.

The DPSA convinced the ANC to include five disabled people on their electoral list. Our political system is a little bit different from those in, for example, Scandinavia and the United States. In the United States, a candidate can present himself for election, but in our country you must be on the party's list. We five disabled people were in the first eighty names on the ANC list. I was number 76. In talking with a news reporter, I realized that if the ANC garnered 50 percent of the vote, then all five of us disabled people would be elected and become members of parliament because we were in the first eighty names. That in fact happened, and we five disabled people do all have seats now in the South African parliament. Since then, altogether the ANC political party now has nine disabled people on their list who have seats in the parliament. We did have ten at one time; however, one recently passed away, so we now have nine. In addition, we just had local elections in South Africa. These are not elected representatives of the province but rather representatives on the local level. On the local government councils there are many disabled people, but there are no deaf people in the provincial councils.

The ANC is very supportive of disabled people and especially women; 38 percent of ANC representatives in the South African parliament are women. There are more than twenty-six portfolio committees in the parliament; each one of the members is expected to serve on at least two committees. I currently serve on the Communications Committee and the Joint Monitoring Committee on the Improvement of Life and Status of Children, Youth, and Disabled Persons.

The first is the Communications Committee, which I thought was very important for me to be on because it covers issues about broadcasting and national television. Deaf people have limited access to television so I have been vigilant to ensure that provision for captioning and subtitles for most programs as well as sign language interpreters for news are included in draft bills as far as possible. The committee also covers telecommunications, and there is a lot of work to be done in the telecommunications field to improve access for deaf people so that we can make any calls to anyone. There were not many text telephones in our country, but our national telephone company, Telkom, has become involved in the development of Teldem, which is a form of text telephone device. The postal service is also under the purview of our committee.

The Joint Monitoring Committee is the second committee of which I am a member. When the different government departments come and report to us about their activities and account for how they are spending their budgets, we question them intensively about how much of the budget is going to be used for disabled people and what they are doing with programs for disabled people.

There are twenty-six other portfolio committees in the parliament, and ideally there should be a disabled person in each committee because when a bill is drafted before it becomes law, disabled people should monitor the text of that bill to make sure that disabled people are included. South Africa is a little bit different from the United States in that there are not as many highly educated deaf people. Thus, I have a particular responsibility to watch for the rights of deaf people whenever a bill comes up in parliament. In our portfolio committees, we ask the lawmakers what they are doing about including disabled people in the bills and make them think about including disabled people in the provision of services.

I have to remind myself that I am not a deaf advocate. I cannot function like a political activist when I go into the houses of parliament. As a member of the parliament, I am a lawmaker rather than an advocate or activist. When a bill is presented in the parliament in South Africa, individual members of the community are given the opportunity to come and speak before the portfolio committees. We listen to their objections and their suggestions for amendments.

However, the call for people to come to the portfolio committees often has not reached the deaf community in a timely manner. The call for comments does not appear in deaf newsletters, but in newspapers and government gazettes, and so deaf people have often missed the opportunities to comment on draft bills before the portfolio committees. Because there are so many bills, I am not able to monitor the deaf issues in every single committee. Fortunately there are other disabled members—and even some nondisabled members whom I have educated on issues about disabled individuals—that assist in monitoring the treatment of disabled people in our legislative processes.

There also is an office called the Office of the Status of Disabled Persons (OSDP), which is now in the office of the president of the ANC. President Thabo Mvuyelwa Mbeki established that office when he was deputy president, and when he became president that office moved directly under the office of the president. He is very interested in and supportive of disabled people. He has a big heart and an open mind about our issues. There are disabled people working in the OSDP within the president's office, but I have to admit that there is no deaf person on the staff yet. There is a deaf person who works in the OSDP on the provincial level in the provinces, but not on the federal level.

Deaf people still have a long way to go to fight for our rights and for equal access in South Africa. Each member of the parliament has a constituency office; when the parliament is in recess, members of the parliament generally go to their offices in their local area to talk with their constituents. Because I consider my constituency to be the deaf people all over the country, I asked for special consideration from the ANC not to have a constituency office in my local area in the city of Cape Town, but to spend my time during recess traveling around the country, explaining to deaf people all over South Africa about my role in the parliament and the parliament's role in government, understanding deaf people's issues, and discussing what deaf people can do to get involved. That unique dispensation was granted to me, and I spent my recess time traveling around the country, talking with deaf people, finding out what their needs are, and bringing those needs to the attention of the members of the parliament with suggested solutions.

Deaf people have asked me what achievements we had managed to push through the parliament and what I can do as a member of the parliament. People in the country cannot come and speak before parliament; only a member of parliament can speak on the floor in parliament. As a deaf person, I need to speak in parliament with an interpreter, but the rules of parliament did not allow an interpreter to be on the floor of the parliament while I was speaking. On the second floor, there is a television studio, and in the beginning my interpreter was required to be up on the second floor in the television studio watching me on a monitor and translating into a microphone, not even in the same room where I was. I absolutely refused and said that I must have an interpreter with me on the floor in order to have two-way communication. Of course everything is political; I asked the members of my party, the ANC, if they could support me in getting my interpreter on the floor with me in parliament. We knew the opposition party was going to object. However, just before I made my first speech in parliament, the deputy speaker of the house announced to all of the members of parliament (MPs), "I have granted permission for the interpreter to be on the floor of the chamber." There was silence from the opposition. I was the first person to use sign language and an interpreter on the floor of the parliament. Even if I have done nothing else, that is really a significant accomplishment. After the speech, I got support not only from my own party, the ANC, but also from the opposition party, whose members came to me and thanked me for my speech. Some of them had disabled or deaf people in their families. In South Africa, many disabled and deaf people are locked away and hidden in homes, and information about what to do and how to help deaf and disabled people has been minimal. After my speech, some MPs asked me what we could do to enhance their lives.

In the United States, you have the Americans with Disabilities Act (ADA). In South Africa, we have a white paper, which is a policy document called the Integrated National Disability Strategy (INDS), endorsed by the government in November 1997. Every department within the government must follow the guidelines in the INDS. It is not law yet, but it is still mandated for government departments; we are hoping that it will eventually become law.

Many people think that once MPs who are deaf or disabled are in office, then changes in the country will occur very fast. However, it does not happen overnight. We have a long way to go, but we have to be aware of the need for change and be persistent until the desired change occurs. It is important that deaf people, not just a deaf MP but all deaf people, become involved in politics. You can become involved in your political party, ask for interpreters, and start building good, solid relationships with the political parties in your country. Deaf people simply must be aware of what is going on in their parliament or congress in their country. When a bill is submitted in the parliament, deaf people need to know how to advocate for their rights before the bill becomes law, including how to raise amendments and how to comment on bills.

The ANC slogan over the years has been "the work to make a better life for all our people continues." This is also true for deaf people—we cannot give up; we have to continue.

World Deaf Leadership Project Enhances Deaf Empowerment in Thailand

PEOUNGPAKA JANYAWONG

I was born and grew up in Phayao, a northern province of Thailand. Before I participated in the World Deaf Leadership (WDL) project, I was a seamstress. The National Association of the Deaf—Thailand announced that Ratchasuda College was accepting applications for admission in an eighteen-month Thai Sign Language Teachers' Certification Training Program, which was a WDL program. I became interested in seeking a new career, and so I applied and was accepted into the program. In the fall of 1998, I started to attend classes at Ratchasuda College. My professors were James C. Woodward, Mike Kemp, Jean Gordon, and Sam Weber. Upon completing the program, I immediately began to teach Thai Sign Language at the Department of Employment Services, the Ministry of Labor, and Ministry of Social Welfare under the auspices of the Thai government. Of course, when I got my first assignment, I became anxious and nervous. My teachers told me not to worry too much and just do my best. I put every effort into teaching Thai Sign Language. Ever since my first assignment, I have taught Thai Sign Language classes at various schools for deaf people throughout the Kingdom of Thailand. Each time I taught a new class, I gained more self-confidence than before.

James Woodward moved to Vietnam to set up a similar program for deaf Vietnamese. He and Mike Kemp asked me to teach Visual Gestural Communication twice, in October 2000 at the Lac Hong University and in October 2001 at the Cao Dang Su Pham (a teacher's college) in Bien Hoá City, Vietnam, which is about one hour northwest of Ho Chi Minh City.

Because of my participation in the WDL project, I have improved my self-esteem and I feel good about my progress in this new professional career. I became empowered. Before that I was merely a seamstress, with no high aspirations. Currently, I am an undergraduate student at the Ratchasuda College seeking a degree in Sign Language Linguistics. I will complete my undergraduate studies in about two years. After my graduation, I hope to empower many individuals within the Thai Deaf community.

In December 1996, the Nippon Foundation awarded a $3 million grant to Gallaudet University to establish an endowment for the Nippon WDL to enhance the

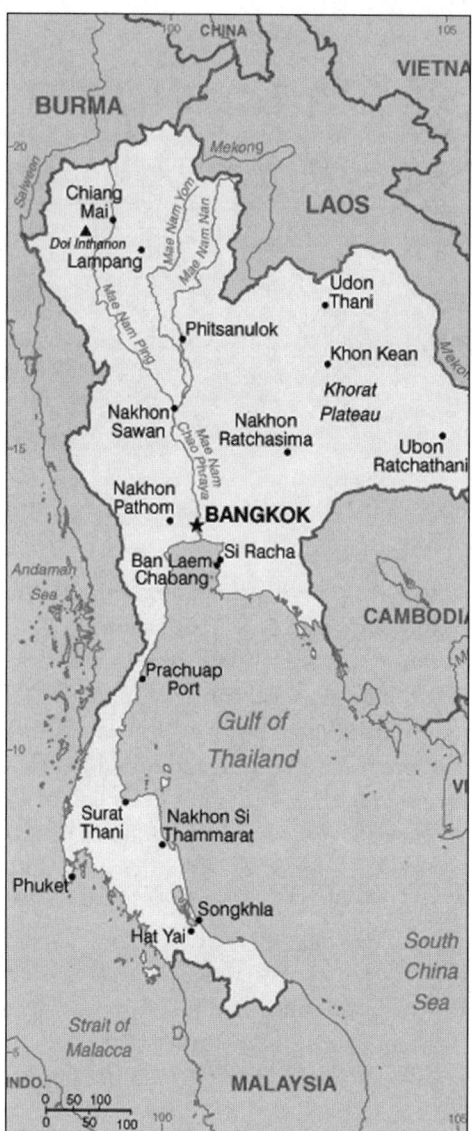

quality of life for deaf individuals in selected developing countries. Thailand and South Africa were the first two countries identified, and I discuss the WDL project in Thailand.

Thailand neighbors countries such as Myanmar, Laos, and Cambodia. The planning and operation of the WDL project involved an active partnership of three organizations: the National Association of the Deaf in Thailand, Gallaudet University, and Ratchasuda College of Mahidol University, along with support from the Nippon Foundation and in cooperation with La Trobe University of Australia.

Her Royal Highness Crown Princess Mahachakri Sirindhorn is a great benefactor of disabled people in Thailand. It was her dream and commitment that led to the founding of Ratchasuda College in 1992, where deaf and disabled people can study at a university, by consenting to give her name and patronage to Ratchasuda Foundation for the establishment and operation of the college. Poonpit Amatayakul was charged with establishing Ratchasuda College on a twenty-acre campus across the street from Mahidol University's campus, which was intended to be fully accessible to all students. Ratchasuda College is located nearby to the west of Bangkok, the capital city of Thailand. For many years since then, on behalf of the college, Jitprapa Sri-On worked to educate, research, and provide services for Thai people with disabilities.

Ultimately, the WDL project was effective in resolving the communication gap between deaf and hearing people in Thailand. This communication gap had adverse effects on the lives of deaf Thai people. They are often isolated from family life. They have limited opportunities to acquire professional jobs and education. There are very few interpreters of sign language in Thailand. Deaf people are not treated equally in Thai society. Many teachers of the deaf in Thailand do not sign well, and when they do, use only basic sign vocabulary. This creates a problem of communication. Most members of the deaf community in Thailand are unemployed; the few that work are in manual trades, such as basket weaving, manual production of handicrafts, carpentry, and so on. They do not have access to or given opportunities for professional occupations. Such jobs pay a subsistence wage. For example, seamstresses often get paid on a piecework basis. People in these jobs have no access to or opportunities to obtain white-collar or professional jobs.

The WDL project had two strategies in Thailand. First is to train deaf teachers of Thai Sign Language. The second strategy is to involve members of the broader deaf community in sharing new ideas and to mobilize them to work in partnership with the sign language teachers to promote the Thai Sign Language.

Let us now look further into the WDL project's first strategy. The certificate in teaching Thai Sign Language has a curriculum in which students learn about sign language teaching methods, assessment of sign language skills, sign language research, and other things. Here is a list of the many courses that we took in the program learning to become sign language teachers:

- Introduction to Sign Languages and Deaf Communities,
- Methods of Teaching Sign Languages,
- Curriculum Design and Materials Development for Sign Language Instruction I and II,
- Introduction to Structure of Thai Sign Language,
- Practicum I and II: Teaching Thai Sign Language,
- Research in Sign Languages in Thailand, and
- Methods of Evaluating Sign Language Skills.

James Woodward taught linguistics and helping us to analyze Thai Sign Language. He was also the WDL project codirector in Thailand along with Charles Reilly at Gallaudet. Mike Kemp taught methods of teaching Thai Sign Language. Jean Gordon taught evaluating skills in Thai Sign Language. They were instructors from Gallaudet University. Members of the local deaf community who saw what was happening at Ratchasuda College became excited about it and got involved in learning the new things.

The second strategy of the WDL project was to involve and mobilize the greater deaf community in promoting the Thai Sign Language. Thailand has roughly one hundred thousand deaf people, and many of them are living in very remote places, in rural areas without access to education or modern communications. They do not have pagers or text telephones, so it is very difficult to contact them. It is fortunate that we have a deaf association of with four branches, located in the four regions of the country.

The leaders of these branches are involved in various activities with their membership. Under the WDL program, leaders of the regional branches of the association gathered to talk about how they can distribute the new ideas and knowledge to the greater deaf community in Thailand through an informal education scheme using videotapes and visits.

For example, one of the messages is that deaf people can be proud of their Thai Sign Language, that this sign language is distinct from spoken Thai language and has its own grammar, and that regional variation of the Thai Sign Language is fine and acceptable. It does not all need to be the same, and these regional variations should be preserved. These are the kinds of things that were being shared with the broader deaf community.

It is important to remember deaf children. The WDL program tried to have the sign language teacher trainees become role models for children, and we had a program of visiting the schools. We would tell the children that they can study at a university when they grow up. I told them I am studying at a university, and the children would say, "I can?" It was important for the children to see that they could become like these successful deaf university students.

There are several positive outcomes of the WDL project. The first is teaching Thai Sign Language to a variety of groups, including teachers, deaf and hearing parents, and deaf and hearing children. The second outcome is that the Thai government has recognized Thai Sign Language as the language of Thai deaf people. The third is a partnership between deaf sign language teachers and leaders of the Thai deaf community to work together.

Many Thai deaf people are living in rural areas, are very isolated, and have not been to school. They have not had the opportunity to learn Thai Sign Language before, and so they are brought together in classes. Under the WDL program, new sign language teachers are collaborating with the rural deaf clubs to create courses in Thai Sign Language. The clubs are learning how to design small-scale projects to teach sign language in rural areas; for example, in Nakon Sri Thammarat in southern Thailand, twelve local people were trained as mentors for families with deaf children, from newborns to three years old. It is very important that children learn the Thai Sign Language as early as possible.

Before the WDL program, deaf people were not in a positive situation. They were living from hand to mouth on subsistence wages. After they were involved in the WDL program, you see a very different, more positive situation.

The Thais have learned a lot and have great success from this project. We are interested in collaborating with our neighboring countries, such as Cambodia, Laos, and Myanmar. We have already become partners with Vietnam; we are helping Vietnamese deaf people to learn how to teach their sign language. I have been there twice to run workshops. I hope in the future we will be able to collaborate with other neighboring countries such as Laos and so on. I am very appreciative of the support that we have gotten, and it has allowed us to improve our lives. Again, I express great appreciation to Her Royal Highness of Thailand, the National Association of the Deaf in Thailand, Gallaudet University, La Trobe University and Nippon Foundation for making all of this possible.

Through the WDL program, our lives have changed, and now deaf people are becoming role models in working with deaf children and gaining a new sense of what they can do in their lives. This is truly deaf empowerment, and it is especially important that deaf people work together to enhance our aspirations and opportunities.

Communication, Sign Language, Culture, and Education as Human Rights

YUKATA OSUGI

I am the executive director of the head office of the Japanese Federation of the Deaf. The Japanese Federation of the Deaf is a long-established organization whose history dates back fifty years. As you know, there are countries that do not consider the needs and rights of Deaf people. Governments consisting of hearing people make decisions for us, but we have been protesting this. We have to represent our own views. The Japanese Federation of the Deaf has been very active in conducting such movements. We have been disseminating information about Japanese Sign Language throughout the country.

We recently published a new book that contains the signs of the names of the countries of the world. It contains the signs of the names of 140 different countries. They are not the signs that we use in Japan for those countries but the indigenous signs of the countries themselves. The Japanese Federation of the Deaf would not have been able to compile this book alone. There was one very important person who supported us in this project, Tomas Hedberg. Tomas, who is from Sweden, has been doing a tremendous amount of work on collecting signs of the names of countries and towns. He is an expert in this field. It was only with his support that we were able to complete the book. Unfortunately, it is only in Japanese at the moment. However, the board of the Japanese Federation of the Deaf has discussed and agreed to make an international version of the book to disseminate this information. I hope that the World Federation of the Deaf (WFD) board will take up this project and print the book in English, so that many of you will be able to benefit from it.

As you know, we do not all use the same sign language throughout the globe. American Sign Language and Japanese Sign Language are quite different. Let me give you an example. In the United States, there is an offensive sign that in Japan is the sign for *brother*. Signs are related to the culture of the country. The American sign for *name* relates to your perception of the word, which is written. In Japan, the culture associated with the word is different. We use stamps with our names engraved in Japanese characters, and so the sign for *name* is quite different. What is important is that we identify the innate cultural characteristics of the signs. It is essential to demonstrate that culture is an integral part of sign language. It is impossible to separate culture from the language of the country. That is also the case with sign language. When I speak of culture here, I am referring to Deaf culture. What we perceive with our eyes influences the way we produce our sign language.

I have conducted research on many different sign languages, but now I will discuss the sign language of one very small location—a group of very small islands close to Japan known as the Amami Islands. Many of the people who live on this island work as fishermen. It is a very tiny island. There are many intermarriages, and accordingly, many children are born Deaf. There is no school on this island, but the children mix with the Deaf people on the island, as well as with many hearing people, who all use a form of sign language. Is it the same as the sign language used in Japan, to the north of the islands? No. It has evolved from the essential communication needs of those who live on these islands. No one came to these islands and taught sign language. The sign language evolved from the communication needs of the people of the islands. The sign language that they use has an incredible number of lexical items and variations. Take squid, for example. By the way, do you have a sign for *squid*? I see you finger spelling it. Probably many of you have never eaten squid, but in Japan, we love to eat squid. We have three different types of squid. I would use the same sign for all of them. They are all squid, and I can eat them all. However, the Deaf people in the Amami Islands have a completely different sign for each of the three types of squid. They use three different locations for the sign SQUID. I found that quite amazing. It was difficult to distinguish them at first, but as I worked more and more with the islanders, I began to distinguish the different characteristics. I was brought up in Tokyo, and I am not a fisherman. We buy fish in the markets and eat them. I did not know there were three kinds of squid. They look and taste the same, so one sign is enough for all. However, for the islanders, it is very important to distinguish the three different types. Why? Because for those employed in the fishing industry, the type of squid that they catch influences the market economy. One is expensive. That is the one they should concentrate on catching. These will yield high income, and that is why it is important to have this clear distinction.

Language and culture cannot be separated. I have just discussed the three different signs for squid. In literal concepts, we can see why there should be distinctions. But would there be a difference in signs for abstract concepts? For example, take the American sign for *year*. Now, do you think there is a sign for *year* in the Amami Islands? It is an abstract concept. When I worked with the islanders, I could see that they had developed their own sign for year. It was signed KILL-TEAR. I thought this to be very strange. YEAR-PIG-TEAR—at first, I could not understand how these words were connected, but eventually, I managed to work it out. There are pigs on the island. At the end of the year, on the very last day, New Year's Eve, they kill the pigs, chop them up, and cook them. On New Year's Day, they make rice and roll the rice into small rice balls. That is their New Year celebration meal—pork with rice. The four individual signs related to this meal are PIG, KILL, TEAR, ROLL. Over time, they have been reduced and amalgamated into two signs. They have been incorporated to form this lexical item. Thus, you do not see all four signs, but only two signs for the abstract concept *year*. This is something that has been created by people with no education. They have used what they see, what is part of their culture, to create a sign that meets the needs of that culture and that community.

In the Amami Islands, we see that there are a number of different signs for literal concepts and for abstract concepts. We see that the culture, the food, the way of living, and the way Deaf people perceive with their eyes enable them to create and develop a signed language system of communication that meets their needs. Initially, these signs and concepts were very long, but over time, they have obviously been reduced, but there is still enough information to encapsulate the entire concept. I would not call it sign language, but it is a form of sign communication that has many of the characteristics required of a language. It is not quite at the level of a full-fledged language yet. Now let us consider how we can make this sign communication become a full-fledged language.

What is crucial and essential is education. Deaf children have the right to learn, to be educated, and to know about their rights. They have an educational right. If they receive education, they can be creative and develop their own language. When Deaf people marry Deaf people and have Deaf children, they should be informed that there are schools where their children can access education. In the Amami Islands, there is no school. However, if they are told that there are schools on the mainland and knew that their children have the same rights to education as hearing children, they would send their children to school. Such children would go to school, eventually graduate, and return to the island. They might get married to a Deaf person on the island and create another family. Then, we would begin to see a transition. It will be the start of a great evolution process of an indigenous sign language for the island.

The right to learn, the right to education, is essential and of critical importance. Another essential factor is legislation. We know that governments should recognize, respect, and promote our sign languages. Deaf people who wish to be part of mainstream society can do so if there is the provision of sign language interpreting services. Today, in the Amami Islands, sign language classes are available for hearing people who wish to learn, but the problem is that the signs that they are taught are the signs from the mainland of Japan. These potential interpreters are not learning the sign language of the islanders. We should be much more aware and sensitive to the needs of the islanders. Teaching potential interpreters the sign language of the mainland results in conflict. There will be a potential breakdown in communication. However, the teaching system is still in its early stages, and we very much hope that things will be rectified.

In my work in the Amami Islands, I have selected a couple of things that I feel are very important. I stress again that it is essential that Deaf people are enabled and empowered to be creative in the development of their sign language. To enable this to happen, there must be good education. This education must be ensured as a right and given in their own language. I have been discussing the Amami Islands, but now, I will discuss other parts of the world.

Let us take a bird's eye view of the global situation. We see from the WFD statistics that there are 70 million Deaf people in the world. Eighty percent of these Deaf people do not receive any education. Twenty percent may have received education, but the number is incomparably small. Eighty percent, an enormous majority, have no education at all! Let me explain a little more. Among the 80 percent that do not receive any education, there are those who are not able to access a school for the Deaf. Even if there is a school for the Deaf in the country, it may be so far away that some Deaf children are unable to attend it. They may have to travel by boat or by horse or donkey over mountains. There are places where there are no roads. For some, the journey may be shorter, but they may not have the money to travel even a short distance. The school may have residential facilities, but to stay in residence at the school requires money to pay for bed, board, and food. They may not have this money, which results in the 80 percent.

Let us look at the 20 percent that are supposed to have access to education. I am not so sure that this is correct. I think this is a questionable factor. Yes, they may receive some form of education, but many educational establishments still regard education as something to be transmitted using the spoken form of language, either orally or to support a sign language. It may well be that Deaf children are educated in the mainstream hearing schools. In such schools, there are far more hearing children than Deaf children. There may even be only one Deaf child in the whole school. These Deaf children will be getting a hearing perspective on life. Where are these children going to get the Deaf cultural input? This is why I believe it is a questionable factor. There are problems with the 80 percent with no education as well as with the 20 percent who supposedly receive an education. Both are in need of education and linguistic rights. Without these rights, how can we assert our basic human rights? We have no basic human rights. As a Deaf person, I cannot be denied such rights.

The United Nations and governments around the world must ensure that Deaf children are provided with an educational medium enabling them to learn. That is, of course, through sign language. If Deaf children can use sign language, they can develop and learn. They can develop their cognitive and emotional abilities by seeing Deaf adults. Without such input, this development is not possible. If governments of each country do not provide Deaf children with the proper educational environment, the Deaf children will not be able to exert their maximum potential. It is as if we will be dead inside if we do not have this cultural linguistic input as our basic human right. I do not want to see that.

The United Nations and many national governments are introducing the new concept or philosophy of inclusion. Do you think it is possible? How can those with physical disabilities, those who are hearing, those who are blind, those who are Deaf, and others be educated in the same place? Well, they may be able to associate with each other. Governments, particularly those which are restricted financially, seem to like this idea. It costs less than providing special schools for Deaf children. They will put everyone into one educational establishment and will justify this cost-saving system by calling it *inclusion*. However, we have seen that Deaf children who are included in an education system with hearing children, or those with physical or other sensory disabilities, have no communication. They cannot gain language competence. It is very difficult. Learning, receiving an education, would be extremely difficult in such an environment. The concept of inclusion may become an appropriate concept in future, but I do not think we are ready for it yet.

Before we can realize an ideal form of inclusion, we need to focus on early intervention. What do I mean by early intervention? If we identify a child, an infant, as Deaf, we must immediately provide the child and parents with support, cultural learning, and sign language. We have to bring the parents in contact with a wide range of Deaf people—Deaf people who received a cochlear implant, Deaf people who use speech, and so forth. We need to provide all this information as a well-planned early intervention program so that the hearing parents can be fully aware of all the things that make up a Deaf person within a Deaf community.

At present, parents of Deaf children do not have the opportunity to receive all the information they need, or they receive it too late. We Deaf people, we in the Deaf community, must consider ways to enable hearing parents of Deaf children to access early intervention services as quickly as possible, so as to be able to explain to them what is needed. We must help to provide this support. If they need sign language, we must enable the parents to learn it. This is the kind of system or methodology we should be introducing. We are not ready for inclusion yet. Early intervention is what we must focus on now.

Instead of going into more detail, let me go back to the bird's eye view of the globe. Let me go around the globe and discuss two good examples of schools educating Deaf children. One good school is the Rocky Mountain Deaf School in Colorado in the United States. I was very impressed by what they are doing there. This is a Deaf school located within the campus of a larger hearing school, but the Deaf children do not receive their education in an integrated way. They are educated separately. Those in the Deaf school are educated in sign language, and, of course, those in the bigger hearing school are educated in spoken language. In the evenings or after classes, both groups mix together. The hearing children can see how the Deaf children behave and what their culture is like. Likewise, the Deaf children can learn about the hearing children, so they have this exchange of cultures. For the education curriculum, they are kept apart. I think this is a model of a good school system.

Another excellent example is in Nepal. I found this impressive example in a very small town with a very small Deaf association. There was a government-supported Deaf school nearby, but this school had many problems. There were financial problems, the teachers were not trained, and there were many other problems. The Deaf association saw this unhappy situation and decided to build a new school—their own Deaf association school. In the new school, they teach using sign language and they have Deaf teachers. Gradually, all the children moved from the government school to the Deaf association school, and the government school is left with no children attending it. Because the Deaf school has been established by empowered Deaf people with the Deaf association, they are teaching in sign language and using education methods that the Deaf people believe in and that the Deaf children can benefit from. I have seen many other examples of good schools around the world, such as the one here at Gallaudet. I know that there will be many more new initiatives in years to come. The important thing is to reconsider the concept of inclusion. If we do not share opinions and discuss these concepts, then we will never develop our beliefs and understanding. Gallaudet University and Deaf Way will enable such sharing of opinions and discussions.

I cherish the thought of all Deaf children learning through sign language. This will enable our sign languages to flourish and our human rights to be firmly established. We have our Deaf rights. I studied here in America for ten years, and I have to thank many in America for the support they gave me. However, it was one man whom I met here who opened my eyes to what Deaf culture means and how I must fight to preserve it. After returning to Japan, I received the saddest news of the loss of Lou Fant. I was heartbroken. I dedicate this essay to his memory.

Hands across the Pacific: Partnerships for Progress

JAN FRIED, NANCY BRIDENBAUGH,
AND LINDA LAMBRECHT

Hands across the Pacific: Partnerships for Progress is a collaborative project involving the American Sign Language/Interpreter Education Program, the Gallaudet University Regional Center for the Pacific at the University of Hawai'i-Kapi'olani Community College, the University Center for Excellence (UCE)—Pacific Outreach Initiative (POI) at the University of Hawai'i Manoa, and several departments of education throughout the Pacific. The project's Pacific partner is the Federated States of Micronesia (FSM), which consists of four different island states: Guam, Palau, American Samoa, and Fiji. To establish successful programs and services for deaf children in these remote locations, it is important to form partnerships. At each locale, administrators, teachers, community members, students who are deaf or hard of hearing, and the students' families are involved with the goal of improving the state of deaf education for their community.

This article illustrates the activities that were implemented and the successes, challenges, teaching strategies, and long-term goals that occurred in two specific areas: FSM and American Samoa. It is important to note the kinds of services for deaf and hard of hearing children that were available prior to the partnership and the significance the partners' physical location had on these services. The widespread island nations of the Pacific are either independent and fall under the Compact Agreement of Independent States or they are U.S. territories and are required to comply with federal statutes such as the Individuals with Disabilities Education Act (IDEA). Limited resources make compliance difficult and necessitated the hiring of outside consultants. For the collaboration to be successful, however, it was critical that these consultants not only had a respect and an understanding of island culture but also experience living on an island. It made sense, then, that the consultants came from their closest resource, Hawai'i.

Up to this point, the programs that were available on these small islands in the Pacific lacked appropriate resources. The people who were working within the Department of Education on the islands did not have the expertise to teach deaf or hard of hearing children. In some cases, the personnel working with the students not only lacked fluency in American Sign Language but also had limited language proficiency in English. They did not have sufficient opportunities to access additional training and professional development.

The professional development model that was pervasive prior to the implementation of the project contracted consultants to conduct one-time trainings and then leave. This hit-and-run type of training was neither consistent nor successful. Hands across the Pacific wanted to provide training that would be sustainable. The collaborative efforts of the Hands across the Pacific project have been able to provide the type of resources and training necessary to improve education and services for deaf children on the islands.

With the partnerships and need established, it is important to explain how this project was funded. The University of Hawai'i (UH) succeeded in receiving several federal grants from the U.S. Department of Education. The funding was applied to implement a new program called the Pacific Outreach Initiative (POI). POI's goal is to improve services for children with disabilities in the Pacific region. Grant money was also received for technical development and to train related services assistants (RSAs) to work with children with disabilities. Funding from Rotary International allowed one of the project members to travel and provide training in FSM for three months. Through their initial efforts, the University of Hawai'i POI programs found that the services provided to deaf and hard of hearing children were not adequate and that they did not have the appropriate personnel to provide the necessary training to effect change. It was at this point that the coordinators of several POI projects contacted the programs at Kapi'olani Community College (KCC) because the personnel at KCC already had extensive experience working with deaf and hard of hearing students throughout the Pacific.

A key aspect of the training was the importance of a deaf and hearing team approach. KCC wanted to ensure that local deaf people had the opportunity to access the training and learn the language and culture directly from a deaf role model. As a result, local deaf adults could become role models for the deaf community on their home islands. Additionally, the deaf teammate became an example to families of the levels of success their deaf children could attain. Because of this, it was agreed that each training would be conducted with a deaf and hearing team.

Although the University of Hawai'i performed the initial identification of need, it was important to do an on-site assessment of the students' and staff's language skills, the current program status, the cultural differences, and the level of administrative support.

The deaf person on each team did an on-site observation to determine the current language need. The assessment was done by meeting with the students and teachers in their classrooms. Many of the children knew some sign language already, but it was a mixture of signed English, a local sign dialect, and home signs. The students were primarily using Signing Exact English (SEE) because of the earlier influence of missionaries who taught SEE. They also had developed their own native signs and were using some similar structures found in ASL. Several of the outlying areas had their own sign dialects, and the team did not want to lose that aspect of the native language. It was important to respect the native language and culture that already existed. For example, on Pohnpei in FSM they were alternately but naturally using their native sign for breadfruit and the SEE sign, which uses two separate signs, BREAD and FRUIT. They wanted to know which sign was correct. The team explained the differences between SEE, ASL, and their native signs and encouraged them to preserve their native signs.

Another part of the assessment was to observe the classrooms to evaluate the current status of the educational programs serving deaf and hard of hearing students. The team immediately recognized the impact of using SEE signs for this population. It quickly became apparent that the children were memorizing the signs and did not understand the concepts behind them. One girl was asked to read a particular sentence from one of her books. She signed each word correctly: ONE . . . DAY . . . THE . . . SUN . . . CAME . . . UP. She was then asked to tell the meaning of that sentence, and she signed it again using SEE: ONE . . . DAY . . . THE . . . SUN . . . CAME . . . UP. Her ability to sign the sentence correctly was commended, but she was asked again if she knew the meaning of what she had read and signed. Finally she shrugged her shoulders and admitted that she really did not know. That girl was nineteen years old. She was shown the sentence signed in ASL as the sun coming up and raising up in the sky, and she was amazed to finally understand the concept behind the string of words that formed the sentence.

The team recognized that the children could benefit conceptually from understanding ASL structure. All along their teachers naively thought that using SEE meant students were learning and understanding English, but in reality students did not understand the concepts behind what they were signing. They were not using English at home with their families. At home, the families use the spoken native language of the island. Most students cannot speak their native language, but some of them can lipread it from their parents or siblings.

The team also observed there were insufficient materials in the classroom—not enough books or resources to guide the learning process. Several of the teachers were using an ASL dictionary as their only source of educational materials to teach the students language, word for word. With this method the students were learning individual signs for English words but not developing language at all because their learning had no real-world relationship. They would read books and stories and memorize how to phrase them in sign, but they had no idea what they meant.

Another part of the initial assessment was to find out what the administrative expectations were for the team and what they expected of the teachers and of the students themselves. What was the current attitude and philosophy? In most cases the administration was very supportive. As mentioned earlier, there may have been a lack of real understanding of how to educate deaf and hard of hearing children, but the administrators supported the efforts of the team and raised their expectations for their personnel.

The team also needed to assess the number of deaf students being served in the classroom as well as the number of deaf adults in the community and the level of community support. The participants on each island truly valued the deaf community experience that was shared with them because they had not developed a deaf community in their locality. One of the goals was to form a deaf community using their own local resources as models.

After completing the assessment, the team reviewed the curriculum to determine how to best match their needs with the services the team was able to provide without forcing a Western culture on their community. The curriculum was modified to meet their existing needs.

To improve students' literacy skills, the team used a curriculum that was obtained from the Laurent Clerc National Deaf Educational Center. This curriculum, the Shared Reading Program or SRP, has been used effectively in many other communities and teaches hearing teachers and hearing parents how to read to their deaf child. One critical component of the SRP program is having deaf tutors help the parents learn to read aloud to their deaf child. For the project to be effective, local deaf adults who were knowledgeable, had the reading skills, and were fluent signers were needed to function as tutors. Unfortunately these resources did not yet exist on the islands; therefore the program was adapted to be used as a teaching tool. The program was modified to teach eighteen- and nineteen-year-olds how to read specific stories first, so that they could then become the tutors or teachers, as well as role models, for young children. This served the dual purpose of teaching literacy skills to the older children while developing role models and tutors for the reading project geared toward the younger students. Each teaching strategy was similarly adapted to suit the cultural needs in varying situations. The team members modeled teaching strategies, interpreting, deaf community involvement, and language.

The following situation is a poignant example of the effect a Deaf role model who is fluent in ASL has on a community where Deaf adults are not readily visible. When the team presented a three-week ASL intensive training for educational personnel and community members in Pohnpei, several deaf children also attended. Among them was Willy, who was seven years old at the time. For the two years prior to the workshop, he had been attending a mainstream program at a private school. In class, he spent most of his time copying work off the board or from a classmate seated next to him. He did not have interpreters, and no one was able to sign with him, including his teachers. His mother and grandmother participated in the ASL training because they were unable to communicate with him and were concerned that Willy did not have language. The Deaf team member suspected that Willy could easily pick up ASL if he was exposed to it, so she showed him a videotape of Bernard Bragg, a well-known deaf mime and actor, signing a story about an eagle flying. Willy watched the videotape and immediately started copying Bernard's signing, capturing his expression and the intention of the story. It was at this point that Willy transformed from passively sitting and drawing during the workshop to becoming actively engaged in learning ASL, hungrily consuming everything the Deaf trainer was teaching. In the afternoons, the Deaf trainer privately worked with him in sign language to increase his ASL fluency and reading comprehension using SRP strategies. His progress over the three weeks was remarkable; his family was reassured that he could acquire language and communicate when given the opportunity. They came to understand that continued exposure to ASL was the key to Willy's future and that he could achieve his dreams like the Deaf workshop instructor.

After the curriculum was established and adapted, the team determined the best methods for delivering the services. Three different approaches were used for providing services. The first approach was on-site training, which meant flying to each island and providing training within their community and schools. The second method was to host a regional conference in Hawai'i where the Pacific Islanders came to get training and to meet other professionals with the same needs. Third, training was provided through distance education.

The on-site portion of this program occurred in FSM and American Samoa. Historically, students had been isolated in programs on different islands because IDEA promoted their inclusion in mainstreamed settings. The educators in these programs often did not sign themselves and were not sure what do with deaf students who had no communication in classes. Classmates who could hear did not sign, and the deaf student was primarily relegated to copying work off the board or from another student. As a result of the on-site visits, the team was able to work with administrators, parents, and teachers to successfully get a class of deaf students together or at least bring the deaf students together once a week for socialization and literacy. The team provided ASL classes and instruction on teaching strategies during one-week intensive visits to the islands. Through these classes, the community became better able to communicate with the deaf students and became more knowledgeable on how to teach them.

To ensure that a positive change would occur, regular meetings were held with administrators to update them on the progress and changes that had been implemented. The team also made contact with the local government officials to ensure they would support their department of education's endeavors for positive changes. Beyond that, the team made contact with state and federal officials to guarantee that the changes would legally provide the most appropriate education for deaf students as mandated by IDEA. It was important to get families and communities involved with the process and familiar with the desired outcomes. All of this support needed to be in place before the team could effectively provide on-site training. The goal of the on-site training was to train the personnel on the islands to become trainers for the others in their community so that the progress would be sustainable. On-site training, workshops, and visits occurred in the classroom, at a family's house, and at public sites for the community.

For the regional conference, the Pacific Islands personnel came to Hawai'i to share experiences with others in their situation. By hosting the conference in Hawai'i, the participants were within reach of various resources, could immerse themselves in the language, and could observe the teaching strategies.

Distance education through videoconferencing has been an effective way to share information because it is accessible to ASL users. The personnel on the islands could easily share ideas or questions and get answers with the visual support. ASL classes were also offered via videoconferencing on one of the islands. Another form of distance education was the use of video letters. Students from the deaf school in Hawai'i sent video letters to the children in FSM and Samoa, and they sent video letters in return. This was beneficial for both groups because they learned about each other's way of life and were exposed to another group of ASL users.

In closing, the results of the work over the past three years in American Samoa and FSM showed that the following goals of the project were accomplished:

❖ A large pool of interested personnel, co-workers, family, and community learned basic sign language skills.
❖ Personnel working with deaf students acquired advanced signing skills and enhanced teaching strategies.

- ❖ Resources were established for continued development.
- ❖ Local service providers and educational administrators became more aware of issues facing deaf students.
- ❖ Deaf Awareness Week was established.
- ❖ Partnerships developed within the community and across the Pacific.

Also, the team was able to stay long enough to set up the necessary foundation and resources that would enable the local people to continue running the program by themselves. The next step for the Hands across the Pacific project is to implement this model in other locations.

Partnership in the Irish Deaf Community

KEVIN STANLEY

A well-established Deaf community is based on the strength of its leadership and unity. Effective advocacy reinforces the fundamental principle of sign language and Deaf culture. This can be achieved through a partnership among the wide variety of people within the Deaf community. The absence of partnership could cause fragmentation of the Deaf community and lead to a monopoly of services by paternalistic organizations, as has happened in Ireland. Besides a lack of partnership, our greatest obstacle in Ireland is misconceptions of the Deaf community by the general public and apathy from Deaf people.

Historically, members of Deaf communities suffered oppression because of who they were, particularly by the infamous Milan Conference in 1880 where oralism triumphed over manualism and the ideology of eradicating Deaf communities through "science" such as eugenics. Deaf people went through decades of cultural and linguistic suppression before society began to accept our culture and language.

The Irish Deaf experience is no different, but it has lagged behind the rest of the Western world. Irish Deaf people only began to advocate their equality in the 1980s. Paternalism was rampant in Ireland, and the Deaf people had very little input in policymaking. In the Irish tradition, the Irish Deaf community was overwhelmed by a rigid religious ethos, led by the Catholic Institute for the Deaf (CID) since 1846.

Irish Deaf people, through their Catholic upbringing, would not dare to criticize the CID about how it managed the Deaf community. Notwithstanding CID's authority over the Deaf community, Deaf people actually rejected the recommendations of the 1880 Milan conference but mainly for economic reasons rather than teaching philosophy. Irish Deaf people enjoyed a freedom from oralism until the 1940s; a few exceptions were short-lived private schools for Deaf students where a method of oral teaching existed.

The Deaf community's apathy and religious fear allowed the introduction of oralism to Ireland through the Dominican sisters, who visited Deaf schools in the United Kingdom. Interestingly, these nuns acknowledged the superiority of Irish education through Irish Sign Language (ISL) over oral education in the United Kingdom. However, they were concerned about the rapid increase of middle-class Irish Deaf Catholics attending Deaf schools in the United Kingdom. The idea for the introduction of oral education was to prevent Irish Deaf children from attending U.K. Deaf schools, regardless of teaching methods.

As oralism progressed, throughout the 1950s, the CID perceived this as an opportunity to extend their supremacy over Deaf education when the Irish government funded the development of Deaf education. The CID continued to dominate the Deaf community with separate Deaf clubs for Deaf men and Deaf women, similar to the separate schools for Deaf boys and Deaf girls. It meant that many Deaf adults never interacted with the opposite sex, resulting in a low rate of Deaf marriages.

Some Deaf men and Deaf women defied this gender segregation by meeting up in landmark locations, such as pubs or restaurants. Deaf people were able to run Deaf clubs but still under the eyes of the CID, where the Catholic ethos remained with regular religious services, prohibition of alcohol, and display of religious icons.

While the status of sign language and Deaf empowerment surfaced in many Western countries in the 1960s and 1970s, the Irish Deaf community remained in the doldrums. In 1964, oralism advocates established an organization for Deaf people, the National Association for Deaf People (NADP), to push for the education policies based on oralism. They succeeded in 1972 when the Irish government rubber-stamped the organization. Deaf people were not consulted at any stage.

Toward the end of the 1970s, frustration among Deaf people became evident when some Deaf people attempted to get involved with the NADP to ensure Deaf input, but they were frequently thwarted with paltry promises that never materialized. Deaf people took this matter into their own hands by forming their own group called Deaf Action Group (DAG). It was the first time that a national Deaf organization, at a political level, was lead by Deaf people.

Early progress included campaigns for

- ISL in Deaf education,
- improved broadcasting and telecommunication access, and
- interpreters' service.

In 1983, DAG became the Irish Deaf Society (IDS), which skeptics suggested would be short-lived and described it as bunch of nuisances. Fortunately, the IDS soldiered on throughout the 1980s at a steady pace with representation on the international front, leading to IDS membership in the World Federation of the Deaf and the European Union of the Deaf. The IDS contributed on an international basis to the European Deaf Culture festival, International Junior Summer Camp, and European Deaf Empowerment Project.

The emergence of the IDS altered the general public's outlook on the Deaf community especially in terms of ISL, the capability of Deaf people, and the flaws of oral education. An increasing number of Deaf people became more self-confident and independent. Deaf leadership brought further establishment of Deaf-run organizations with special interests such as women, youth, ISL, technology, arts and culture, gays and lesbians, and so forth. The religious fear among Deaf people receded, though some retained strong Catholic traditions.

The Irish Deaf community encountered tensions due to the lack of leadership, because they were used to hearing people looking after their needs. A deep division among Deaf people arising from their personal conflicts emerged. The Irish Deaf community was fragmented because more than 80 percent of the Irish Deaf population were clustered into urban areas to avoid the risk of isolation from living in rural areas. These problems played into the hands of paternalistic organizations in fortifying their stronghold of the Deaf community by manipulating the Irish government to fund their control over the Deaf community.

In the mid-1990s, the IDS embarked on a major organizational transformation to prevent the continuing trend of division and paternalism. The IDS began to reunite with local Deaf organizations, forming a national council as an umbrella body directed by the IDS to share the philosophy and priorities of the Irish Deaf community. This lead to a series of spectacular achievements, such as

- legal recognition of ISL in education;
- introduction of the Model School for the Deaf Project, based on a bilingual philosophy;
- initiation of the Centre for Deaf Studies;
- establishment of an ISL interpreters' agency;
- state support of the Deaf Adult Literacy Project; and
- increased technological advancement.

They increased awareness of the significance of ISL, Deaf empowerment, Deaf culture, and augmentation of support from hearing people, especially hearing parents. We cooperated with other disability groups to promote the legal rights of people with disabilities—for example by supporting the United Nations Standard for Equalisation of Opportunities of Persons with Disabilities.

However, we still lag far behind the rest of the Western world. Discrimination in Irish society remains, leaving us marginalized with the following problems remaining:

- a meager number of ISL interpreters,
- slow rate of improvement in Deaf education,
- limited broadcasting and telecommunication for Deaf people, and
- lack of access to various vital services.

Our objective of full human rights could still be obstructed by paternalistic organizations, especially the CID and the NADP, that hold the vast bulk of assets and funds designed for the Deaf community. Apathy among Deaf people may be thinning, but a number of Deaf people continue to receive paternalistic services. They are reluctant to organize their life independently and are happy enough to receive freebies, which is understandable. However, Deaf people have two choices: strive to maintain their empowerment and independence or accept paternalistic services, thus reducing their independence.

On the other hand, we perceive more Deaf people challenging the CID's role in the Deaf community and the NADP's monopoly. There are an increased number of hearing people who support the Deaf community being led by Deaf people.

This partnership with the Deaf community's partnership could bear fruition in the form of enhanced living standards inline with our counterparts in other parts of the Western world within the next ten years.

Only through Irish Deaf people, community through partnership, and democratic empowerment can this be achieved. Destiny is in our hands!

References

Crean, Edward J. 1997. *Breaking the silence: The education of the Deaf in Ireland 1816–1996.* Dublin: Irish Deaf Society.

Department of Education. 1972. *The education of children who are handicapped by impaired hearing.* Dublin: Government Publications.

Department of Equality and Law Reform. 1996. *A strategy for equality: Report of the Committee on the Status of People with Disabilities.* Dublin: Government Publications.

Department of Health. 1995. *Towards an independent future: Report of the Review Group on Health and Personal Social Services for People with Physical and Sensory Disabilities.* Dublin: Government Publications.

Irish Deaf Society. 2001. *Fourth National Congress: Irish Sign Language, our language, our culture.* Dublin: Irish Deaf Society.

Ladd, Paddy. 1991. The modern deaf community. In *Constructing deafness*, ed. Susan Gregory, 35–39. London: Open University Press.

Lane, Harlan. 1984. *When the mind hears: A history of the deaf.* New York: Random House.

Matthews, Patrick A. 1996. *Survey report: History of education, language, and culture.* Vol. 1 of *The Irish Deaf community.* Dublin: ITE.

National Association for Deaf People. 2001. *Report of services.* Dublin: NADP.

Swan, Ethna. 1994. *Report of the study on the Dublin School for the Deaf.* Dublin: Catholic Institute for the Deaf.

Deaf Empowerment in Greece

VASSILI KOURBETIS AND KOSTAS GARGALIS

The main purpose of the Deaf Empowerment Project was to provide young deaf children access to the Greek Deaf community and Deaf culture during their school years. We believed that this would help them develop a solid identity as Deaf people early in their lives.

Only a few parents of Deaf children can communicate effectively with their child, and Deaf children have limited contacts with other Deaf people when they are young. They first come in contact with each other at school. Many Deaf adolescents are communicatively isolated at home, at school, and in the neighborhood (Foster 1989). The reality of access to communication for Deaf people with disabilities is reported as severely disadvantaged even within the Deaf community (Turner, Traynor, and Harrington 2000). Kourbetis, Adamopoulou, and Ferentinos (2001) reported that Deaf children are isolated from other Deaf people, their parents do not know and do not learn their natural language (Greek Sign Language, GSL), they are forced to use a language they cannot naturally comprehend (spoken Greek), and they are deprived of story-telling experiences. In Greece there is still a climate of pathological approach to deafness. Deaf people are still called deaf-mutes, the educational system has mainly been oral, and even though GSL was recently recognized and its use is mandatory (Law 2817/2000), it is not yet widely used for educational purposes. There are laws still in effect that describe Deaf people as people with lower levels of capabilities and responsibilities (Kourbetis 2000).

Holcomb (1997) argues that healthy, realistic expectations for Deaf children, positive reactions to deafness, and exposure of Deaf students to Deaf role models will better develop a bicultural identity and form healthy relationships with Deaf and hearing people alike. Acquiring a bicultural identity is crucial for most Deaf people in developing a productive and rewarding life. Hearing parents of Deaf children will benefit from early contact with Deaf adults in terms of understanding and accepting deafness and Deaf culture (Lane, Hoffmeister, and Bahan 1996; Moores 1996; Mahshie 1995; Woodward 1989).

Projects that involved Deaf adult mentors in teaching, interacting, and sharing their personal knowledge of deafness with young Deaf children and their families resulted in those children having greater language gains and higher scores on measures of communication and language than children who had no such interaction (Watkins, Pittman, and Walden 1998).

Rutherford (1987) has argued that folklore reflects the culture of a people, serves as an educative tool, and establishes and maintains group identity. The value of group narrative to the community provides avenues for creative expression, releases aggression, and relieves minority group anxieties.

Theaters of the Deaf play an important role in Deaf communities all over the world. They usually start as an amateur theatrical company, where certain individuals, who are mainly Deaf, join forces to create a fully professional acting company that achieves national and in some cases international recognition. The theater of the Deaf has developed its own unique style, related to cultural, linguistic, and worldview factors that makes it an essential part of Deaf culture (Baldwin 1995; Rutherford 1987). The Greek Theatre of the Deaf does not differ from other theaters of the Deaf and demonstrates all of these characteristics.

The Deaf Empowerment Project included three main activities: a series of informative and counseling workshops, theatrical educational workshops, and a Deaf festival.

The Hellenic Federation of the Deaf (HFD) implemented the project. The main objective of the HFD is the support of the needs of the Deaf community in Greece in all aspects of life. The organization's aim is to empower Deaf individuals and their families to lead productive and fulfilling lives.

The project was implemented for thirteen months, from December 1998 to January 2000. The majority of the people involved in the project were Deaf. Only a handful of hearing people were involved in the execution and follow-up of the program. This has never before been done in Greece, where usually hearing people design and execute programs for Deaf people with little or no involvement of Deaf people. We consider this the most innovative approach of our project and hope to set the standards for others to follow in the future.

Goals and Objectives

Every activity was targeted to empower Deaf children and adults and also their families (hearing or Deaf). Specifically, the goal of the group of Deaf animatures and the theatrical group was to learn and acquire the ability to transfer their internal experience and knowledge about deafness to both Deaf and hearing people, to enrich the materials they possessed about certain topics, and to familiarize themselves with new subject matters. To achieve these goals, the group of Deaf animatures was advised by a Deaf person who had an acknowledged outstanding leadership role in the Deaf community and a wealth of experience, the president of the National Federation of the Deaf and coauthor of this essay.

Because this was a pilot project for Greece, the transnational experience of our French and Danish partners was of great value. Two people, one hearing and one Deaf, who worked on training of Deaf animatures participated in this project. They offered a lot both in theory and practice and especially discussed the advantages and disadvantages of similar projects in France and Denmark.

Informative and Counseling Workshops

Our partners from Denmark assisted us in developing the material for the specific issues and offered knowledge from their experiences in similar activities. The Greek

Deaf animatures visited their organization to gain knowledge of and experience with counseling and empowerment of the target group.

The workshops addressed specific issues about Deaf culture and its effect on human development, education, and social functioning in addition to the status and importance of GSL in the lives of Deaf people. They offered emotional support for parents and Deaf people by discussing the idiosyncrasies and strengths of the community along with information on services and rights of Deaf people and their families as they already exist in the Greek and European social and legal system.

Theatrical Educational Workshops

The Greek Theatre of the Deaf has been working with Deaf children for more than a decade now and implemented theatrical educational workshops at the National Institute for the Deaf. The workshops included dramatic play, GSL instruction, expressive communicative techniques, and theatrical communicative skills.

The Deaf Festival

The Deaf Festival was a two-day long festival that focused on what Deaf people can do, not what their handicap is. The festival was contacted in GSL with interpretation in spoken Greek and International Sign. It included a crafts fair showcasing the works of Deaf children from schools all over Greece and the partner countries, storytelling from older Deaf adults, an arts exhibition of works of European Deaf artists, a photography exhibition, a book fair, and International Sign storytelling. All participants signed a petition for the recognition of GSL as an official language by the Greek Parliament. The grand finale was a play by the Greek Theatre of the Deaf in collaboration with the International Visual Theatre of France.

Methodology of Evaluation

The results were evaluated in three different ways: internal evaluation with semi-structured interviews with the beneficiaries of the project, external evaluation of the program by a Deaf scholar not involved in the program through qualitative and quantitative observation and analysis, and a public opinion poll at the Deaf Festival using interviews and short questionnaires.

Evaluation Process of the Project

The evaluation of the project was a long process that included observations, discussions, and questionnaires. The evaluation of the project was both quantitative and qualitative and lasted throughout the duration of the program. This has resulted in changes that improved the effectiveness of the project in all aspects of implementation.

Achievement of the Program

It appears that through such programs the Deaf community can set aside the stereotypical notion of "people with a pathological medical condition" and project themselves as people of a cultural and linguistic minority. Deaf people are seen as a resource of information and support and not as a problem.

From the informative and counseling workshops, Deaf people and their families gained the necessary empowerment to face the difficult challenges our society has set up for them. It helped build a positive image of the Deaf community in the hearts and minds of the members of the community. The widely accepted belief that hearing parents need not involve Deaf adults early in the life of their Deaf child was proven wrong.

In general, the parents were both satisfied with and eager to continue with the project. The workshops started with sixteen people attending on a weekly basis. Attendance increased to a high of twenty-nine with an average of eighteen people per session. Deaf people were used for the first time in the counseling process, an area that has been dominated by hearing professionals. This resulted in the upgrading of the services provided by hearing professionals and the social and professional integration of both the hearing and the Deaf communities.

Parents expressed their satisfaction with their exposure to Deaf adults and their life experiences as well as the acquired knowledge and information about deafness and Deaf culture. There is no evidence to support many professionals' fear of establishing contact between Deaf adults and parents of Deaf children. Parents expressed their need for the continuation of such programs and the establishment of permanent workshops, especially for young parents, using a parent-to-parent model. They found the involvement of Deaf parents of Deaf children to be very helpful.

Parents can become empowered through cooperation with Deaf adults and other parents of Deaf children and work together toward common goals. Empowered parents express what they want and gain the knowledge and skill to act upon their wishes.

The theatrical educational workshops offered a rare opportunity to children in schools for Deaf students to be involved in an educational practice unknown to the majority of schools for Deaf students. It was a rare opportunity for Deaf adults to have full responsibility for the outcome of the project. Several day students at the residential school traveled back to school in the afternoon to attend the workshops. The number of the students per group was two to three times larger that a typical school class. The age spectrum of the groups varied, as well as their communicative competence. Despite all these factors, the students demonstrated different behavior than their behavior during their day classes. Their attendance was voluntary, and they usually arrived in class before their instructor. Many times it was difficult to get them to transfer to other activities or leave the school. They had a lot of zeal and enthusiasm throughout the project. A physical disaster, the earthquake of September 1999, deprived the members of the workshop, children and adults, of showing the result of their work to the general public at the Deaf Festival. The members of the National Theatre of the Deaf gained valuable experience setting up and operating educational theatrical workshops. As a result, they plan to set up a permanent workshop for school-aged children.

The festival gave members of the Deaf community the opportunity to design and implement a social event for them and the hearing community. It supported the acceptance of Deaf people by their families and the hearing community on the basis of equality and their strengths. This helped the public to form a positive opinion about

Deaf people and helped depathologize deafness to a degree that it has never happened before in Greece. It supplied a forum for political action for the recognition of GSL, a long-standing demand of the Greek Deaf community. The minister of education attended the festival as well. GSL was officially recognized five months later (Public Law 2817/2000).

Our activities helped change the situation of Deaf people for the better. The community seemed to accept Deaf people as having a cultural and linguistic identity and embraced the depathologized approach that is more accepted in the rest of Europe and the United States. Our activities empowered Deaf people to take charge of their destiny and show the world what they can do and not what they cannot. We demonstrated that for Deaf people to be successful, productive, and happy, they do not need to be hearing or behave as hearing.

Finally Deaf people, not hearing people, designed, implemented, and executed activities that focused on Deaf people. This practice was innovative not only for Greece but for numerous other countries of Europe and the world. Both in their content and methodology of implementation, such activities have been limited in Greece or never have been done before.

Problems, Solutions, and Suggestions

There is a great wealth of educational tools such as written material, GSL material and a general curriculum for such projects. The material used by the professional staff should be available to other professionals for similar future projects and a certain budget should be provided for material development.

The use of hearing professionals to work with Deaf people seemed to be a problem in the beginning of the project but none existed in the end. Three Greek hearing professionals (a psycholinguist, a psychologist, and an art teacher of Deaf students) participated. All have long-standing experience of working at different organizations of and for the Deaf population.

The use of Deaf professionals working with the hearing parents and professionals seemed to be a problem also but an asset in the end. It is necessary for the good of the community as a whole to expose both hearing and Deaf people to common activities for the solution of this long-standing problem.

It is necessary to use professionals who are well accepted by the community, know and use GSL for their everyday communication, and know and accept the idiosyncrasies of the Deaf community.

We believe that this was an important project that has to be continued. Deaf people should be trained in various areas. There is a need for in-depth training and specialization in the fields of early intervention, schooling, vocational rehabilitation, and social services for the Deaf population.

We highly recommend the implementation and support of similar projects in the future. These projects should be carefully planned, organized, supported, and implemented to utilize fully the strengths of the Deaf community for the well-being of both the Deaf and hearing communities. Parents' organizations as well as professional organizations should team up with the Deaf community to implement such projects to achieve the unity the community desperately needs.

The festival should be a biannual event that should take place in various cities of Greece with the involvement of local Deaf organizations. The workshops, both counseling and theatrical, should be set up in every school for Deaf students nationwide and should involve parents of children of all ages. We believe that we empowered the Deaf community in Greece and the partner countries with holistic involvement in the activities. This project could not be implemented without the European Commission's and the Prefecture of Athens' financing. To effectively generalize this practice, continuous financial support from the Hellenic Federation of the Deaf is necessary.

References

Baldwin, S. 1995. *Pictures in the air: The story of the National Theatre of the Deaf*. Washington, DC: Gallaudet University Press.

Foster, S. 1989. Social alienation and peer identification: A study of the social construction of deafness. *Human Organization 48:* 226–35.

Holcomb, T. 1997. Development of deaf bicultural identity. *American Annals of the Deaf 142*: 89–93.

Kourbetis, V. 2000. *Noima stin ekpedefsi*. Athens: Pedagogical Institute (in Greek).

Kourbetis, V., A. Adamopoulou, and S. Ferentinos. 2001. *From disabling to enriching the Deaf world: Forms of discrimination Deaf people are faced with in Europe*. Athens: Hellenic Federation of the Deaf.

Lane, H., R. Hoffmeister, and B. Bahan. 1996. *A Journey into the Deaf-World*. San Diego: DawnSignPress.

Mahshie, S. 1995. *Educating deaf children bilingually*. Washington, DC: Gallaudet University Press.

Moores, D. 1996. *Educating the Deaf: Psychology, principles, and practices* (4th ed.). Boston: Houghton Mifflin.

Rutherford, S. 1987. A study of American deaf folklore. PhD diss., University of California, Berkeley.

Turner, G., N. Traynor, and F. Harrington. 2000. Problematising "minimal language skills." Poster presented at the Seventh International Conference on Theoretical Issues in Sign Language Research, Amsterdam, July 23—27.

Watkins, S., P. Pittman, and B. Walden. 1998. The Deaf Mentor Experimental Project for young children who are deaf and their families. *American Annals of the Deaf 143*: 29–34.

Woodward, J. 1989. How you gonna get to heaven if you can't talk with Jesus? The educational establishment vs. the Deaf community. In *American Deaf culture: An anthology*, ed. S. Wilcox, pp.163–72. Burtonsville: Linstok Press.

A Model in Accessing the Community for Deaf-Blind Adults

MARICAR MARQUEZ AND ILISSA RUBINBERG

Can you imagine relying on others to assist you with simple tasks such as food shopping, reading mail, or explaining to you what is happening at a basketball game? As Deaf, hard of hearing, or hearing and sighted individuals, we freely access transportation, navigate our surroundings, make phone calls, and enjoy local cultural events. Envision what it would be like if you often had to depend on others to assist you with these activities. A Deaf-Blind person may encounter these challenges every day. A Deaf-Blind person may use a support service provider (SSP) to access their community and overcome these obstacles.

Let us clarify the role of an SSP. An SSP plays an integral role in the life of a Deaf-Blind person. SSPs are people who provide assistance to Deaf-Blind individuals in attending to life's everyday tasks. SSPs can provide assistance for recreational activities, errands, reading mail, visiting friends, or making a simple phone call. An SSP facilitates communication between a Deaf-Blind consumer and the outside world regardless of the communication method. An SSP can provide transportation for a Deaf-Blind individual as long as the SSP is accompanying the Deaf-Blind individual for the duration of the assignment. It is not the SSP's role to provide only transportation by dropping the Deaf-Blind person off at a particular destination. Similarly, SSPs cannot be utilized for personal care, housecleaning, or food shopping if the Deaf-Blind is not present. If an SSP and a consumer go to the mall to purchase an article of clothing, the SSP would be responsible for describing the item's color, texture, and price. If the Deaf-Blind consumer asks for an opinion, then of course the SSP can respond. However, the ultimate decision to purchase the item is solely up to the Deaf-Blind person. It is not the SSP's role to make decisions for the Deaf-Blind person. The ultimate responsibility of an SSP is to promote the independence and autonomy of the Deaf-Blind person in a respectful and supportive manner by providing access to visual and auditory information while empowering the Deaf-Blind individual.

Although we are aware that interpreters and SSPs have different roles, often it is desirable that there be some flexibility within each role. For example, when I (Maricar) was a graduate student at New York University, an interpreter would graciously show me the way to a vending machine and assist me with purchasing a snack or guide me to the restroom during a break.

We discuss several programs and services provided at the Helen Keller National Center (HKNC) in this essay. The first program is called the PATH program (Person-Centered Approach to Habilitation). The consumers in this program require a great deal of assistance with mobility, eating, and grooming skills. They learn and develop needed skills in a variety of environments in a one-to-one situation. This program does not utilize SSPs.

The next program is called the traditional program, in which students have a schedule of classes to attend on a daily basis. A variety of support and training for students in this program is provided to meet their needs and abilities; however, they can function independently. In this program, the consumers frequently use SSPs. The traditional program is a comprehensive program that provides training to Deaf-Blind consumers in a variety of areas such as Braille, sign language, speech and language services, audiology services, case management, counseling, vocational services, and independent living skills.

There are several known causes of Deaf-Blindness including Usher syndrome, congenital rubella syndrome, CHARGE syndrome, premature birth, and age-related hearing and vision loss. *Deaf-Blind* does not necessarily mean being totally blind and totally deaf. Usher syndrome, which I (Maricar) have, is quite common in the Deaf-Blind community. An individual with Usher syndrome typically starts off with night blindness developing into tunnel vision before the vision deteriorates to partial or total blindness. The degree of blindness and deafness varies from one individual to another, and one's communication preferences vary as well.

The SSP program was established at HKNC in 1995 for the benefit of the students residing at the center. HKNC is a comprehensive rehabilitation and training facility working with Deaf-Blind youths and adults located on Long Island, New York. This program was modeled after the SSP program established and utilized in Seattle, Washington, through the Deaf-Blind Service Center. We allow some out-of-state individuals to come here and get SSP training. Mostly they live in the surrounding area such as New Jersey or Connecticut. At this time the SSP program at HKNC is not funded and relies on volunteers, grants, and donations.

It has been a challenge recruiting individuals into the SSP training program. Fortunately, there are many ASL classes and interpreting programs in the New York City metropolitan area, and we are able to recruit a good number of individuals from these programs. Many times we give presentations and spread the word about HKNC at various colleges, universities, schools, and other Deaf events to enhance public awareness of the SSP program. We also advertise our program through a local newsletter that is sent out via e-mail to subscribers.

HKNC provides SSP workshops three or four times a year. Initially, we hosted the training during the weekday evenings but had limited success because of the small number of attendees. We then started to provide workshops during the weekend, and we were able to attract a large number of people to the workshops. It has been quite successful.

HKNC requires that SSPs attend a six-hour training workshop before serving a consumer. This workshop covers basic sighted guide techniques, a brief overview of Usher syndrome and etiologies of Deaf-Blindness, modes of communication utilized by people who are Deaf-Blind, a cultural perspective of Deaf-Blind people, a consumer panel's expectations of an SSP, and an explanation of the roles and responsibilities of the SSP. Also included in the training is a hands-on experience where the SSPs have the opportunity to wear a blindfold and earplugs while eating lunch. This helps them to understand what it may be like to not hear or see. The SSP program at HKNC emphasizes the opportunity to learn about a different community and culture of people. The workshop is intended to educate interested individuals about our SSP program. It is hoped that these individuals will learn the skills necessary and gain the desire to serve the Deaf-Blind community as SSPs. At the completion of the workshop, an SSP certificate is given.

We are also in the beginning stages of setting up an internship/mentoring experience where the trainees attend and observe the already existing relationship of an SSP and a Deaf-Blind person, for example, a weekly shopping trip, dining out at a restaurant, or going to the bank.

To be an SSP at HKNC, you do not need to be fluent in American Sign Language (ASL). There are consumers who utilize SSP support that communicate via spoken language as well as those who communicate via sign language. Students of ASL can use this time to improve their communication skills while at the same time assist Deaf-Blind people in accessing the community. There is reciprocity in this relationship—the student enhances their sign language skills and the Deaf-Blind person is able to have access to visual and auditory information to fully participate in daily life activities. Also, previous knowledge of Braille and various visual impairments are not necessary. All you need to be an SSP are a positive attitude and determination.

Currently the HKNC SSP program requires consumers who utilize the services of an SSP to be older than eighteen and capable of making effective and appropriate decisions while in the community, thereby not relying on the SSP to make decisions for them.

The Deaf-Blind person's ability to gain access depends a great deal on an SSP who matches that person's communication need. Many times the SSP does not need to be fluent in ASL to assist the consumer with a particular activity. They can use other methods of communicating, such as note writing. However, in some situations it is important to match the SSP with the consumer. For example, a museum trip would require a great deal of detail and description by the SSP. For this situation, we would look at the Deaf-Blind consumer's communication preferences or skills and then find an SSP who could communicate with the consumer. We also look at other characteristics such as gender, ethnicity, interests, and preferred recreational activities. In the past we had a Deaf-Blind consumer who enjoyed running. Therefore, we focused on finding an SSP who also enjoyed running and not necessarily concentrating on their communication skill or level.

At HKNC we do have a special SSP request form that we ask all Deaf-Blind consumers to fill out whenever they want to attend an event. They are encouraged to fill out the form at least two weeks ahead of time, so that we will be able to look around for the most appropriate SSP. Once we receive the request, we start making phone calls and sending out e-mails asking SSPs if they are interested. We try our best to accommodate any requests made on short notice, such as a last-minute trip to the grocery store, but it all depends on the availability of the SSP.

It is important to note that Deaf-Blind consumers need to learn how to best work with the SSPs as well. We developed a curriculum designed to teach the Deaf-Blind users to understand how to best work with an SSP successfully.

A few cities, including Seattle, Boston, and Minneapolis, have SSP programs and services. Many states do not have any SSP program and many Deaf-Blind individuals come to HKNC from various states to learn as much as they can about the SSP training program and services. However, when they return home they experience difficulties and frustrations in setting up programs and services because of lack of funds in many states.

In closing, we discussed the role of an SSP, the services provided, and what an effective SSP training program entails. For additional information later on, please feel free to contact the HKNC.

Improving Development Assistance from American Organizations to Deaf Communities in Developing Countries

AMY WILSON

In this essay, I discuss how American organizations, such as church groups, nongovernmental organizations, and American federal agencies, offer assistance to Deaf people in developing countries. I share how and why I think we need to discuss this topic and propose what I believe Deaf organizations in developing countries should expect and require from American organizations offering them development assistance.

The Importance of Deafness and Development

I became interested in how Americans brought "help" to Deaf people in developing countries when I began traveling the world twenty-five years ago. As a teacher, I was able to travel to more than thirty-five different countries during my schools' summer holidays. I often made an effort to meet the Deaf community or visit the schools for Deaf students and was struck by the great number of Deaf people I met who never attended school. I also encountered Deaf people in rural areas who did not belong to a Deaf community and had no Deaf friends. These Deaf people were not getting the services they deserved and needed. Yet, occasionally I would find programs established by concerned American church groups or development agencies or even independent American individuals working alone, which attempted to meet the needs of Deaf people in developing countries. Initially I was quite impressed that these Americans were making an effort to help others so far away from their own countries, but then became concerned when I observed some disturbing situations:

1. While sitting at an open-air café in the Philippines, I observed a group of Deaf children signing to each other using signs from American Sign Language and not from their native Filipino Sign Language. I learned that they were students

at a nearby school run by American missionaries. These children did not know their native sign language and said they had only met a few Deaf adults and those adults were the teachers' aides who worked at their school. They had never been introduced to their native language nor given any exposure to their native Deaf culture.

2. A handful of Deaf adolescents were the first Deaf people in their South American city to attend high school with an interpreter. They studied subjects never studied by Deaf people in that area before, so many of the words they learned had no matching Brazilian signs. During the weekly local Deaf Association meetings, the students taught the Deaf adults (many who never attended school) the new vocabulary. As a group, the association then created signs for the words, as a Deaf artist drew the new signs for a sign language book the association was compiling. An American volunteer had financially supported this Deaf Association for many years, and the Deaf members felt obliged to follow her request that their weekly meetings concentrate on creating Biblical signs for her catechism classes. For many months, the Deaf Association put aside their project of creating new signs for the Deaf students in high school and created Biblical signs to please their benefactor. Interest soon lagged, and the weekly meetings creating new signs disbanded.

3. One day, an American volunteer arrived at a rural Brazilian school for Deaf students carrying a video camera. His intention was to engender the sympathy and collect donations from Americans by showing them a film of the poor conditions of the school. The Brazilian parents and teachers were proud of their school and were embarrassed to be portrayed as being pitiable, needy, and unable to support themselves. Yet, they allowed the filming because they did not want to insult or anger the American, because they needed donations to keep the school running.

4. I observed an American volunteer bringing curriculum from the United States to a small rural school for Deaf children in South America. Although her American system of teaching was much different than the educational system of the country she lived in, she insisted on training the teachers in the "new way." She did not think to ask the teachers for their input, ideas, or opinions.

5. In several countries I have seen well-intentioned Americans giving children used hearing aids. Yet, after the Americans leave, often there is no one available to service the hearing aids, make ear molds, teach the proper care of the aids, or give adequate audiological assessment of the children's hearing losses. Yet, because the aids were technology from the United States, the parents were convinced the hearing aids were essential and forced their children to wear the improperly working aids. When I lived in Brazil, a mother begged me for money to buy medicine for herself because she had spent her money to buy her Deaf daughter overpriced and very expensive hearing aid batteries. The irony was the hearing aid did not fit correctly, and the daughter would rip out the hearing aid when not in sight of her mother, forgetting to turn it off, and the batteries would wear down.

6. I met a North American high school history teacher sent by a North American nongovernmental organization to a developing country to act as a teacher-

trainer of teachers of Deaf students because she knew some American Sign Language. She had never studied Deaf education or had any background in Deaf culture and knew no Brazilian Sign Language. She was frustrated, the teachers were frustrated, and the Deaf community was frustrated.

7. In several countries I have met American volunteers who fly into a developing country for short periods of time to build schools and churches for Deaf people, yet never spend any quality time with the Deaf community or learn about the native Deaf culture. Many Americans leave with misconceptions about the local Deaf people, feeling sorry for them rather than questioning why Deaf people are denied rights in their home countries. The volunteers are not encouraged by the American sending organization (usually a church group) to consider other ways to offer assistance that would be a means to empower the native Deaf people rather than to care for them as needy and helpless.

8. In many countries I have seen American organizations send development assistance to native agencies run by hearing people who help Deaf people rather than send development assistance directly to the native Deaf Associations themselves. This can lead to the hearing organization holding power over the Deaf community.

These situations are not uncommon when well-meaning Westerners try to meet the needs of the poor and underserved in developing countries (Ajuwon, 1996; Chambers, 1983; Cheru, 1988; Hoy, 1999; Mittleman & Pasha, 1997; Thomas & Thomas, 1998; Williams, 1995). Instead of teaching Deaf people empowering skills necessary to live full and independent lives, thoughtful Americans are unknowingly oppressing those they have come to serve (Ogoki, 1999; Wilson, 2000, 2005; Wilson & Kakiri, 2005; Dunn, 1999; Lane, 1992). How then, can American organizations improve their services to Deaf people around the world? What can Deaf people expect and require from American organizations when they work with American groups?

Eight Factors of Effectiveness

There has not yet been research done to determine what is the best way for American organizations to work with Deaf communities in developing countries. However, I propose eight factors of effectiveness in the general field of disabilities and development that could improve the effectiveness of development assistance from American or any international organizations to Deaf communities overseas (Heumann, 1997; Hurst, 1999; Schneider & Segovia, 1999; Stone, 1999; Metts, 2000; National Council of Disability, 2005).

1. The American provider employs Deaf workers in their own organization who associate with the overseas program. Deaf adults in developing countries, as well as hearing people, are often surprised to learn about Deaf professionals in the United States who are doctors, lawyers, and teachers. Deaf people understand other Deaf people best, and the American Deaf workers would be an inspiration and excellent role models for Deaf children, parents of Deaf children, and the community as a whole. Unfortunately, in the world of interna-

tional development, it is rare to find people with disabilities from industrialized nations working with people with disabilities in developing countries (Schneider & Segovia, 1999). Also, few Deaf people today are trained to do international development overseas and need to be trained for this work, although the Graduate School of Professional Programs at Gallaudet University now offers courses in international development focused on working with Deaf people and those with disabilities in developing countries.

2. The American provider supports and works with indigenous Deaf organizations. Although hearing indigenous organizations are well-intentioned, from my observations around the world, they are not always transparent in financial matters. Because money is often channeled from the American organization to a hearing organization that works with Deaf people or to a school board that controls the schools and its finances, Deaf people are wary of how the funding is spent. Although well-meaning Americans donate thousands of dollars to charitable organizations earmarked to assist Deaf people overseas, the Deaf people themselves rarely have input as to how the money is spent or know where the money goes. They argue, too, that hearing organizations are not aware of Deaf peoples' needs and desires and waste the money on invaluable or weak programming.

3. Indigenous Deaf people are involved in the planning, implementation, and evaluation of the program. Deaf people themselves know best what their needs are but may not possess the knowledge of how to plan, implement, or evaluate a program. American workers can teach them those skills as they design programs together. Later, the American can leave, knowing that Deaf leaders have been trained to plan, implement, and evaluate on their own.

4. The provider has an understanding of Deaf culture and issues that surround communication, language, and Deaf education. If the provider lacks knowledge in these areas, how can it provide quality services to the constituents who receive their services? American missionaries in one Jamaican Deaf school were depressed and frustrated that they could not offer what the Deaf community wanted because they had no background in Deaf education, sign language, or Deaf culture. Instead, the Americans taught what they knew, which did not necessarily match what the Deaf children or adults needed or wanted. This mismatch can be avoided if the provider understands Deaf culture and the various issues surrounding communication, language, and Deaf education.

5. There is an understanding by the provider about how their employees and their American culture respond to deafness. Americans heading overseas must first understand how they perceive and construct deafness themselves. Some Americans I have interviewed who work with Deaf people overseas referred to Deaf people as if they were objects or children. Some referred to Deaf people as the "deaf/mutes." The provider should also be in tune with the legal, political, and cultural issues existing within the American Deaf community. One must have their own house in order before venturing forth to help someone else set up theirs.

6. There is an understanding by the provider of how different cultures respond to deafness and construct deafness/disability in the developing country's

society. Deafness is looked upon differently throughout the world, from deafness seen just as a difference in a person to deafness being caused by the "evil eye." It is essential in planning to know what Deaf people have learned about themselves from their own culture in order to work with them more effectively. In a South American community, Deaf people tried to hide their signing because they were told they looked like monkeys. That same community believed that the "evil eye" caused pregnant mothers to have deaf babies and thus they shunned their Deaf children. Working in communities such as this, for example, requires that the provider gently challenge the folklore and myths of the community and build up the self-esteem of the Deaf people themselves. Venturing into a foreign community without this sensitivity could cause undue conflict and misunderstandings.

7. The American provider is accountable directly to the people who support and sent them and to the Deaf people they are serving. Americans who make donations to organizations often never receive a detailed description or an evaluation of how their money is spent overseas. They may receive glossy brochures of smiling Deaf children with little substance of what actually is being accomplished. It is questionable if Americans would continue to donate money to help Deaf people if they knew how upset Deaf people were with the American programs that do not meet their needs. The indigenous Deaf community also has the right to know how American money, earmarked for the benefit of the Deaf community, is spent.

8. The provider networks and shares with others who work in the field of deafness and development. At the moment, there is only a very small network of organizations working in the field of development and deafness. Good resources that do exist on the Internet are the Enabling Education Network (www.eenet.org.buk), Disabled People International (www.dpi.org), and the World Institute on Disability (www.wid.org). Because there is such a dearth of information concerning this field, it is important that best practices concerning working with Deaf people in developing countries be shared among American organizations, other industrialized nations' organizations, and indigenous Deaf organizations. Grassroots organizations can work with one another within a country or between countries.

Conclusion

As our world becomes smaller, more American organizations are generously reaching out to Deaf communities overseas as they become aware of the difficulties Deaf people in developing countries must face. Despite good intentions, some groups may be unaware that their goal of enhancing the integrity, growth, and independence of Deaf people may not occur because of a lack of appropriately trained personnel, a lack of knowledge about deafness and issues surrounding deafness, and a lack of accountability. Deaf people from developing countries can suggest, demand, or request that the American organizations they work with exhibit all or some of these eight factors of effectiveness.

References

Ajuwon, Paul. "Educational and Rehabilitation Aspects of Visual Impairments in Developing Countries," in *Beyond Basic Care: Special Education and Community Rehabilitation in Low Income Countries,* ed. Roy Brown, David Baine, and Alfred Neufeldt, 183–99. (North York, Canada: Captus Press, 1996).

Chambers, Robert. *Rural Development: Putting the Last First.* (Essex, U.K.: Longman Group Limited, 1983).

Cheru, Fantu. "The Garden of Eden Revisited: Why has African Development Gone Wrong?" *Food Monitor* (Spring/Summer 1988): 10–12.

Dunn, Lindsay. "A New Model for the 21st century: A case for Partnering with International Relief Agencies." *World Federation of the Deaf News* (July 1999): 4.

Heumann, Judith. "Keeping the Promise: Reflections on a Global Workshop on Children with Disabilities in Developing Countries," in *Report of the Global Workshop on Children with Disabilities in Developing Countries* (Washington, DC: Academy for Educational Development, 1997).

Hoy, Paula. *Players and Issues in International Aid* (West Hartford, CN: Kumarian Press, 1999).

Hurst, Rachel. "Disabled People's Organisations and Development: Strategies for Change," in *Disability and Development,* ed. Emma Stone, 25–35 (Leeds: Disability Press, 1999).

Lane, Harlan. *The Mask of Benevolence: Disabling the Deaf Community* (New York: Knopf, 1992).

Metts, Robert. Disability Issues, Trends and Recommendations for the World Bank. Social Protection Discussion Paper Series, No. 0007, 29–38 (Washington, DC: World Bank, 2000). Retrieved from http://siteresources.worldbank.org/DISABILITY/Resources/Overview/Disability_Issues_Trends_and_Recommendations_for_the_WB.pdf.

Mittleman, James, and Pasha, Mustapha. *Out from Underdevelopment Revisited: Changing Global Structures and the Remaking of the Third World* (New York: St. Martin's Press, 1997).

National Council of Disability. *Future Policy Directions Needed for People with Disabilities in the Developing World,* 2005. Retrieved from http://www.ncd.gov/newsroom/testimony/2005/durocher_04-08-05.htm.

Ogoki, Aristotle. "Development Assistance: No Strings Attached Commitment or Is There a Hidden Agenda?" Paper presented at the Thirteenth World Congress of the World Federation of the Deaf, July 1999, Sydney, Australia.

Schneider, Estelle, and Segovia, Hector. "Development of Community Rehabilitation in Nicaragua: Training People with Disabilities to Be Trainers" in *Cross-cultural Rehabilitation: An International Perspective,* ed. Ronnie Leavitt, 191–206 (Philadelphia: W.B. Saunders, 1999).

Stone, Emma. *Disability and Development: Learning from Action and Research on Disability in the Majority World* (Leeds, U.K.: Disability Press, 1999).

Thomas, Maya, and Thomas, M. J. "Controversies on Some Conceptual Issues in Community Based Rehabilitation." *Asia Pacific Disability Rehabilitation Journal* 9 (1998). Retrieved from http://www.dinf.ne.jp/doc/english/asia/resource/apdrj/z13jo0100/z13jo0105.htm.

Williams, Leonard. "Rights not Charity," in *Disabled Children and Developing Countries,* ed. Pam Zinkin and Helen McConachie, 214–18 (London: MacKeith Press, 1995).

Wilson, Amy T. "Considerations for Western Educators Working with Deaf Children in Developing Countries: Community Development in a Rural Brazilian Town." Paper presented at the Nineteenth International Congress on Education of the Deaf and Seventh Asia-Pacific Congress on Deafness, July 2000, Sydney, Australia.

Wilson, Amy T. "The Effectiveness of International Development Assistance from American Organizations to Deaf Communities in Jamaica." *American Annals of the Deaf.* 150 (2005): 292–304.

Wilson Amy T., and Kakiri, Nickson. "Improving Overseas Development Assistance to Deaf Communities in Developing Countries." Paper presented at the Supporting Deaf People Online Conference, February 2005. Direct Learn Service: Cheltenham, U.K.

PART TWO

Economics

How We Can Better the Lives of Deaf People in Developing Countries through Business Investment

ADEBOWALE OGUNJIRIN

My first point is that we need to get together in form of a group to look at how we can start making more investments in different countries that have not grown to the status of other countries. For example, Nigeria, like several other African countries, is a developing country. We want to find solutions to those problems through business investment. There are several topics I cover in this essay, and I give some examples and background information.

In Nigeria as well as in other developing countries in Africa, most of the needs of people are resolved among themselves. The government leaves people alone. If there is no telephone in a town in Africa, then there would be individuals who would go out and contact telephone companies or services outside of the country, obtain the needed telephone equipment and infrastructure, bring them in for use in Africa, and make profit for themselves while at the same time helping people get the desired access to telephone service.

Using the same principle, deaf people from all the African countries need to get together to share their ideas on how to help improve their situation and go out of the country if necessary to obtain the needed investment and infrastructure. In many of these particular countries, there is very little respect for deaf people, and they always work at the very lowest jobs, never at the top. Some of the problems of the deaf people exist because there is no good regulatory body available to watch over them. For example, on the international level we have the World Federation of the Deaf, but on a national level in our country the deaf leadership is very weak. We have a very good structure in place, but we do not have much power. This is not because deaf people do not want to do it but rather because somehow they do not have the means to accomplish it.

Let us look at the current situation in the area of education. In these countries is education has been stagnant and the level of education remains low. This is due to a lack of encouragement or incentive, a lack of motivation in the whole educational field. In Nigeria, for example, the curriculum is not well thought out and not well planned for deaf people. No serious attention is given to providing appropriate education and support to deaf children. Right now most of them are mainstreamed with all of the hearing students but have no support services.

There is also a lack of job opportunity and job satisfaction. Deaf people in developing countries do the same kind of work for many years and never move up. They might get small raises from time to time, but the money they earn is not as significant to their well-being as job satisfaction. Many of them want to be able to move up and improve themselves. Employers or people on the outside may view deaf people as not being able to perform a certain job at a high level whereas deaf people themselves know that they can do it.

The first time I came to America was the first time that I ever saw a teletypewriter (TTY), a pager, or an alarm clock designed for deaf people. I felt silly myself and wondered why I did not know anything about them. These are things that we could use in Africa to enhance our independence and opportunities in many different situations.

There is a lack of investment capital in developing countries in Africa such as Nigeria. We have a lot of talented people, but they do not have the capital to get started on something they want to do. Most of them are working in low-level jobs, but if they had the capital, they would be able to establish their own businesses. Thus, most of them are stuck and remain with their other employers for many years with no opportunities for advancement. They have to accept it, unless they decide to move to another country with better opportunities.

We could discuss several possible solutions to our problems, but my goal is to obtain business investment so that we may have the capital to improve the situation in a variety of ways.

There is a very old system that is still in use for education, in spite of workshops given by outsiders. In Nigeria, like other African countries, people prefer doing things by and for themselves. They do not want to be told what to do. Instead, they would welcome training to empower deaf people and to teach them what they need to do to get services they need. For example, training could be provided so that they could come up with recommendations to make closed captioning possible. I believe this is part of educating people to do things for themselves in Nigeria and other parts of Africa.

There might be a new technology, such as wireless communication devices, that would be useful for individual businesspeople to make contacts with customers and arrange shipments sent to Africa. This would be a new market, and I hope one of us would be able to work with foreign partners to set up the needed infrastructure so that these people can help themselves and get jobs. It also would be great if we could get such wireless devices or pagers for deaf people in Nigeria so that they would have additional opportunities.

So who can help us out? We do not really know. I think we need to come together as a group, involving myself and others from Nigeria and people from America or any other developed country around the world. We welcome anyone who is motivated to help deaf individuals in Nigeria to get together and work on the possibility of providing funds to deaf businesses or to work as investment partners in setting up deaf businesses to improve the lives of deaf people.

Remember, in Africa, we view ourselves as deaf people first, regardless of other individual characteristics. We believe we are deaf people just like other deaf people all over the world. If we choose to use business to help the deaf community in solving these problems in developing countries, we believe there will be a subsequent impact on other disabled people. This is because once other disabled people see what we deaf people are doing, they are going to follow our steps and do something to get better jobs for them.

We know a deaf person is able to run a school, and we wish there would be one so that it would show that deaf people can accomplish it. Then we might have a deaf principal at many other schools. However, the way things are now has been very hard for deaf people to move up. In fact, if there is an important government meeting, and different directors are called together to have a meeting on certain issues, deaf people are not represented there. We would like to see business investment made to provide the educational exchange and training we need.

I have touched on all these different areas, and I hope that we are able to get together and share information and ideas with each other to help deaf people anywhere in the world, whether in developed countries or not. Perhaps while we are here, developed countries such as America can discuss the concept of business investment and may find some good ideas that people from developing countries can take back home so they can raise their standards and have a good life.

As I return to Africa, it is going to be hard for me to communicate with most of my friends. We need to see the day when we can use the TTYs and the Internet real soon. I urge that you think about our need to access to these telecommunications technologies and come up with viable solutions so that we can achieve improved education, services, and job opportunities.

Successful Entrepreneurship in Third World Countries

ALOK KUMAR KEJRIWAL

I was born in Assam, India, and received my early education there. I came to Gallaudet University in 1986 and received a bachelor of science degree in 1989. When I returned to India from the United States, I was shocked to see how discrimination was widely practiced against deaf people at all levels in many areas, particularly in education and employment. In contrast, I have observed that deaf individuals in America can pursue many opportunities in a wide variety of careers and professions.

They say that life is what you make of it, deaf or otherwise. So, I decided to learn to live with what I have and to make the best of it that I can.

When I first joined my family's export business, I was often sidelined from participating in meetings. I could not participate in any discussion because of lack of communication, but I did not give up. To overcome this, I decided to teach ASL to my office staff so that I could communicate. I also taught them about the importance of an interpreter for use in meetings or in making calls. I was so intensely involved and dedicated in my work that gradually I raised to the position of an export director of our family's company. As the director, I had the responsibility of looking after the export procedure, the shipments, timely deliveries, and so forth. I also deal with our foreign clients directly to get new orders with the assistance of an interpreter. Currently we are one of India's leading manufacturers and exporters. We have factories producing glass ampoules, and we also export vials, pharmaceutical packing materials, closures, caps, and machinery. We regularly export to the Middle East, Africa, the Far East, South Africa, Latin America, North and South America, and Denmark. We have international affiliates or agents in many of these countries. Running a business involves dealing with a variety of people: customers, manufacturers, government officials, transporters, and so forth. They are all hearing people, and you need to be able to communicate with them.

Lots of technological advancements are available in India but are primarily for use by hearing people. Unlike the United States, we do not have telecommunications access available for deaf people at this time. That is, we do not have text telephone (TTY), telephone relay service, and closed captioning on television. Practically no support services for deaf people, particularly in the area of communications, exist.

In the United States, deaf people get a lot of access support because of the mandates of the Americans with Disabilities Act of 1990, the Telecommunications Act of

1996, and other laws. Telephone relay service enables deaf people to communicate with hearing people and vice versa. My answer to relay service was to use an interpreter for phone conversations. I bring an interpreter with me when I go to meet government officials. Some are shocked at seeing a deaf person at a meeting, but they get used to me. At times, my deafness works for me. The government officials, after their initial discomfort, feel obliged to go out of their way to help me. That is fine with me.

Group meetings are always a problem even with a very skilled interpreter. The interpreter is always a few sentences behind and this lapse time is very crucial in a business meeting. So, I often stop people and remind them to please wait for the interpreter to complete interpreting to me in sign language. That is their signal that I have "heard" the end of their conversation. This allows me to participate in discussions equally. However, admittedly, there are times when in the heat of discussion, people kept on talking at high speed without waiting for the interpreter to finish. This is a common problem everywhere.

I must say I have been fortunate that I got support and encouragement from my family members, right at the beginning, in spite of difficulties in communication within the business environment. It is because of their confidence in me that I was able to enter the hearing world with a positive attitude and belief that I could do anything on my own initiative. That is, I started to believe that nothing could stop me from working toward a top-level management position in our highly successful company in India.

From my experience working in India and communicating with successful deaf businessmen in the United States, I have learned that the key to success is positive attitude. You have to believe in yourself and have faith in yourself. You have to focus on your strengths and also work on your weaknesses. Instead of complaining about problems, one needs to tackle the problems and resolve them. At any given situation, you need to work to achieve communication access at the workplace and to gain trust and confidence from your co-workers or colleagues on the basis of your performance. Once you have the feeling that you are going to succeed and are willing to work hard, nothing can stop you.

I believe that businessmen such as myself in third world countries would like to be part of a network of some kind to provide support to each other. I suggest that we get together and form an organization so that we can help each other. Many of us have learned a lot in isolation, and it is time for us to start sharing our knowledge with each other. We can also then provide support to up-and-coming future business leaders or owners.

Successful Strategies for Deaf Business Professionals

EMILIA CHUKWUMA, RONALD SUTCLIFFE, JIM MACFADDEN, YURI MAXIMENKO, DAVID BARBER, AND BERNARD BROWN

EMILIA: Many of us want to know how to set up a business. Some of us have tried and failed, and so we would like to hear from people who have successfully set up businesses. My name is Emilia Chukwuma, and I teach business as well as accounting courses at Gallaudet University. I next introduce Ron Sutcliffe, who is the moderator for today's discussion. Throughout the course of discussion, we will get to know our panelists and what led them to success. I am not going to introduce them. To save time I leave the introductions to each panel member.

RON: I know many of you are very involved in businesses or interested in setting up businesses at some point. We have four very successful businessmen here, both in the United States and overseas. We have Jim Macfadden, who is from the United States. We have Yuri Maksimenko, from the Ukraine. The next person is David Barber from Finland. Finally, here is Bernard Brown from the United States.

JIM: I am Jim Macfadden, president of Macfadden and Associates, Inc. We began in 1976. We do mostly computer functions, developing computer software and managing programs for the federal government. We win contracts by open competition. We have roughly eighty people in my employ. All have college degrees, and we are doing just great!

YURI: I represent the Ukraine Deaf Society. The society is sixty-nine years old. For sixty-nine years our society has been engaged in business because our society owns its own factories. In the factories, 75 percent of the workers are deaf. Thus, in our factories, deaf people have been running a business for a long time. We have forty-two factories altogether all over the Ukraine. In twenty of these factories, we do various kinds of sewing, including suits and outfits for workers. We have eight factories involving furniture, furniture for offices, and furniture for schools; twelve factories make electrical gadgets; one factory makes paper products; and one factory makes nails.

DAVID: Hello, I am David Barber. I grew up in Georgia. I graduated from Gallaudet in 1996, and I moved to Finland. My wife is from Finland. I am a course-building specialist and have set up a number of recreation courses like Outward Bound kinds of courses. I have been in this kind of business for about a year and a half, and the business is doing well.

BERNARD: My name is Bernard Brown. We set up a business that specializes in house renovations. We also built five new houses. We started with that, and we found out that remodeling homes was better because we had more income and better cash flow from remodeling existing homes as opposed to building new homes. We have been in the remodeling business since then. I am still with my partner in this business. However, he is out there working while I am here enjoying being on the panel.

RON: Please briefly explain how you started your business and how you got to where you are now. We can start with Jim.

JIM: I worked for about ten different private companies over a series of years before starting my own business. I had a lot of frustrations with managers in my previous employ. I wanted to be a manager. I wanted to take control, and that is just me. I had a lot of experience with federal government contracting, so I decided to go into business based on my experience, and that is how it led me to where I am today.

YURI: It was different for me. When our society was founded, the deaf people did not have money, but the deaf people needed jobs. At that point, the government helped us create our own factories, and we started working for the factories and eventually started making money. When we were making money, we did not need the government's assistance anymore because we were able to sustain ourselves. In the past few years, of course, things are a little different and a little worse. But we know how to do business.

DAVID: When I was young I knew I wanted to start a business. Here in the United States, there were a lot of different opportunities. I knew I wanted to do something with the outdoors and with wilderness adventure. I had done something like that in Virginia in terms of setting up camps and different activities. Also in Virginia, there was a company from which I was able to gain experience. When I moved to Finland, I saw there were opportunities for different outdoor experiences, but there was no professional organization involved in the kind of business I had in mind. I decided to set up that kind of business because I saw a need, as well as to fulfill my lifelong dream. I went from there.

BERNARD: I was an accountant, my partner was a machinist, and we did different kinds of work together previously. We always talked about setting up our own business, but we just talked and did not do anything. Finally in 1985, we looked at each other and did it. We knew we needed some kind of financial backing. We had our own homes, so we drew money from our own homes using our home equity lines of credit and built our first house in Connecticut. It was a risk because if we did not pay back that money we owed, the bank could take back our homes. We had to make regular payments on this money we owed. We sold the first house we built, and the rest is history. We built additional homes but then decided not to build new homes anymore, because like I mentioned earlier, the cash flow was not really that great with new homes. Instead, we decided to do home rebuilding.

When we tried to sell our first house, we met many new faces. We were new faces ourselves, like the new guys on the block. It was hard when we first started. We had to sell ourselves, kind of like the door-to-door salesmen where you had a lot of rejection before you get your first sale. We finally did sell our new house—our first house.

When we started remodeling, we did deck work, we did bathrooms, we did roofing, and we did all kinds of home improvement. Again, there were initial frustrations with trying to obtain remodeling contracts, in spite of our strong background. My partner and I were good with handiwork. We had had experience building homes. We got one out of twelve in terms of sales to marketing.

Eventually we built a network of people. Word spread fast from the work that we did, and word-of-mouth gets around. Today, in terms of sales to marketing, we get four out of five. It becomes easier in terms of selling because of networking. People would say, well, I have found your name. At this point we do not need to advertise and do marketing because we already have lots of remodeling jobs lined up. If other people spread word through word-of-mouth, then we can go from there. We work a lot through word-of-mouth because people know the kind of product we sell. When we meet with new clients we show them a book where we can show our product and the kind of finish work that we have done, and people are amazed by the kind of work that we are able to do. From that we are able to sell by showing the kind of product that we do.

That was the strategy that led to our success, convincing clients to buy from us. Some people might ask if we have a lot of deaf clients. Actually, a very small percentage, maybe 2 percent, of our remodeling jobs is done for deaf clients. That is, a large majority of our jobs are for hearing customers. We have been in business for about twenty years now.

RON: You are all deaf. You are dealing with the hearing world. Are there any specific strategies that you used in terms of grasping opportunities? Were there challenges that you confronted? Bernard said that it was difficult to start originally, and can you talk about that, Jim?

JIM: First, I had to spend time doing the necessary applications and paperwork to be certified by the United States Small Business Administration as a minority business. It was a way to help smaller minority businesses, for women, black people, people with disabilities, or disadvantaged groups, get some contracts from the government to get them started.

Then I developed a network of people. I got my reputation out there for doing good work. I also put good people underneath me. As Bernard said, your reputation is everything. If you have a reputation for doing good work, people will have faith in you. I get the work, I do a good job, and I keep in mind that as I pull more good people in our company, the business will continue to grow. I have kept that philosophy more than ten years. All of these different elements of my business have grown because people who we do business with really appreciate the work and the price, too.

Right now I would say about eighty people are in our company, and almost all of them have degrees, with a variety of different experiences and expertise.

YURI: Communication has been our biggest issue both at home and at the factory. There are deaf people who can talk well. They do not need as much help when communicating in various situations. There are deaf people that are not able to talk that well or at all, but they can interact with hearing workers through an interpreter. At each one of our factories, the society has a regional organization providing an interpreter so that hearing and deaf workers can communicate. Interpreters are also useful for deaf people in varying social and medical situations in Ukraine. I cannot say that we are 100 percent successful in resolving communication issues. Obviously, our communication technology is lacking, but we are hoping to see great improvement in available technology so that deaf workers can become independent and able to make contacts and calls by themselves.

DAVID: Finland has many recreation companies, and they have some technology infused with what they do in building courses. For the past thirty years, they have had used different approaches in building courses and often relied on Americans for assistance. They had hired Americans to come and build the courses, and it has been quite costly for them. When I approached them, they could see that I was an American with the needed experience. Because I am already there in Finland, this translates into reduced cost for them.

Inspection for durability and safety is necessary for any recreation course being built. There may be a wire hanging about fifteen feet high between two different trees for people going through this course between the two trees on the wire. We need to be sure that the wire will not break or fall, because it can cause serious injury or loss of life, and then the companies can get sued. They have a big interest in making sure that I would install the course in a way that has safety built in.

There are many variations to consider for the construction of a recreational course. What I have done is to show them pictures of different recreation courses that I have created. They would select some features to include, and then we go from the pictures and make adjustments in customizing a recreation course.

The business I have is freelance work. I have been in business for only a year and a half. My company does not have any other permanent employee at this time. When I get a contract to build a course, then I will pull in one or two freelancers who have experience not only in course building but also in building houses or other kinds of skills that I need. That is the way I run my business.

RON: What advice would you give to people who want to go into business for themselves?

JIM: Originally when I set up my business, I had to have a specific road map. I needed to know how to get there. But barriers always come up, and whenever a barrier comes up, you have to find a way to do something to get around it. If it is in relation to price competition, you have to do something to remain competitive. If there is improvement you need to make, you cannot stay complacent in business because then you would be a guaranteed failure. You need to always take refresher or enrichment courses, do things in terms of business, do better things with people, and study the market.

My job as the president is always looking out for tomorrow. I do not care about today. Today is doing just fine. I am looking at tomorrow, next year, two years. It is always important to have a road map for them. That is the only way to make your business successful.

YURI: There are two ways to look at businesses. One way is setting up and running a business for the benefit of an owner or a number of partners. The other way, like what we are doing with our factories in Ukraine, is to set up a factory (as a business) with an important objective of helping other people get jobs.

To be your own boss and to be able to create money and jobs to give to other deaf people, you have to know a lot. My friend says, correctly, you have to learn a lot. You have to know the economy. You have to know how to organize jobs and manage them.

You need to know overriding civil policies and international politics and work within their framework. You have to know a lot. The head and leaders of the firm should have that kind of knowledge or at least be able to access it. When we go out to look for leaders to work with us, we look for people who have some of this knowledge.

Through marketing, we get orders for these factories that we have and what to produce. Here we do that in several different ways. First we study the market ourselves and try to find our niche. We go to larger firms and ask them if they have work for us. If we have to, we try to get jobs from government. We would find a niche for products that we can supply to the government.

There have been challenging barriers to overcome because Ukraine is under growing pains of a new, independent nation. We need to check whether there are laws for deaf people through which we can find our niche. I repeat, we always continue to look for ways to find a new niche under changing times. We always ask ourselves whether we should go and take this road—or the other road—toward success.

I have been asked we why are we keeping our factories. This is because they also serve as very good schools for the training of deaf people. Not everyone can go to school and get higher education, but if they come to our factories, they can start somewhere and go from there. At the factories, even if they start at the bottom, the ambitious ones often rise up to more important jobs. In the process, they learn and take on larger responsibilities. The more knowledge they gain, the more they can provide us with help in searching for new business areas. We even send them to schools to get a higher education and then they come back to help us.

Our responsibilities are to find jobs for the deaf. Maybe you have a different system. Your system is probably good for you. Our system, for Ukraine, works very well. It has the advantages of serving the economy of the nation and our citizens.

DAVID: I had done work in Virginia for a company, so I learned the important things in their field, involving needed equipment, work that is to be done, and building a client base. I made sure I had a thorough understanding of those areas and then transferred that knowledge when I went to Finland.

In Finland, I did my homework and learned what their culture was and what was important. One of the things I did was to go through a telephone book, and if I saw there were too many companies under one heading or subheading, then I would not get into that field. Eventually I was able to find my particular niche and proceeded to set up a business accordingly.

BERNARD: When I set up my business using all the parameters that were involved at that time, I would continually observe how well things are doing against these original parameters. If I see that some or all of these parameters have changed for me, then I would stop and make adjustments. I have made adjustments throughout the many years I have been in business. If I had not done that, then I surely would have failed along the way. I had to follow the course of emerging technology. I had to keep in mind new, fresh ideas and be open to these ideas.

I am going to share a secret with you. Just last week, I was talking with my partner and learned that next year, there is no pressure-treated lumber allowed. We use it for the foundation on the decks. That is going to stop. But we already have it. Why is this going into effect? As we understand it, it is because of a new law that was enacted in Pennsylvania. So what are we going to do? We have to get ready. We have to know what is going to be happening. Stores are going to stop selling pressure-treated lumber, so we have to be ready for that. We have to be one step ahead.

We look at our competition. We cannot know everything they are doing, but we know we have to follow technology and what is happening. There was the invention of the personal computer, and we had to observe how that would affect business. Other competitors might say, oh, what do I need that for? I can breathe. I can eat. I am doing fine. No problem. But based on our observations, we went ahead and learned and used new computing technology, which proved to be very beneficial.

Others might not have, but we always wanted to stay abreast of what is new, and we would adapt to what we needed. Here is an example about gutters. They are expensive, so we had to figure out time and materials involved to get the job done. It would be difficult to do the job cheaper than a specialized gutter company that has all the updated equipment and machines. What we did was to contract out the work in this area. We looked at market trends and found that other remodeling firms did the same thing.

Is this bad? No. But it makes sense economically. We have twenty subcontractors. That means they are not our employees. They are the subcontractors we hire to do certain jobs. We get profit for the work they do. How? When we write a bid for a remodeling job, we include overhead costs for ourselves as well as the actual costs for the subcontractors to do the job. We get paid a total price for a complete job, including overhead costs, and then we give a portion of that money to the subcontractors for them to do the work. It is a common business practice.

So, you have to keep an open mind and be creative in terms of seeing what your plans are and keeping one step ahead. For example, if you already have a contract to install pressure-treated lumber for a deck, then you need to be sure there is enough lumber in stock. Otherwise, you better run and get that pressure-treated lumber before they stop selling it or before the price goes up drastically.

AUDIENCE: I am from Canada. I have a comment and then a brief question. You know the concept of a job coach. Why not have a business coach or a business coach club? There are deaf individuals who are skilled in different lines of work, but they do not know how to network or find the needed resources to set up a business. They do not know what the law requirements are or how to write business plans. There might be individuals seeking guidance in finding appropriate government agencies or other entities with available start-up money. Is there any interest and experience in setting up business training in this area? What about follow-up support with the provision of a business coach for mentoring purposes? Are there any skills they need to develop? Are there resources available for them?

BERNARD: I was a visiting professor at Gallaudet University last year, and really the students had to learn accounting. It really is a pipeline, but you need to think more broadly. You do not need to look only at accounting. You need to look at different aspects of business. One person might be interested in working in a church setting, and they will need accounting because accounting is involved with someone becoming involved with the ministry. Someone else might say, well, I am going to be involved with the church. I do not need business skills. However, you do need business skills in terms of budget, in terms of fiscal management. It is important within a church group to have this kind of skill, because if not, then you would have to hire out for this kind of help. This is just an example. Learn as much as you can about business. Take business courses. Learn about different aspects of business.

RON: Jim Macfadden, John Yeh, Louis Schwarz, and I, the four of us, had worked together to implement the National Deaf Business Initiative. It is an organization, working through different deaf institutions, with the goal of providing training for deaf people who are interested in setting up businesses, including opportunities for internships and working with mentors.

A Comparative Investigation of Entrepreneurship among Deaf Populations in Developed and Developing Countries

ISAAC O. AGBOOLA

This study investigates, at an exploratory level, entrepreneurship activities among deaf populations in developed and developing countries, with emphasis on environmental barriers to entrepreneurship and how deaf entrepreneurs cope with and overcome the barriers. Specific sources of environmental adversity investigated include education, economic, market, technology, and societal attitudes toward disability. A qualitative quasi-deductive approach with convenience sampling was used to conduct the study. This approach was chosen because of the explorative nature of the investigation and the difficulty of obtaining empirical data from sources in developing countries.

The study was based on data collected through in-depth, semistructured interviews with sixteen deaf business owners. The interviews were conducted over a two-year period and include on-site visits to selected businesses. Nine of the businesses in the study are located in countries classified by the United Nations as developed, whereas seven are in countries classified as developing. Additional data were obtained through literature review, Web-based sources, and statistical abstracts.

The Deaf Entrepreneur

Deaf people have always engaged in entrepreneurial activities, and many have done and continue to do so successfully (Lane 1984). However, the rate of entrepreneurship among deaf people is typically much lower than the rate for the general population. Adverse factors such as lack of access to capital, communication barriers, and competition present formidable obstacles to aspiring deaf entrepreneurs. Characteristics of deaf entrepreneurial activities such as motivation, methods of entry, types of business activities, and mode of operation are discussed in the following sections.

Motivation for Entrepreneurship

Deaf people are motivated to start their own business by the same factors that motivate the general population to do so: an entrepreneurial spirit, desire for independence, increased financial rewards, and as an alternative to a tight job market (Morrison, White, and Van Velsor 1992). In developing countries, the lack of jobs is a primary motivation for deaf people to turn to entrepreneurship as a means of economic survival. However, because of lack of capital, inadequate education, limited access to markets, and other environmental factors, the business activities that deaf entrepreneurs in developing countries engaged in are largely at a subsistence level. By contrast, deaf people in developed countries have greater access to jobs and generally tend to engage in business for reasons other than subsistence.

Methods of Entry

Most deaf business ventures start out as sole proprietorships begun from scratch. Less frequently, an existing business is purchased or leased. In rare cases, a deaf person may take over the family business, gain control of a part of the family business, or attain an executive-level role in the family business. Startup capital might be raised through savings, contributions from relatives, bank loans, government grants, or grants from charitable organizations. In many cases, more than one of these sources were used to start the business. In developed countries, aspiring deaf entrepreneurs have the opportunity to raise substantial capital through savings, contributions from relatives, bank loans, and government grants. Deaf business owners in the United States, for example, have the opportunity to obtain government-backed loans through the Small Business Administration program. In developing countries, lack of startup capital is a primary obstacle to entrepreneurship. The level of poverty is often such that an aspiring deaf entrepreneur would find it difficult to raise the necessary capital through savings or contributions from relatives. Economic conditions in developing countries also often mean stringent requirements to obtain a bank loan and little or nonexistent government assistance for startup capital.

Types and Scope of Entrepreneurial Activities

Although deaf entrepreneurs engage in a wide variety of business activities ranging from personal selling to manufacturing, the size and scope of the business operations tend to be relatively small even in developed countries. In the United States, where conditions for entrepreneurial success are perhaps more favorable for deaf entrepreneurs than anywhere else in the world, no deaf-owned business is large enough to rate a mention in the various annual surveys of the largest national or regional corporations. The vast majority of deaf-owned businesses are sole proprietorships with fewer than twenty-five employees. Deaf business owners in developed countries are able to engage in a wider variety of business activities than their counterparts in developing countries whose business activities are generally limited to crafts and basic services. Types of business activities in developed countries include medical and dental practices, small-scale manufacturing, hotels, restaurants, real estate investments, consulting services, financial planning, interpreting services, publishing, and, in recent times, Internet-based commerce. In developing countries, however, the prevailing types of deaf-owned business are craft based, and they tend to be on a smaller scale than in developed countries.

Modes of Operation

Deaf entrepreneurs generally adhere to the same basic business principles as any other business, such as attention to quality, customer satisfaction, cost controls, and marketing. However, deaf business owners in developing countries are generally not as well educated or as exposed to standard business practices as their counterparts in developed countries. Therefore they are more likely to make unsound business decisions and less likely to apply proven business practices. In developed countries, most deaf-owned businesses are single proprietorships, as is the case in developing countries. In developing countries, deaf business ownership may also take the form of a business cooperative. A business cooperative may comprise from two to as many as fifteen or more members, each in specific roles from management to employee. A cooperative may be affiliated with a school, charitable organization, or deaf association.

Environmental Adversity to Entrepreneurship

Environmental adversity presents a constant threat to entrepreneurs everywhere and discourages new entrants. Sources of environmental adversity to entrepreneurial activities include competition, economic conditions, market characteristics, government regulations, and lack of capital (Miller and Friesen 1984; Zahra 1996; Slater and Naver 1994). For entrepreneurs and aspiring entrepreneurs who have a disability, some aspects of environmental adversity are magnified and present more formidable obstacles to success. For example, Deaf entrepreneurs are further subject to additional adversity such as societal attitudes toward deafness and communication barriers between the deaf business owner and potential clients. In the following sections, major barriers to deaf entrepreneurs, as determined through interviews with deaf business owners, are examined.

Lack of Capital

Interviews with deaf business owners in both developed and developing countries indicate that they perceive the difficulty of obtaining startup capital to be the most serious and intractable obstacle for aspiring deaf business owners to overcome. Deaf entrepreneurs in developed countries generally find it easier to raise business capital than their counterparts in developing countries. In developed countries, aspiring deaf entrepreneurs can raise money from their savings, obtain bank loans, secure government assistance, or be supported by relatives or a spouse while they get the business off the ground. By contrast, these resources tend to be severely limited for aspiring deaf business owners in developing countries. The high rate of unemployment among deaf populations in developing countries is also a major reason for lack of startup capital. In some cases, foreign donors have stepped in to provide startup capital to deaf communities in specific countries. One notable example of this is the efforts of a consortium of European charitable organizations that provide financial and other support, including training, to deaf organizations in developing countries.

Economic Conditions

Among respondents from developing countries, unfavorable economic conditions ranked second to lack of capital as a perceived major barrier to deaf business ownership. Unfavorable economic conditions present obstacles on two fronts: limited resources to start a business and a limited market for business products or services. Respondents in developed countries ranked economic conditions lower as an obstacle, ranking communication barriers as the second most serious obstacle to starting their business and staying competitive. This disparity in perception of the impact of economic conditions on entrepreneurship is to be expected, because access to both capital and markets is considerably easier in developed countries than in developing countries. In the depressed economies of developing countries, deaf entrepreneurs also have to contend with stiffer competition from mainstream business for the limited customer base.

Communication Barriers and Societal Attitudes

All respondents considered societal attitudes toward disability and the difficulty of communicating with hearing customers as major obstacles. The negative impact of these two factors seems to be less severe for deaf business owners in developed countries than for those in developing countries for the following reasons:

- existence of a ready niche market of deaf customers with considerable economic means, providing an alternative to total dependence on hearing customers;
- availability of alternative means of communication with hearing customers such as relay services, e-mail, and the Internet;
- resources to hire employees who either work full-time as interpreters or who combine interpreting duties with other duties in the business; and
- opportunity to partner with established name brands and gain access to mainstream markets.

Skepticism concerning the ability of a person who is deaf to successfully operate a business was cited as a major reason why banks and other traditional sources of business capital are reluctant to extend business loans to deaf entrepreneurs. Such skepticism was also cited as a major obstacle to attracting new customers and getting business accounts. As a result, most deaf entrepreneurs interviewed reported that they had to use personal savings and contributions from friends and relatives to start their business. Societal attitudes and communication barriers also force deaf entrepreneurs to focus, at least initially, on the deaf niche market as their primary market segment. However, the deaf niche market tends to be both too small to support a small business and to be geographically fragmented. Still, in developed countries at least, the deaf niche market is often large and economically strong enough to successfully support some types of business such as medical practices, law practices, financial services, home improvement, crafts, and retail sales of technological devices for deaf people.

Deaf entrepreneurs in developing countries often have fewer means of dealing with communication barriers and societal attitudes toward individuals with a disability than their counterparts in developed countries. High unemployment and underemployment is a common characteristic of deaf populations in developing countries, so a deaf niche market, which could nurture an initial business effort, is often nonexistent. As a result, the level of entrepreneurship among deaf populations in most developing countries is much lower than in developed countries. The rate of venture success also tends to be much lower for deaf business owners in developing countries.

Overcoming Adversity

Clearly, deaf and other entrepreneurs with disability, regardless of where they live, face a greater level of adversity in starting a business and staying competitive than the average business owner who has no disability. The negative impact of adversity is generally greater for deaf business owners in developing countries than for their counterparts in developed countries. However, the existence of so much environmental adversity has never completely stifled the entrepreneurial spirit of deaf people, even in developing countries with grinding poverty (Gannon 1981; Lane 1984). Individuals with an entrepreneurial spirit also tend to possess a high degree of persistence, courage, creativity, and other personal qualities that they draw on when faced with environmental adversity. Some of the strategies employed by deaf business owners to contend with environmental adversity include seeking alternative sources of capital, concentrating primarily on the deaf niche market, forming cooperative associations, lobbying the government for favorable laws, hiring hearing employees for positions where interface with customers is critical, taking advantage of technological innovations, and engaging in e-commerce.

The relative success of deaf entrepreneurs in developed countries provides useful insights into successful strategies to overcome barriers to business ownership that deaf business owners in developing countries could emulate, if local conditions are right. Obviously, not all the successful strategies are applicable globally because of local factors such as economic conditions and availability of technology.

References

Gannon, J. R. 1981. *Deaf heritage*. Silver Spring, MD: National Association of the Deaf.
Lane, H. 1984. *When the mind hears: A history of the Deaf*. New York: Random House.
Miller, D., and P. H. Friesen. 1984. *Organizations: A quantum view*. Englewood Cliffs, NJ: Prentice-Hall.
Morrison, A. M., R. P. White, and E. Van Velsor. 1992. *Breaking the glass ceiling: Can women reach the top of America's large corporations?* Reading, MA: Addisson-Wesley.
Slater, S. F., and J. C. Naver. 1994. Does competitive environment moderate the market orientation–performance relationship? *Journal of Marketing* 38: 46–55.
Zahra, S. 1996. Technology strategy and company performance: Examining the moderating effect of the competitive environment. *Journal of Business Venturing* 11 (3): 189–219.

PART THREE

Education

Deaf Education: Whose "Way" Is It?

LAURENE SIMMS

Deaf education: whose way is it? That is the question. Is that a political question? Or is it a moral question? There are a variety of ways to view the question. I focus on Deaf education as a civil right to be given to deaf children. On September 11, two planes crashed into the World Trade Center in New York City. Many of you know the story, and you have heard it time and time again, but that story has had impact on people around the world. It made us step back and reevaluate what our lives are all about. We realized that we needed to be closer to our families, to appreciate ourselves as human beings, and to see one another as such. Now, how does this impact Deaf education?

Why does Deaf education still fail? We talk about two hundred years of history, and still Deaf education fails. This failure has been demonstrated through studies that report low reading ability. For instance, Allen presents statistics in his 1994 report that show that most deaf high school graduates can only read at a fourth-grade reading level. In this report, he noted that only two deaf children out of one hundred go to college, and high school graduates cannot read the newspaper. This is a question that has come up time and time again throughout the ages. Why? Why does it still fail? As deaf people, we see our classmates and schoolmates, our friends, struggling to receive an appropriate education, to develop literacy skills, and to do their schoolwork. We have seen this type of frustration from generation to generation to generation. I share that frustration. We have to rethink: why does Deaf education still fail? We think about all the different educational systems around the world and how different people here in America have thought throughout the educational system. I have chosen two specific groups whose educational history parallels ours: that of African American and black children and that of Native American indigenous people.

In black education, the case of *Brown v. Board of Education of Topeka*, which you may be familiar with, was a landmark case. It was one of the most important cases presented before the U.S. Supreme Court having to do with unequal education. People at that time got together and fought to improve the educational status of their children. How did it happen? What was their inspiration? Who was behind the movement? Who led the protests? How did the fight start and carry all the way to the Supreme Court, whose unanimous decision, passed in 1954, outlawed school segregation? That case had to do with unequal education. As we study that case, how can we apply what was learned there to deaf education? Another historical parallel relates to Native Americans who have fought fiercely to keep their culture. What can we learn from them, and how can we apply the principles of equal education and preservation of culture to deaf children?

I begin with the parallel to Black education. Many schools for black children were in disrepair and not adequately equipped. The seats were crowded, and some were broken. There were not enough books and materials for each child. Black children had to walk to school, and as they walked along that dusty road to the schoolhouse, they saw buses go by with white children seated in air-conditioned comfort on their way to school. The school building that the white children went to was nice, and they had comfortable chairs. They had plenty of textbooks and other materials. They had rooms that were air conditioned, with a heater for the winter as well. They had all the comforts, whereas the black children went to schools that were crowded. Again, black children had to walk a long way to school; they arrived tired and had to struggle to stay awake to study, and then to walk all the way back home afterward.

Why was there inequality in education for black Americans? The answer is white supremacy. The white supremacists believed that negroes were inferior beings and of an inferior race. As such, they were unfit to associate with the white race, either in social or political relations, and they had no rights to education. As a nonwhite person, I have had a hard time understanding that concept. I cannot fathom this type of white supremacist thinking.

So, how does black education parallel with Deaf education? What do I mean by unequal education access? I have two examples. The first is a student by the name of Frankie McClendon. He was from the state of Alabama and won a major lawsuit against the Alabama Department of Education. Frankie was a black student who was deaf and who did not receive appropriate education throughout his school years. He was put in a classroom of mentally retarded children for years. In that class he would show up for school every day and color pictures until he was sixteen years old. His mother fought his case all the way through various courts, all the way up to the state level. The state decided that school administrators had to hire someone to work with Frankie. The teacher that they hired was Anne Peterson from Alabama. After being taught by Amy on a one-to-one basis for one year, Frankie's learning had a breakthrough like Helen Keller. When I met Frankie, I was absolutely astounded with the miracle of his progress. Amy shared with me that one day she was sick that she could not come to tutor him. The next day when Amy showed up, she saw that Frankie was upset. He said, "Do not ever again miss a day of school. I want to learn, as I've missed so much. I can't afford to miss one single day of getting my education." He was such a motivated student. Frankie described his experience of unequal education access and about what happened at school:

> "So, tell me about what it was like for you going to school."
> "I didn't do anything in school."
> "Where was your school? Was it a deaf school?"
> "It was a hearing school. And I just used to sit and color in my book."
> "What were you writing?"

"I wouldn't write anything; I was coloring. We didn't have anything like math books or anything like that. So I just had to sit and draw, and other kids used to make fun of me and I used to have to sit there and take it. My mother told me to just focus on my studies. But I would get angry. And I kept telling my mother I wasn't getting any education."

"They didn't teach you to read or write or math or anything?"

"All I did was color."

Frankie is bright and is now eighteen years old. He has been signing for only the past two years and received education only for the past two years. That's what I mean by unequal education access. This happened not long ago, in 1998. How many more children like Frankie are in a situation where they are receiving unequal education access?

Let us now talk about the next example of unequal education access. This particular teacher is a well-spoken researcher sharing information with all of the students in her class. There is an interpreter who is interpreting to the deaf student, but as you can see the student is not getting much information. The information flow is not the same from the hearing teacher directly to her students as through the interpreter to the deaf student. The teacher has two masters' degrees; she has a background in teaching and has taught for five years, whereas the interpreter completed only high school and has no college degree, no training as an interpreter, and no certification as an interpreter but has been working for three years. Do the parents know about situations like this? No. Does the principal know about situations like this? Is the teacher aware of the interpreter's profile? No. What about the student? I doubt it. That is what I mean about unequal access, and it is something that continues from year to year. Who evaluates people in that program? Who is out there doing the research about programs like that where students receive unequal education access year after year? No one. That is why I say it is unequal access to education.

There is a parallel with black education and how that fight for equal education compares with equal education access for deaf students, such as the case of Frankie from 1998 and students in mainstream programs in the year 2002. In the twenty-first century, unequal access still remains.

The majority of American professionals think that mainstreaming Deaf children will normalize them and that they will become normal children. But is that true? Does deinstitutionalization lead to normalization? No. The students' needs for social and language development are ignored.

There is a parallel with another group, the Native American community. The book that you see here, *Making and Molding Identity in Schools* by Ann Locke Davidson, was a book that I read during my doctoral study. The author is an anthropologist in education. It is full of children's narratives about their own experiences, not only Native American children but also Latino children, Asian children, and children of other cultures, talking about being raised in the American system and being molded to fit in with the white American. Although there are no narratives from deaf children in this book, the stories are quite riveting.

One clip from the documentary film *Teaching Indians to be White* describes how Native Americans' hair was cut. It also explains how they were not allowed to wear their traditional clothes and that all of their cultural values that they held dear they had to leave behind to assimilate into this world. They were forced to suppress all their cultural values that they passed on from generation to generation—their heritage. Captain Richard Pratt was a famous man who went out into the frontier, rounded up Indians on horseback, brought enslaved Indians to the forts, made them clean up and bathe, cut off their hair, and then forced them to become acculturated and molded into white Americans. Yet people said he was a great captain. Well, maybe he had the best intentions. Maybe with his heart he wanted to mold the Indian into a man that could be respected and seen on par with white Americans.

What is the parallel between the Native American community and the Deaf community? The parallel is that our deaf children are molded as well. Deaf children were often seated with their hands restrained. It was a painful experience to be forced to sit in a chair for hours on end, to try to follow what others were saying, to try to read their speech patterns, to have to restrain the natural use of language, to have ear phones on your head as you sat for hours practicing and hoping that you would hear that tone just so you can get a piece of candy. That type of molding of deaf children continues to this day.

It has been a long battle. Our battle parallels that of both the African American and Native American communities who fought to make desired changes, and they were both successful in their fight: the Native Americans and the fight to have their culture respected and African Americans and their fight for equal access. We in the Deaf community have been involved in this battle for a long time. It seems hard for us to come to some agreement as to what exactly can be done to improve the state of education for deaf children today. We have gone a full cycle.

The three separate cultural groups—African Americans, Native Americans, and Deaf Americans—have something in common. Each group is bonded to culture and has a fighting spirit. However, for hearing parents who have deaf children, their experiences are different—there is not one of pride, but rather one of pain, of grief, of having a deaf child and not knowing what to do with him or her, and of having a deaf child but really wanting the child to have normal hearing. They do not have any fighting spirit; they do not have that instilled in them. That is why they are different from deaf parents with deaf children. I am not saying that hearing parents or their ways of parenting are wrong. They often do not have access to the right information; what they do is out of love, and they believe that they are doing the best for their child. They often do not see success as part of their child's future; rather they only see pain and suffering in the future of the child. That is why the battle about Deaf education continues.

Like the Native American and black communities, I want you to fight for our children and talk about what we will do as far as the system is concerned. Yes, there is a system that we face. Think about the words of Frederick Douglass, the civil rights advocate and a great abolitionist: "O! had I the ability, and could I reach the nation's ear, I would, to day, pour out a fiery stream of biting ridicule, blasting reproach, withering sarcasm, and stern rebuke. For it is not light that is needed, but fire; it is not the gentle shower, but thunder." We need to be heard loud and clear. We need to fight for our civil rights, as Frederick Douglass did. Thunder is the only way that we're going to get people to pay attention to the issue of civil rights for deaf children. How can it be done? How did black people give out thunder? How did Native Americans become thunderous in their roar for equality?

This is a true story about Ruby Bridges that happened about forty years ago. This little girl was six years old. She courageously, bravely marched into the schoolyard surrounded by marshals. Behind the marshals were adults who spit at her, literally. They spew words of hate at her and threw things at her, yet she continued bravely, step by step, into this school building. She only wanted to go to school. She just wanted to learn. What is wrong with somebody who wants to be literate and to learn to read and write? Why could they not accept that at that time? Why could they not allow black children and white children to go to school together? What was wrong? I thought about that again and again. When we think about the answer, we think about the media, television, newspaper, and the fact that African Americans use the media again and again to make the point that they would not accept "separate but equal" education because it was unequal. The same goes with Native Americans. They went to the media to make the point again and again that they would not accept the destruction of their culture and their people. Yet the Deaf community sits in silence, and we did not get media attention, either. There are very few books about us and very few articles about us. We are not talking to people outside of the Deaf community about issues that need to be faced.

Professional development is also a key consideration, because often you find that dedicated teachers want to make changes and to be progressive in the education they provide. However, they are fearful that by pushing too far they will get fired or demoted by administrators with the plantation mentality. Now deaf people think we have to acquiesce, we cannot make any changes, and we cannot make waves—or else possibly face adverse consequences. That has got to change. We have to do what is needed. We have to become politically savvy. We have to figure out how to work our way through this educational system, as the African Americans and Native Americans did. There must also be collaborative efforts.

In conclusion, this is a story that happened exactly ten years ago with my hearing son. I asked my son what he learned in school today. This was something that he told me that I have held on to ever since:

> A long time ago, there lived a king. He was a very wise king. Any riddle that was proposed to him, he could answer without a doubt. Any problem brought before him he could solve it. It happened one day that the queen of another country thought that she had a riddle that she could pose that would stump this king. What she did was to have a courtyard of flowers planted; they were all artificial flowers except for one real flower. She asked the king to come and she said in this courtyard of flowers there's only one real flower. Find it, and see how wise you are. And he thought about it, thought about it, and suddenly it came to him that he should open the window. A cool breeze passed through and a bee went through the window. The bee flew from flower to flower until it finally found the real flower and sat on it, pollinated it, and then flew out the window. And the king went over and picked up the flower and said, this is the real flower. And people were absolutely astounded and amazed with the wisdom that he presented.

We have gone through the system feeling frustrated, knowing that oppressive thinking and misconceptions are not the right way for the education of my child. This is a struggle that has been going on for centuries. Finally, we see our natural language and culture, and we know the child will be best able to learn in that environment because that is our flower.

References

Allen, T. E. 1994. Who are the deaf and hard of hearing students leaving high school and entering postsecondary education? Unpublished manuscript, Gallaudet University Center for Assessment and Demographic Studies, Washington, DC.

Davidson, A. L. 1996. *Making and molding identity in schools: Student narratives on race, gender and academic engagement*. Albany: State University of New York Press.

Signs of Literacy: Naturalistic Inquiry into ASL/English Bilingualism at Home and at School

CAROL J. ERTING, CYNTHIA NEESE BAILES,
LYNNE C. ERTING, CARLENE THUMANN-PREZIOSO,
AND MARLON KUNTZE

> [Literacy is] a set of social practices associated with particular symbol systems and their related technologies. To be literate is to be active; it is to be confident in these practices.
>
> —Barton, 1994, p. 32

The Signs of Literacy research team is an interdisciplinary team of Deaf and hearing researchers and teacher-researchers at Gallaudet University.[1] Our ethnographic studies seek to understand the sociocultural context of ASL/English bilingual Deaf education in the United States as well as Deaf children's individual pathways toward becoming bilingual and biliterate (C. Erting 2003). In this chapter, we present an overview of our emergent theoretical framework on Deaf literacy, discuss some of the methodological issues involved in videotaping in naturalistic settings, and briefly introduce three of the lines of research we are pursuing: (1) indigenous Deaf bilingual pedagogy and practices, (2) case studies of Deaf children becoming bilingual, and (3) indigenous Deaf bilingual parenting practices.

Theoretical Perspectives: The Deaf Way of Literacy

There is a need for a paradigmatic shift in the conceptualization and study of deaf children acquiring languages and literacies. We argue that attempts to apply methods of teaching deaf children literacy guided by theories developed on the basis of research on hearing/speaking children learning to read and write English in the United States have not achieved the desired results for the majority of deaf children (Traxler 2000). Instead of blaming the low test performance of deaf students on the students themselves or their teachers, we suggest that theories of literacy development that do not derive from processual research in naturalistic Deaf settings are misleading and inadequate at best. Why? In the United States, English-speaking hearing children

---

1. In this chapter we have utilized the D/d distinction that has become conventional to differentiate members of a cultural group (Deaf) from reference to the audiological condition of hearing loss (deaf).

are already familiar with the language they will learn to read in school because they arrive at school having had extensive experience with English through everyday interactions at home and in the community. When these children approach the task of reading and writing, the teacher mediates that learning through spoken English, reminding them of what the written words sound like. Their linguistic resources allow them to map the English they see in print with the English they use in their everyday talk. Once they have begun to read, they continue to learn English through reading and through interaction in spoken English, in and out of school.

However, Deaf children have not had full access to any spoken language by the time they are expected to begin reading and writing. But, if they have acquired American Sign Language (ASL), a natural language completely accessible to them through vision, they do have a powerful linguistic resource that can be used to support learning to read and write English. Despite the myths and misconceptions about ASL, we know it can support English language acquisition because research has begun to demonstrate the relationship between proficiency in ASL and English (Prinz 1998), but also because there have always been large numbers of bilingual Deaf people who have never heard English spoken. Theories of literacy development dependent upon the learners' access to the phonological system of English cannot explain the success of these proficient Deaf readers, and that means we need a new theory.

Toward that end, we are examining Deaf parents and Deaf teachers supporting Deaf children's ASL/English bilingual development in naturalistic settings in the U.S. context. We want to know what is happening when these adults and children interact in ASL during literacy events in the home and preschool classroom. What can we learn about indigenous Deaf practices in both settings, practices that use ASL to support English literacy development? Once we begin to discover what Deaf teachers and Deaf parents do and how Deaf children learn to read and write English, we will have taken a step forward in our ability to fashion a theory that helps explain Deaf literacy. Our ideas and findings may apply to contexts outside of the United States as well, but we want to be clear that they are based solely on data collected in the American educational arena.

We began collecting data for these studies in 1987, before the current research team was constituted, when Thumann-Prezioso and C. Erting began monthly videotaping of Deaf families interacting in their home environments (C. Erting, Prezioso, and Hynes 1990/1994; C. Erting, Thumann-Prezioso, and Benedict 2000). Literacy activities between Deaf parents and their preschool Deaf children interacting in ASL were prominent in these videotapes. The second phase of data collection took place from 1994 to 1996 when we expanded our team, included teacher-researchers, and began collecting data in ASL/English bilingual classrooms. In addition to videotaping classroom activities for an entire morning biweekly in each classroom, we also conducted ethnographic interviews with teachers and aides and collected teacher journals (written and/or videotaped) and classroom artifacts. Our goal was to understand both what was happening in the classroom and how teachers were thinking about what they were doing and experiencing. The six classrooms were in a day school for Deaf children where the Deaf and hearing preschool teachers themselves had decided to follow a bilingual approach. Eleven teachers (five Deaf and six hearing) and sixty Deaf children from diverse backgrounds participated in this phase of data collection. The third phase of data collection is under way—following up five children from our original preschool population who differ from each other in theoretically important ways. These case studies will document the ASL, English literacy, and academic achievement of the target students to understand how home and classroom environments as well as individual histories might influence the course of each child's developing bilingualism.

Challenges of Videotaping in Preschool Classroom Settings

Our research questions dictated the use of video for data collection because we wanted detailed documentation and description of teaching practices and student learning in Deaf bilingual (visual) classrooms. Furthermore, video recordings allowed researchers and teacher-researchers to view and analyze classroom interaction together, a condition necessary for the insider/outsider collaboration central to an ethnographic approach. The videos also provided teacher-researchers with opportunities to reflect on their teaching practices and the progress of their students, gaining insights for immediate application in the classroom. Limited space prevents us from describing our research methodology in depth, but we discuss some issues related to videotaping naturalistic interaction in preschool classrooms. Two principles guided our data collection strategies: (1) capture activity in the classrooms as comprehensively as possible without sacrificing detail of the video images necessary for analysis and (2) when studying sign language discourse, the video image must be framed so that it includes face, body, hands, and referents. These principles led to the decision to use three cameras operated individually by three researchers with a fourth researcher acting as coordinator, observing and directing focus. These researchers needed to be taught to see with what we called "Deaf eyes" to capture essential behaviors and referents, often requiring rapid decision making during framing.

Along with the benefits of videotaping, there were several logistical challenges. Video equipment in the classrooms included three cameras, VCR carts, and cables, resulting in decreased flexibility in the arrangement of classroom space and the presence of four additional adults. Being observed by outsiders and the creation of a permanent video record contributed to some anxiety on the part of the teachers and was a distraction on occasion for the children. However, the research plan had been developed collaboratively, and there was a commitment from all participants to work together as a team to overcome the difficulties. In addition, all were committed to the principles of bilingualism and full accessibility to communication and agreed that the children's welfare took precedence in decision making. Flexibility, mutual trust, and the designation of one researcher to serve as the principal liaison between the teacher-researchers and the research team all contributed to the success of the team building and collaboration.

Study 1: Using ASL to Mediate Book Sharing

Our preschool classroom study focuses on describing the multiple ways that the teachers used ASL and English in an early childhood setting to promote bilingual development and learning. Noting differences in children's responses to her book sharing and that of her Deaf colleagues, teacher-researcher L. Erting investigated the book-sharing practices of two Deaf teachers, each sharing two different books with a total of thirteen deaf children from diverse linguistic and cultural backgrounds. (See L. Erting 2001 for a detailed accounting of this study.)

Book sharing, a widely researched school event, is an optimal context for linguistic, cognitive, and literacy development in children when done regularly and over time (see Dickinson and Tabors 2001 as one example). Yet, there have been few studies investigating the book-sharing practices of effective deaf teachers with Deaf preschool children. Our findings suggest studies investigating the practices of skilled Deaf teachers engaged in book sharing with their young children are crucial for the understanding of optimal preschool practices. We found, for example, that the Deaf teachers used the same set of strategies for constructing meaning that hearing teachers use with hearing children: modeling, explaining, translating, expanding, questioning, and problem solving. However, *how* they applied these strategies were unique to the ASL/English bilingual context. Understanding these differences is important for the linguistic, cognitive, and literacy development of young deaf children.

For this chapter, we highlight the strategy of *translating*. In applying this strategy, the teachers translated English texts into ASL, mindful of the need to make the language conveyed in the book visually accessible and meaningful to their diverse groups of students. Translating in this context is a complex phenomena; not only did the teachers need to convey the meaning from a printed language to a visual-spatial language, they had to consider the ages of their children and translate the text into a developmentally appropriate register of ASL that was understandable to their students while also varying the linguistic complexity of their translations to extend their students' understanding of the story and development of ASL as a language. Ms. Chris, for example, in introducing a new book, *One Zillion Valentines*, by F. Modell (1981, New York: Mulberry Press), extended her students' understanding by adding questions and elaborations that tapped her students' prior knowledge:

> [Points to the word one in the title] *One valentine? No! How many valentines?* [Counts quickly] *1-2-3-4-5-6-7-8-9-10-11-12* . . . [Responds to a student's interjection] *Ok, seven? Fine.* [Continues] *A zillion valentines! That is the title: One Zillion Valentines.*

During translation, Ms. Chris was guided by her Deaf cultural knowledge to use child-directed signing (CDS), a simplified, easily understood register of ASL that Deaf adults use to attract and hold the visual attention of deaf infants and young children. CDS, like its counterpart in spoken languages, is marked by special features and in ASL include expressiveness, redundancy, exaggerated sign size, expanded sign space, exaggerated facial expression, and rhythmic movement. As Ms. Chris continued to introduce the story, she signed FRIEND back and forth between herself and each of her students in a rhythmic and playful way in an extension of the idea of exchanging cards. The teacher employed this type of rhythmic signing throughout this book-sharing event in the process of translating text to ASL, eliciting a sense of excitement around book sharing and literacy.

We offer but a brief glimpse of this detailed, in-depth study from which complex and multifaceted Deaf ways of book sharing emerged. Findings illuminate indigenous cultural practices that have a profound effect on the development of language, cognition, and literacy of young deaf children—native and new signers alike.

Study 2: Alternative Paths to Deaf Bilingualism

In our longitudinal case studies, we regard paths to bilingual development as paths formed by the history of the student, the social contexts available for learning, and the support the children receive to engage with a variety of topics and texts in both ASL and English (Moll and Dworin 1996). A brief look at two of the students is illustrative. The first is a Deaf child we call Rita, born into a nonsigning family with no previous experience with Deaf people. The second we call Ann, the second Deaf daughter born to signing Deaf, bilingual parents. Both Rita and Ann were reading on grade level when they were tested at third grade.

Rita's Pathway to Bilingualism

Rita's parents discovered that their daughter was deaf when she was three months old and decided almost immediately to learn to sign to ensure communication and language development. They enrolled Rita in an early education program at five months of age, bought ASL dictionaries, and began taking sign language classes. Rita's parents began signing with Rita immediately even though their signs were not perfect because they considered communication with their daughter paramount. They also realized the importance of Rita becoming involved with the Deaf community because they knew that other Deaf people would be a big part of her world. Rita's parents decided very early that they wanted her to be bilingual in ASL and English and that they wanted her to achieve at an above-average level in school. They clearly had high expectations for their daughter.

When we analyzed Rita's development in ASL at six years, one month of age, we saw her using primarily simple sentences with some complex structures in ASL, approximately two years behind her native Deaf signing peers. She could participate appropriately in discourse with peers and adults about diverse topics. Rita could use ASL effectively for a variety of purposes and demonstrated metalinguistic awareness through sign play, discussion of lexical preferences, and correction of others. When we analyzed Rita's English literacy development at this age, we saw behaviors supporting her mother's statement that Rita had loved books from an early age. Our data showed that she interacted with books for extended periods of time, pointing to pictures, matching her handshape with drawings of handshapes, and mouthing the names of labeled pictures. She also observed and participated in extended conversations around texts in the classroom. She could read and write her own name as well as the names of her peers and other short words, and she created stories with invented spellings, using support from environmental print, signs, and finger spelling—typical literacy-related behavior for children this age. What was clear to us, too, was that she was a confident communicator, a confident learner, and a confident reader.

Ann's Pathway to Bilingualism

Ann's parents expected her to be Deaf, a member of the fourth generation of Deaf people in her family. Because ASL and written English were the languages of the home, Ann's parents signed to her from birth and exposed her to written English through books and other environmental print. They were actively involved in the Deaf community, providing Ann with frequent opportunities for interaction with Deaf peers and adults. They enrolled her in an early education program by seven months of age, and, like Rita's parents, they had high academic expectations for their daughter, expecting her to become bilingual and achieve at above-average levels.

When we examined Ann's ASL development at five years, six months of age, we found her using complex grammatical structures, common ASL idioms, code-switching between ASL and contact sign, and controlling a variety of registers and genres. Her discourse skills were well developed so that she could maintain conversations with adults and peers over multiple turns. Pragmatically, she used ASL for a variety of functions, and there was evidence of considerable metalinguistic awareness in discussions about finger spelling and formational features of signs as well as in sign play. Ann's English literacy development is evident as she interacts with teachers and peers during book sharing, participating actively in the discourse surrounding the text. She, too, loved books from an early age according to her mother. Videotapes show her finger spelling words from the text, reading and writing her own and others' names and short words, and using invented spellings. Ann is a confident communicator, learner, and reader who demonstrates metacognitive awareness in lengthy discussions of reading and writing with her peers.

Study 3: Literacy Acquisition through Scaffolded Interactions in ASL

In the previous section, we described Ann as a confident five-and-a-half-year-old child immersed in language and literacy. Increasing evidence of the importance of experiences prior to preschool (Hart and Risley 1997, 1999) led us to question what experiences in Ann's ASL/English bilingual home contributed to her language, cognitive, and literacy acquisition and learning that prepared her for subsequent school experiences. To investigate this question, we drew on three years of video data collected during home visits that began a few weeks after Ann's birth and ended just before she began preschool at the age of three.

One of the primary findings was the depth and breadth of scaffolding the parents used during interactions with their daughter. Ann's parents, like most parents, did not explicitly plan to teach her language and literacy. Rather, within authentic social and collaborative contexts, they guided Ann's engagement and responses in ways that mediated learning within implicit, subtle, and intuitive communicative exchanges that were culturally rooted and complex (Hart and Risley 1997, 1999). Ann was born into an unusual linguistic environment for Deaf children, and her parents, drawing upon indigenous knowledge and practices, were immediately able to interact with her in ways that scaffolded her emerging and rapidly developing language, cognition, and literacy.

We found evidence of scaffolding in the first home videotape of Ann at six weeks, and the data was rich with examples thereafter. We present evidence in four age-based stages. In the first stage, from six weeks to twelve months, the parents scaffolded to establish and maintain Ann's attention, her eye gaze. Initially, they optimized the short periods of time when Ann watched them to name objects and people. As Ann became older, they increasingly elaborated their naming routines, extending with descriptions and explanations. At seventeen weeks, Ann's mother, while feeding Ann her first breakfast, followed her eye gaze, and signed: Do you like it? It's your first breakfast. Your first . . . Do you like it? Yes? Do you want more? Do you want more? Do you want it? When Ann shifted her attention to the cereal bowl in her mother's hand and back to her mother, she continued: It's a red bowl.

In the next stage, from twelve to eighteen months, the parents' shifted the focus to eliciting responses from Ann. This is not to say the parents did not previously attempt to elicit responses nor that they no longer attended to eye gaze. Rather, once Ann began signing, her parents mediated her comprehension of and responses to various language constructions tied to environmental stimuli. This scaffolding took place around routines established by both parents. Ann's parents explicitly invited Ann's participation in routines, modeled responses, and elaborated on constructions as Ann responded to them. For example, Ann's father initiated a routine, asking Ann: *Where's the sock?* He repeated his question, modeled responses (*There's the sock!*), and when Ann began to respond (*There!*), he elaborated with a new language construction: *Give me the sock!* A variety of routines emerged during this stage, including book sharing as a labeling routine: *What's that? What is it? What is it?* [Mother pauses.] *It's a car.* [Ann signs CAR.] *Yes, that's a car!*

At the eighteen- to twenty-four-month stage, Ann's parents shifted their focus to elaborating on language constructions and concepts with which Ann had become familiar. As one example, Ann's father initiated a routine of naming puzzle pieces. When Ann responded to his prompt by signing DUCK, her father confirmed and extended by nodding and then pointed to a picture of a duck on the wall, signing: *Yes, a duck, and that's a duck, too!* In extending TEAPOT, he tapped into Ann's prior knowledge, explaining teapots were for pouring hot liquids. This stage was replete with scaffolded interactions characterized by routines to explain, verify, elaborate, and clarify Ann's increasing knowledge.

By twenty-four to thirty-six months, Ann had acquired age-appropriate language and knowledge about the world and showed a rapidly increasing control of this knowledge. Her parents responded by stepping back and allowing Ann to guide their interactions. In a book-sharing episode with the mother, Ann pointed to the picture of a dog and the number one and signed: DOG! ONE! Her mother then guided her to the word *Dog*, pointing to each letter in turn, asking her: *What's that?* Ann could readily identify the capitalized first letters, and then she looked to her mother to guide her in identifying the lowercase letters that followed. Ann noticed features of print and tried to make sense of them, and her mother instinctively picked up on and extended her approximations. Arriving at the page with the number nine, Ann noted it looked like the number six. Her mother manipulated the book, turning it upside down and right side up to explain the similarities and differences, signing in part: *This one is six and that one is nine. See this is six and if I turn the book it is nine. Six is nine upside down. You are right, they look little bit the same, but they are different.*

Through active involvement in mediated interactions, Ann gained confidence in the social practices of her home and community. This in turn led to language acquisition, communicative competence, and emergent literacy learning, and, thus, readiness for the requirements of schooling.

Toward a Deaf Theory of Literacy Development

What is the relevance of this kind of research for gaining a better understanding of what we mean by the Deaf way of language and literacy? This body of research is unique for a number of reasons. As far as I know, both in the American and international research landscape, this is the only research group looking at both home and school environments, interpreting findings from the two environments, and investigating how they interact with each other. The study is unique also in that there is a large database of more than two thousand hours of videotaped data in authentic ASL/English bilingual home and school environments over a significant period of time—an unusual wealth of data. The success of the research project depends a great deal on teamwork of Deaf and hearing individuals—not only the researchers but also the parents and teachers and recognizing the importance of all participants in capturing this emerging knowledge about the Deaf way of doing things. Such an ambitious research project requires the dedication of the research team to render this knowledge available to the research field as well as to parents, teachers, and others with a vested interested in Deaf way practices.

Evidence from this research presents a compelling argument for a sociocultural framework of a Deaf theory of literacy development. Through the evidence presented, we find meaning within the everyday practices in naturalistic home and school settings in response to such questions as these: How do members of Deaf families interact at home? How do Deaf teachers communicate with children in preschool classrooms? How do parents and teachers behave when they are interacting bilingually? How are the variations and complexity of ASL and English being used? Longitudinal studies following children from home to school, and continuing as they progress through school, help us understand that English literacy does not start with schooling. We gain insights about what competent members in each of home, preschool, and school settings do and how do they interact with one another. We suggest that there is not *a* Deaf way or *the* Deaf way but rather a number of Deaf ways. Ethnographic studies grounded in the authentic everyday lived experiences of the participants will help us understand these Deaf ways better.

References

Barton, D. 1994. *Literacy: An introduction to the ecology of written language.* Cambridge, MA: Blackwell.

Dickinson, D., and P. Tabors, P., eds. 2001. *Beginning literacy with language: Young children learning at home and school.* Baltimore, MD: Brookes Publishing Co.

Erting, C. 2003. Signs of literacy: An ethnographic study of American Sign Language and English literacy acquisition. In *The young deaf or hard of hearing child: A family-centered approach to early education*, ed. B. Bodner-Johnson and M. Sass-Lehrer, 455–67. Baltimore: Brookes.

Erting, C., C. Prezioso, and M. Hynes. 1990/1994. The interactional context of deaf mother-infant communication. In *From gesture to language in hearing and deaf children*, ed. V. Volterra and C. J. Erting, 97–106. Berlin, Germany: Springer Verlag (1990); Washington, DC: Gallaudet University Press (1994).

Erting, C., C. Thumann-Prezioso, and B. Benedict. 2000. Bilingualism in a Deaf family. In *The deaf child in the family and at school*, ed. P. Spencer, C. J. Erting, and M. Marschark, 41–54. Mahwah, NJ: Lawrence Erlbaum Associates.

Erting, L. 2001. Book sharing the deaf way: An ethnographic study in a bilingual preschool for deaf children. *Dissertation Abstracts International* 64 (12), 4031 (UMI No. 3035993).

Hart, B., and T. Risley. 1995. *Meaningful differences in the everyday experiences of young American children*. Baltimore: Brookes.

Hart, B., and T. Risley. 1999. *The social world of children learning to talk*. Baltimore: Brookes.

Moll, L., and J. Dworin. 1996. Biliteracy development in classrooms: Social dynamics and cultural possibilities. In *Discourse, learning, and schooling*, ed. D. Hicks, 221–46. New York: Cambridge University Press.

Prinz, P., ed. 1998. ASL proficiency and English literacy acquisition: New perspectives. *Topics in Language Disorders* 18 (4): 47–60.

Traxler, C. B. 2000. The Stanford Achievement Test, 9th edition: National norming and performance standards for deaf and hard-of-hearing students. *Journal of Deaf Studies and Deaf Education* 5 (4): 337–48.

Deafness and the Pedagogy of Difference

GLADIS PERLIN

More than a concern for our time, education of deaf people is a crisis that demands innovation in education. Research has been conducted on the struggles of Rio Grande do Sul deaf community, currently organized in FENEIS.[1] With the research, sponsored by FAPERGS and developed in the countryside of Rio Grande do Sul State, the unsustainable situation of deaf education, which my colleagues Ricardo Martins and Wilson Miranda are reporting everywhere, became evident.[2] In the face of this evidence, a proposal for a new pedagogy for deaf people has been put forth. This proposal appears because of problems such as the lack of sign language, identity, and deaf community within the deaf population as well as the presence in the educational system of forms of subjection of deaf people. These problems stem in part from stereotypes of deaf people attributable to poor training of both hearing and deaf professionals about the deaf difference.[3]

Lack of deaf educational professionals and insufficient training for deaf teachers who feel their identity is continuously usurped in their difference as educational professionals also contribute.

In Rio Grande do Sul, the schools for deaf people are mainly in the largest cities, and continuously they change their pedagogy for deaf education. The majority of these schools follows the hearing model; few of them have programs that respect the deaf difference. It creates isolation and does not allow an unified policy.

We are in times of postmodernism that allows us to see the "other," the different alterity, the self as a performer to the difference. We see a trend to new discursive practices, not only in the deaf community but also in the Afro-Brazilian, indigenous, and the rural populations. These times refer to the philosophy of the education that is appearing among deaf people, the manner of teaching deaf culture, and practical alternatives of education. This issue is not only ours; other authors as Bernard Charlot ask for respect of cultural differences in the classroom.[4] The deaf community, in a

---

1. National Federation of Education and Integration the Deaf, a nongovernmental organ with the social, political, and cultural goals of the deaf community.
2. Rio Grande do Sul Foundation to Support Research.
3. My first introduction to this term came from Silva 2000.
4. Paris University professor, in his lecture at the World Education Forum in Porto Alegre.

proposal for differentiated education, worries about the training of their teachers and uses the example of the structure of the communitarian schools. The deaf community is creating sufficiently decisive changes, but these still require improvements.

When Rio Grande do Sul deaf community prepared the document of the V Congress, "What Kind of Deaf Education Do We Want?," few people had any notion of what it meant.[5] However, it was so decisive that many institutions, including the Ministério da Educação, opened the path to sign language and signaled the introduction and formation of the deaf teacher as an educational professional. The deaf community also made the document "Pedagogy for the Difference" in one recent seminar in the city of Caxias do Sul/RS. This document discussed the differences in the education of deaf people.

The Deaf Education Model Today

Which model of deaf education do we have today? Which is the position of the schools? Which is the position of the governmental agencies?

- ❖ Deaf and hearing teachers study at universities where the pedagogy follows the pattern of normality, and it is difficult to find information about deaf difference. This perpetuates the uniformity of the teachers.
- ❖ Research indicated that the deaf teachers (with rare exceptions), in the classroom, follow the methodology of the hearing teachers, which tends to privilege the "regular identity" over the "different identity."
- ❖ MEC national policy, instructor of sign language model, states that deaf instructors are not professionally recognized but are only allowed to teach sign language in the classroom.

The Resistance to Deaf Teacher in the Schools for Deaf Students

Considering the current situation, with rare exceptions, the deaf teacher does not exist. A deaf teaching identity does not exist. Deaf educators who feel capable of guiding deaf education are rare. The lack of deaf teachers in the classroom is due to the resistance. Aspects of this resistance include the following:

- ❖ Resistance to the theory that deaf children need a deaf adult to construct their identity.
- ❖ The image the hearing teacher has of deaf teachers is often reduced to a handicapped educational professional.
- ❖ Deaf teachers complain: "If we say that we are also educators, we are ridiculed; if we run for office, we are considered socially handicapped; the hearing teachers treat us badly."
- ❖ Deaf pupils, with very rare exceptions, do not trust the capacity of deaf teachers.

---

5. Latin American Bilingual Education for Deaf Congress V, UFRGS, 1998.

What Must This Pedagogy of the Difference Contain?

Considering that at the turn of this century a pedagogy of the difference already exists, I mention some questions that would have to be addressed in its constitution:

- ❖ The question of deaf people not being alone but belonging to a culturally different community.
- ❖ The question of the construction of the identities with regard to the difference.
- ❖ The question of frontier collisions, links, and cultural hybridization.
- ❖ The double cultural registration of deaf people.
- ❖ The resistance to the overwhelming predominance of the normal identities.
- ❖ Overcoming the freezing of the identities, construction and reconstruction.
- ❖ Cultural agreement and disagreement.
- ❖ Cultural supremacy.
- ❖ The category of the cultural difference.

Where to Find This Pedagogy of the Difference?

The contents of the pedagogy of the difference must have its basis in the distinguishing valuation of the cultures, in the representation character that considers the identity and the difference. It must do this following things.

- ❖ Be in contact with deaf educators who currently are trying to filter the specific aspects of a differentiated deaf education.
- ❖ Put an emphasis on the cultural aspect of deaf difference and show the critical view and alternatives before the hegemonic culture.
- ❖ Privilege strategies and contents developed in the courses that toggle the question of identity and difference.
- ❖ Work with these questions in the context of subject matter.

Challenges for the Pedagogical Proposal

- ❖ Empathy and understanding from hearing people, accepting the cultural positions of the difference.
- ❖ The actors who take part in the different identity construction and not in the normal one, as is demanded today in issues of deaf education. Also, articulating this specific construction to citizens and communities, and specific points in opposition to the normal identity that deaf people will not achieve.
- ❖ The character of this pedagogy argues, recognizes, and celebrates identity and the difference.
- ❖ Other developing cultural positions that are searching for an approach.
- ❖ The perceived normality of the dominant identities, the dynamic character of formation of teachers, and the confrontation between the formation proposal and the notions constructed in the difference.

Conclusion

From this identity, theoretical dimensions and practical experiences turn toward the formation of the pedagogy of the difference, focusing particularly on the discursive ways identity is formed from this deaf perspective.

The biggest difficulty for the possibility of a pedagogy of the difference in the deaf cultural context is dealing with the view of "normal identities" and the stereotypes that the hearing people have. Another challenge is the construction of thematic alternatives for the formation of deaf teacher. This construction is possible but needs to articulate the knowledge fields with the pedagogy of the difference, thus meaning the adopted theoretical positions in our pedagogy faculties.

An important contribution is to collect the experiences of some deaf educators to see their strategies, contributions, and ideas and to detect emergent doubts and contradictions.

References

FENEIS/RS. *Surdos: um olhar sobre as praticas em educação*, Caxias do Sul, September 27–29, 2001.

Hall, Stuart. 2000. Quem preciosa de Identidade? In *Identidade e diferença: A perspectiva dos estudos culturais*, ed. Tonaz T. Silva. Petrópolis, RJ: Vozes.

Silva, T. T. 2000. A produção social da identidade e da diferença. In *Identidade e diferença: A perspectiva dos estudos culturais*, ed. Tonaz T. Silva. Petrópolis, RJ: Vozes.

Stam, R., and E. Shohat. 1995. *Estereótipo, realismo e representação racial*. Imagens, local, n. 5: p. 70–84, ago./dez.

American Sign Language Curriculum for First-Language ASL Students

HEATHER GIBSON

The past two decades have seen a change from the monolingual model to the bilingual-bicultural model in the education of Deaf students in Ontario, Canada. In response to the Deaf Ontario Now Rally 1988 and the 1989 Ontario Review of Provincial Programs for the Deaf, the bilingual-bicultural policy has been implemented in several schools in Ontario. Subsequently, on July 21, 1993, Bill 4 was passed, authorizing the use of American Sign Language (ASL) and Lingues des Signes Quebecois (LSQ) as languages of instruction for Ontario's Deaf students (Carbin 1993–94).[1] ASL is now used as a language of instruction to teach ASL students.

The Provincial Schools Bilingual-Bicultural Committee in Ontario has realized the value of formally teaching ASL to students, just as English or French-speaking Canadian students take formal courses in English and/or French. This committee recommended to the Ontario Ministry of Education and Training that an ASL curriculum be created to meet this need as a part of the bilingual-bicultural educational program. The curriculum writing team was set up at the provincial schools for the Deaf under the leadership of Heather Gibson. First convening in the fall of 1999, the team is composed of first-language ASL teachers from the provincial schools who have a background in ASL linguistics, ASL assessment, ASL literature and texts, ASL media arts, and ASL culture, as well as a basic knowledge of Ontario curriculum design. The Ontario ASL curriculum continues to be developed, piloted, and field tested. As each grade level of the curriculum is completed in draft form, it is field tested in three Provincial Schools for the Deaf. This process involves ongoing briefings and consultation regarding curriculum issues with the Ontario Ministry of Education Curriculum Branch, Special Education Branch, and Provincial Schools curriculum coordinator. Final review and analysis of the draft is then completed by Marlon Kuntz, the ASL curriculum analyst.

1. Our initial discussions made reference to Deaf culture, but our team agreed that this was a confusing term, because the two groups of Deaf people in Ontario to which Bill 4 applies (one of which uses ASL and one of which uses LSQ) have separate and unique languages, literatures, and cultures. We needed to be clear about this distinction. Therefore, we refer not to Deaf culture and Deaf students but rather to ASL culture and ASL-using students.

Educational Constraints

The Provincial Schools Bilingual-Bicultural Committee came to realize that the average ASL literacy skills among Deaf children were below expectations when compared to "first-language norms" in the bilingual-bicultural educational environment. Students' everyday use of ASL was mainly at a level of conversational language rather than at a level of academically proficient language. Cummins (2000b) reported that according to Corson's work, as students move through the grades at an academic level, they encounter far more low-frequency words; he further reported that when dealing with academic levels of language, students encounter complex syntax and abstract expressions seldom seen in everyday conversation. Compounding this problem in a school for Deaf students is the fact that the majority of ASL-using students do not enter the broad, adult language and cultural community until after they graduate from school, in contrast to hearing children, who are exposed to the larger adult language-cultural community throughout their years of development. As a result, ASL students do not have sufficient opportunity to see the complex uses of ASL as an academic language and to experience sophisticated ASL literary works. To give ASL students the chance to experience the full spectrum of a metalinguistically sophisticated language, an academic level of language proficiency is necessary. Such language is fundamentally different from conversational language in that it demands the application of cognitive, creative, critical, and analytical/synthetic skills. When ASL is used as an academic language, it creates a critical learning and thinking academic environment for ASL-using students and aids their development of complex language and literary skills.

The Bilingual-Bicultural Committee further understood that one of the reasons Deaf ASL students tended to lag significantly in their acquisition of English skills and vocabulary was that they had few if any opportunities to (a) make comparative studies of the structures of their two languages, ASL (L1) and English (L2), and (b) deepen their comprehension and critical study of ASL literary works. Instead, they acquired ASL and English in two separate monolingual processes with *very little understanding of the bilingual relationship between L1 and L2*. Because research has indicated that knowledge of the grammar of one's first language (ASL) and having high L1 literacy skills strongly contribute to competency and literacy in the second language (i.e., English), it was clear that the development of high ASL literacy skills in ASL students would require a curriculum offering (a) the formal *study* of their own language (that is, of the grammatical structure, vocabulary, and pragmatics of ASL, including its discourse, conversational structures, and rules of use, and the stylistic and register forms found in the literature and text of the language) and (b) extensive exposure to ASL and ASL literature, texts, and media arts at the academic level. No such curriculum was available in any form in North America.

In response to this concern, and as a result of the collaborative work of the Provincial Schools Bilingual-Bicultural Committee, the director of the Provincial and Demonstration Schools, the superintendent of the Provincial Schools for the Deaf, and stakeholders such as the Provincial and Demonstration Schools Council and the Ontario Association of the Deaf, a clear and solid rationale for the ASL curriculum was developed. It was agreed that the goals of the ASL curriculum would be to (1) provide learning benchmarks for ASL students' development and demonstration of expected ASL at both academic (comprehensive academic language proficiency, or CALP) and conversational levels (basic interpersonal communication skills, or BICS); (2) contribute to the development of a healthy self-image for ASL students by nurturing a strong first language that would aid in the development of cognitive, analytical/synthetic, and critical thinking skills and would provide a firm foundation for English (L2) acquisition; (3) introduce the formal ASL assessment process [e.g., ASL Proficiency Assessment (ASL-PA) and ASL diagnostic tools] to all principals, teachers, parents, and support staff; and (4) achieve equity in what is offered to ASL bilingual students with regard to the use and study of their own language, literature, media, and culture. The ASL curriculum team used the Ministry of Education curriculum framework in designing the ASL curriculum.

Curriculum Design

The ASL curriculum is designed to develop a range of essential skills in three strands. The committee collected a wide range of resource materials, both text and videotaped, to support instruction in each of the strands.

ASL Grammatical Linguistic Construction and ASL Text and Literature Construction

This strand refers to the skills essential to produce ASL, incorporating its contents and forms effectively for a variety of uses. Students also learn the skills and knowledge necessary to produce ASL texts and literature, including a variety of fictional prose and poetic literary works as well as nonfictional ASL texts reflecting the knowledge base of the ASL language and cultural community.

ASL Grammatical Linguistic Comprehension and ASL Texts and Literature Analysis

This strand refers to the skills essential to comprehend ASL, including its contents and forms used in a variety of contexts. Students will also learn the skills and knowledge necessary to comprehend, analyze, and respond to the variety of ASL literature and ASL texts in the cultural context of the ASL community.

ASL Conversation and ASL Media Arts and Technologies

This strand emphasizes the conversational skills needed for students to understand and interact with others to express themselves in ASL at a sophisticated, even eloquent, level with fluency and confidence. It also pertains to the use of knowledge and skills in ASL media studies to further the understanding and appreciation of ASL heritage and culture for the enrichment of the lives of people in the community at large.

General and Specific Curriculum Expectations

The ASL curriculum includes general and specific expectations that outline the knowledge and skills students must have to complete each grade level.

The Curriculum Must Teach ASL as a Conversational and an Academic Language

Historically, ASL has been used as a conversational language in the schools for Deaf students. It is the language Deaf ASL children use on a daily basis and acquire naturally in both the educational environment and outside the classroom. In contrast, academic language involves the formal *study* of the language (just as English-speaking hearing students engage in the formal study of English), as well as the literary and media works of the language, giving students a firm sense of their linguistic and cultural identity and membership.

The Curriculum Must Have Guidelines and Benchmarks for Monitoring Students' ASL Skills

The curriculum should monitor each child's progress in mastering linguistic structures and metalinguistic challenges. This will ensure continuity in language development and establish that our students' competencies in ASL grammatical linguistic structures and literary skills are commensurate with the standards set forth in the Ontario Curriculum.

Field Testing the ASL Curriculum

To see how the curriculum can be effectively applied in the classroom, field testing is currently being conducted. The major goals of field testing are to (1) observe different instructional strategies and activities that team members use with native ASL students; (2) analyze field test data and formulate appropriate changes to the curriculum draft; (3) eliminate curriculum design weaknesses, and (4) align expectations with appropriate ASL grade-level learning skills. Field testing is focusing exclusively on native ASL students of Deaf ASL-using parents. Field-testing information will be used to train teachers from the Provincial Schools for the Deaf over four consecutive years during an ASL curriculum orientation week in August.

Videotaping

As part of the field testing, the curriculum team is videotaping learning activities employed as the ASL curriculum is implemented in the classroom. This will involve ten- to twenty-minute instructional periods for young children and twenty- to forty-minute periods for older students. Team members will watch and analyse the videotapes, guided by target questions:

- ❖ Are the expectations outlined in the curriculum appropriate for first-language ASL students?
- ❖ Are there significant differences in response to the learning activities from the learners of high, average, and low ability?
- ❖ Do the learning activities appropriately fit the expectations?
- ❖ Do the students find the learning activities engaging or frustrating?
- ❖ Does the number of instructional strategies used provide information concerning the appropriateness of the expectations for a particular grade?
- ❖ Are there sufficient instructional strategies being used to teach the specific skills?

❖ Are there alternative strategies and methodologies that would better meet the expectations?

Field Notes

Field notes taken during the instructional period for students will focus specifically on how students respond to the instruction, recording such information as (1) grade and age of students, (2) description of learning activity, (3) specific expectations for the lesson, and (4) responses by students of varying abilities.

Classroom Visitation and Observation

The ASL curriculum coordinator and peer coaches (ASL curriculum team members) visit participating classrooms and observe students who are engaged in different curriculum-related learning activities. Although not a part of our process in developing the ASL curriculum, team members thought that ideally classroom visits and observations should also be made by an outside curriculum assessor, someone independent of the ASL curriculum team. Each of these observers has specific roles and responsibilities:

ROLES AND RESPONSIBILITIES OF THE ASL CURRICULUM COORDINATOR

The ASL curriculum coordinator is responsible for (1) observing ASL curriculum team members while they instruct students, (2) conducting a one-hour questionnaire interview with each team member, (3) arranging six in-service training sessions, three in the fall and another three in the winter/spring, and (4) providing suggestions and feedback following each session.

ROLES AND RESPONSIBILITIES OF PEER COACHES

ASL curriculum team members may ask their teammates to observe them while they instruct their students. This will give both an opportunity to share their understandings of and perspectives on the ASL curriculum.

ROLES AND RESPONSIBILITIES OF THE OUTSIDE CURRICULUM ASSESSOR

The outside curriculum assessor should be from outside the school and should be a qualified educator not only active in a teaching career but also knowledgeable and skilled in linguistics, literature, ASL assessment, culture, and curriculum design. The outside assessor would evaluate the field-testing data and provide the ASL curriculum coordinator and team members with feedback and suggestions on the curriculum design. Ideally, this assessment/consultation would occur in four sessions a year, two in the fall/winter session and another two in the winter/spring session.

ASL Curriculum Implementation

There are major changes taking place in educational beliefs throughout the provincial schools system in Ontario, Canada. Growth strands, assessment, strategies, expectations, student activities, methodologies, and teaching techniques are all

American Sign Language Curriculum

witnessing dramatic alterations as they are developed and implemented across the provincial schools. To have an effective ASL as language arts program, we need to provide resources, in-service training, and full support in every aspect of the ASL as language arts program.

Resources for the ASL Curriculum

It is extremely important that teachers, support staff, parents, students, and members of the cultural ASL community have full access to a wide range of ASL resources [e.g., videotapes on ASL poetry, ASL stories, ASL texts and literature for different age groups, software, documents, and technologies (video equipment, computer, DVD machine, etc.)]. We also need to take advantage of the resources available in the cultural ASL community. It is also important that we have materials to offer our parents, members of the cultural ASL community, and dorm counselors to support their learning about and using ASL in the communication, language, literature, and text development of our students. It is especially important that we provide them with insight into the value of ASL culture, ASL literature and ASL texts, and ASL media arts, as well as strategies for exposing students to these in the broadest sense (historic and multicultural literary works, ASL poems, ASL humor, science fiction, current events, etc.).

In-Service Training

ASL curriculum team members need to build a common vision of how to develop and implement the ASL curriculum. To develop such a vision and to prepare them to field test, implement, and teach the curriculum, team members will be offered a variety of workshops. Topics will include (1) curriculum design and development; (2) Ontario curriculum and its framework; (3) ASL assessment [ASL proficiency assessment (ASLPA)]; (4) first- and second-language teaching; (5) instructional and learning strategies, activities, and materials; (6) ASL curriculum field-testing and procedures; (7) staff training and ASL curriculum implementation; (8) first- and second-language acquisition and development; (9) conversational and academic languages (BICS and CALP); (10) ASL linguistic structures; (11) ASL literature; (12) metaphors and similes used in ASL; (13) ASL poetry structures; (14) sociology of the community; (15) literature and literacy; and (16) linguistic genocide.

All teachers and support staff need to build a common vision to support the ASL curriculum's implementation in the school system. Because there is no university in Canada that prepares our teachers to use the curriculum, it is imperative that intensive in-service training be provided to help them gain knowledge, skills, and understanding of the theories and practices used in the development of ASL assessment, ASL literacy and learning, and the use of the ASL curriculum.

Those teachers who teach ASL to students in the classroom should be required to know (1) ASL linguistic structures, (2) metaphors and similes used in ASL, (3) ASL number systems, (4) ASL literature (ASL story structure, ASL poetry structure, ASL texts), (5) ASL assessment, (6) ASL curriculum and its framework, (7) first- and second-language acquisition and development, (8) ASL classes (ASL as a second/third language), (9) ASL name signs, (10) first- and second-language teaching and methodologies, and (11) Canadian Deaf ASL culture.

Finally, it is imperative that members of the ASL and hearing communities as well as the parents of our students be kept informed about the development of the ASL curriculum. We had a Parents/Dorm Counselor Information Night to share information relating to the curriculum and how it will be taught to their youngsters. We invited the union president to this information-sharing meeting to assure union support for the project. We also presented our work to the cultural ASL community. Altogether many vehicles for information sharing were used including newsletters, workshops, parent/dorm counselor information night, conferences, person-to-person meetings, staff meetings, school council meetings, principal's meetings, and the Rotary Club.

Conclusion

Having the ASL curriculum used as a guide for the study of ASL as a language and literature will provide our students a better-balanced bilingual learning environment. It will be an important step toward achieving equity between what is offered to ASL students in terms of the use and study of their own language (ASL) and literature and what has, for decades, been offered to their hearing counterparts. They will develop an appreciation of the "power of ASL words" found in their own language and literature. We educators can use the curriculum to provide the learning benchmarks for our students' development and demonstration of expected ASL and ASL literacy skills. For our students, the most important aspect of the ASL curriculum will be the measurable progress our ASL students demonstrate in the development of their own first language.

References

Carbin, C. 1993–94. Ontario's new ASL/LSQ law—PAH! *Gallaudet Today* (Winter): 15–17.
Cummins, J. 2000a. Conversational and academic language. Presentation at Ernest C. Drury School for the Deaf, Milton, Ontario, Canada.
Cummins, J. 2000b. *Language, power and pedagogy: Bilingual children in the crossfire.* Ceredigian, U.K.: Cambrian Printers.
Gibson, H. 2000. ASL curriculum project. *ASL Curriculum in Action Bulletin* 1 (1).
Government of Ontario, Ministry of Education and Training. 1993. Bill 4: An act to amend certain acts relating to education.
———. 2003. 2004 consolidation: education statutes and regulations of Ontario.
Lane, H. 1999. *The mask of benevolence.* San Diego, CA: DawnSignPress.

Asian Deaf Perspectives on Deaf Education

CYNTHIA J. PLUE

This essay presents an exploratory study of Asian Deaf perspectives of Deaf education. The aim of this essay is to explore, investigate, and share Asian Deaf perspectives of Deaf education on the areas of literature review, demographics, common issues, and recommendations for improving the quality of Deaf education.

Who Are the Asian/Pacific Islanders?

Asians are made up of physically and culturally diverse groups with different languages, customs, and values. The category of Asians includes at least thirty-two distinct cultural or ethnic groups (Wong, 1980). Asians have cultural roots from Japan, China, Korea, India, Samoa, Tonga, Fiji, the Mariana Islands, the Marshall Islands, the Philippines, Vietnam, and other Pacific Rim countries. Pacific Islanders are made up of Polynesians, Micronesians, Melanesians, Samoans, Guamanians, and Tongans (Kitano & Daniels, 1995). The only common link that these Asians have is the fact that all may have, at one time or another, in the past or through their ancestors, bathed in, swam in, or touched the waters of the Pacific Ocean.

The term *Asians* covers a variety of national, cultural, and religious ancestries. Although there are many similarities among various subgroups, their differences are the products of different origins, ecological adaptations, and histories (Pang & Cheng, 1998). In addition to the differences among groups, diversity exists within national groups and individuals as a result of their reasons for migration, related hopes and expectations, and reception by the American culture.

Demographics

According to the World Federation of the Deaf (WFD) statistics, there are 70 million Deaf people in the world (Strassler, 1997). Within Asia, there are more than 30 million people with hearing loss. However, there are limited statistical sources on Asian Deaf people worldwide, especially where Asian communities have developed in most large cities.

Because the Deaf community is not characterized nor recognized as an ethnic neighborhood or town, it can be hard to find (Katz, 1996; Lane, Hoffmeister, &

Bahan, 1996). Because the Deaf community is distinctive to its Deaf members, those unfamiliar with Deaf culture can only get access to the Deaf community by meeting other Deaf people. Although exact figures are not available, the Asian Deaf population is increasing with immigration from Asia to America or other countries (Christensen, 2000).

Worldwide, Asian Deaf people have their own culture, history, and sign language. Asian Deaf youth meet other Asian Deaf peers and adults and become acculturated into the Asian Deaf community. They join organizations, marry, and socialize with other Asian Deaf people. They empower themselves with cultural and linguistic knowledge and information to promote themselves in the Asian Deaf community (Lane, Hoffmeister, & Bahan, 1996). The intertwined patterns of actions and interaction that make up groups and societies, which Deaf people have organized, include clubs and other networks of people who come together for political, social, and athletic events. Such Deaf Asian organizations are found in their home countries or America. There are National Associations of the Deaf or Federations of the Deaf in their home countries in Asia, such as Japanese Federation of the Deaf, Taiwan National Association of the Deaf, or the Philippines Federation of the Deaf. America is full of diverse cultural and linguistic ethnic groups such as the National Asian Deaf Congress. Also, many Deaf Asians struggle with discrimination, oppression, and racism issues within the Deaf communities in Asia and America. They found ways to educate and empower their communities: Deaf and hearing Asian and Americans come together to secure those services appropriate to their needs by establishing their social and political organizations.

Language viewpoints

There is a study on language from different viewpoints: language as a problem, language as a right, and language as a resource (Nover, 1995). Language as a problem is viewed as a weakness to be overcome rather than one of the country's greatest strengths. Language as a right is based on a reaction against the language as a problem; a community's language is viewed as a natural, human, moral, and legal right. Language as a resource is seen as a strength for native users in a country, an economic and personal benefit in multilingualism at home, schools, and in society.

Sign Language Usage

American Sign Language is proved to be the American Deaf community's language (Lucas & Valli, 1995; Stokoe, 1960). It has its own phonology, morphology, semantics, syntax, and pragmatics. In other countries, the sign languages are the common language of the Deaf community. They are not universal, but they carry similar principles as other spoken languages. Signed languages have been researched and proved to be used in most countries. In Asia, there are signed languages in Taiwan (Chao, 1994), Japan (Tsuchiya, 1994), Thailand (Suwanarat, 1994), India (Vasishta & Sethna, 1994), Nepal (Joshi, 1994), Pakistan (Shamshudin, 1994), Saudi Arabia (Al-Muslat, 1994), and Indonesia (Branson, Miller, Marsaja, & Negara, 1996).

Multilingual and Communication Skills

What about Asian Deaf people's linguistic skills? Research studies (Lummer, 1999; Lummer & Plue, 2000; Plue, 1997; Plue, 1998–99; Plue, 1999a) proved that there are many Asian Deaf people with multilingual skills (signed, written, and/or spoken). Research studies of successful Asian Deaf adults show that most learned their home language (in written form and sometimes spoken form) first, then moved to United States where they learned ASL (Plue, 1997; Plue, 1998–99). This is true for the Deaf immigrants as well (Lummer, 1999; Plue, 1999b).

Society's Views of Deaf Asians

In general, hearing perspectives of the Deaf world contain paternalism and oppression. The human rights of Deaf people have not been recognized internationally in terms of health care issues, communication accessibility issues, educational rights, employment opportunities, and legal rights. Eighty percent of Deaf people are illiterate (Malzuhn, 1994). Will this apply to the Asian Deaf people of diverse linguistic and cultural homes in their home country where they interface with the cultural, educational, and linguistic barriers while learning in school? That question has yet to be answered.

Asian and Asian American families do not acknowledge their children with disabilities. It is based on the families' language, cultural, and religious attitudes toward Asians and Asian Americans with disabilities, where Asians and Asian Americans with disabilities face double discrimination and prejudice at work, at school, and in society (Lee-Yim, 1994). Family attitudes toward disabilities complicate the task of providing adequate support services. Asian/Pacific Islanders' religious beliefs relating to mind, body, and spirit traditionally emphasize fate controlled by destiny rather than by a person's actions (Sue & Sue, 1990). Many parents may feel guilty about having a Deaf child, or they may believe the family is being punished for the sins of their ancestors (Huang, 1993). Instead of seeking medical help, families may use indigenous faith healers, apothecaries, monks, ministers, acupuncturists, herbal medicine practitioners, and shamans to "cure" the deafness. From an American viewpoint, diagnosis, treatment, and intervention are often delayed while these folk remedies are applied (Cheng, 2000; Monk, 1995; Wu & Grant, 1997).

It is important for international society to gain knowledge about the Asian perspectives on the Deaf education. This led to my exploratory study, which focuses specifically on Deaf Asians worldwide. Interviews with Deaf Asians reveal much about their experiences as Deaf Asians and their outlooks regarding their educational experiences in common areas such as school experience, language usage, Asian Deaf cultural knowledge, exposure to Deaf role models, Deaf identity development, and literacy skills.

School Experience

Asian Deaf people, including students, experience a variety of school settings in Asia and United States: residential schools, mainstreamed programs in hearing schools, or both settings. Not only that, but some of them also have no or limited school experience. For instance, Vietnamese Deaf people have experienced no or limited school because of wars, and thus upon their arrival at U.S. schools, they were faced with cultural and linguistic barriers.

Language Usage

A high percentage of Asian Deaf people experienced oralism and total communication during school days but acquired sign language at a later age. In certain Asian countries, such as Hong Kong, Taiwan, and the Philippines, some of them had limited sign language and/or signing method usage.

Asian Deaf Cultural Knowledge

A high percentage of Asian Deaf people had no or limited Asian Deaf cultural knowledge in academic settings until they met other Deaf Asians, where at Asian Deaf clubs they embraced their cultural knowledge, such as Asian Deaf histories, culture, signed languages, and role models.

Exposure to Asian Deaf Role Models

A high percentage of Asian Deaf people had no or limited exposure to Deaf role models, Asian Deaf teachers or teacher aides, and social interaction with older Asian Deaf people during their educational experience.

Deaf Identity Development

A high percentage of Asian Deaf people had limited awareness and recognition of maintaining cultural pride being an Asian Deaf person or sharing the mutual bonds with other Asian Deaf people.

Literacy Skills

A high percentage of Asian Deaf people had no or limited exposure to sign language, Deaf cultural knowledge, Deaf role models, and Deaf identity development. This leads to poor literacy knowledge and poor quality of life for Asian Deaf people as well as a lack of preparation for educational opportunities, society, and the workplace.

Recommendations

The exploratory study of Asian Deaf perspectives toward Deaf education brought several recommendations to mind: encourage early exposure to sign language, Asian Deaf cultural knowledge, Asian Deaf role models, and Asian Deaf identity development so that Asian Deaf children can develop their social and literacy skills as a part of the language development with their age-appropriate peers; develop partnerships with Asian Deaf organizations in enriching and improving educational/social opportunities; establish a center for families and professionals to learn sign languages, Deaf cultural knowledge, Deaf role models, and family-building development system; set language policy at schools where cultural and linguistic needs can be easily met at home and school in preparation for the wider hearing society; provide youth leadership camps where Asian Deaf youths can be exposed to sign language, Deaf cultural knowledge, Deaf role models, and Deaf identity development; and establish Asian Deaf studies for K–12 and postsecondary educational levels where people can learn more about the Asian Deaf community's complex yet diverse needs.

Summary

Asian Deaf people are still searching for their needs: cultural knowledge, language, exposure to Deaf role models, Deaf identity development, and literacy skills. It is critical to share this study with Asian Deaf students who attend schools that do not have Deaf friendly environments and that emphasize cultures and languages that differ significantly from Asian Deaf cultures and languages. Asian Deaf students may bring to schools a complex diversity of cultural values, historical experiences, assimilation levels, and cultural traditions that conflict with the worldview presented in schools. Thus, Asian Deaf facts are a great asset for increasing cultural and linguistic awareness, which shapes much of the motivation of Asian Deaf youths to be proud of their heritage and Asian Deaf history.

Along with the Asian Deaf organizations as cultural and linguistic sources, Asian Deaf history would help to shape Asian Deaf students as future leaders in Asian Deaf organizations and as part of the larger Deaf community. Thus, the Asian Deaf organizations are indicative of the tremendous support to families of Asian Deaf students with cultural and linguistic sources. We hope that in the future these organizations, along with the broader Asian communities and families, will work together to make sure that Asian Deaf students and adults get the cultural and linguistic access they need to become as successful as their Asian Deaf peers by documenting historical events, people, organizations, and cultural and linguistic events that contribute to the Asian Deaf community as social facts for future use in the schools.

This agrees with the research findings of my previous studies of Asian Deaf students and adults: with their Deaf, including Asian Deaf, peers surrounding them, they will have the linguistic support they need to interact and share their perspectives in a visual language and in a culturally Deaf-friendly and linguistic print environment (Plue, 1998–99).

References

Al-Muslat, Z. A. (1994). The history of Deaf education in the kingdom of Saudi Arabia. In C. J. Ertling, R. C. Johnson, D. L. Smith, & B. D. Snider (Eds.), *The Deaf way: Perspectives from the international conference on Deaf culture* (pp. 275–282). Washington, DC: Gallaudet University Press.

Branson, J., Miller, D., Marsaja, I. G, & Negara, X. (1996). Everyone here spoke sign language, too: A deaf village in Bali, Indonesia. In C. Lucas (Ed.), *Multicultural aspects of sociolinguistics in Deaf communities* (pp. 39–57). Washington, DC: Gallaudet University Press.

Chao, J. C. (1994). Taiwan Sign Language research work. In C. J. Ertling, R. C. Johnson, D. L. Smith, & B. D. Snider (Eds.), *The Deaf way: Perspectives from the international conference on Deaf culture* (pp. 347–349). Washington, DC: Gallaudet University Press.

Cheng, L. (2000). Deafness: An Asian/Pacific perspective. In K. M. Christensen (Ed.), *Deaf-plus: A multicultural perspective.* San Diego, CA: DawnSignPress.

Christensen, K. (Ed.). (2000). *Deaf-plus: A multicultural perspective.* San Diego: DawnSign Press.

Faurot, J. (1995). *Asian-Pacific folktales and legends.* New York: Simon & Schuster.

Huang, G. (1993). *Beyond culture: Communicating with Asian American children and families.* New York: ERIC Clearinghouse on Urban Education.

Jepson, J. (1991). Two sign languages in a single village in India. *Sign Language Studies, 70,* 47–59.

Joshi, R. B. (1994). Nepal: A paradise for the deaf. In C. J. Ertling, R. C. Johnson, D. L. Smith, & B. D. Snider (Eds.), *The Deaf way: Perspectives from the international conference on Deaf culture* (pp. 69–74). Washington, DC: Gallaudet University Press.

Katz, C. (1996). *The history of the Deaf community in Beaumont, Texas* [brochure]. Beaumont, TX: Author.

Kitano, H., & Daniels, R. (1995). *Asian Americans: Emerging minorities* (2nd ed.). Englewood Cliffs, NJ: Prentice Hall.

Lane, H., Hoffmeister, R., & Bahan, B. (1996). *A journey into the Deaf-world.* San Diego: DawnSignPress.

Lee-Yim, N. (1994). A parents' panel: Chinese perspectives on disabilities. In *Access Silent Asia Conference: The Asian Deaf experience.* DeKalb, IL: NIU Publication Press.

Lucas, C., & Valli, C. (1995). *Linguistics of American Sign Language: A resource text for ASL users.* Washington, DC: Gallaudet University Press.

Lummer, L. (1999). *Teachers' perceptions of the academic and language needs of Deaf immigrant students: An exploratory survey.* Unpublished master's thesis, Lamar University, Beaumont, Texas.

Lummer, L., & Plue, C. (2000). *Multicultural Deaf consumers' perspectives of interpreter services panel session* (Interpreter Workshop Series). Aurora, IL: Waubonsee Community College.

Malzuhn, M. (1994). The human rights of the Deaf. In C. J. Ertling, R. C. Johnson, D. L. Smith, & B. D. Snider (Eds.), *The Deaf way: Perspectives from the international conference on Deaf culture* (pp. 45–55). Washington, DC: Gallaudet University Press.

Monk, M. (1995). Asian-Pacific mental health: The importance of sociocultural factors in framing effective interventions. In *Access Silent Asia Conference: The Asian Deaf experience.* DeKalb, IL: NIU Publication Press.

Nover, S. (1995). Politics and language: American Sign Language and English in Deaf education. In C. Lucas (Ed.), *Sociolinguistics in Deaf communities* (pp. 109–163). Washington, DC: Gallaudet University Press.

Pang, V. O., & Cheng, L. (1998). *Struggling to be heard: The unmet needs of Asian Pacific American children.* Albany: State University of New York Press.

Plue, C. (1997). *An ethnographic study of Deaf Filipinos in Los Angeles: Language, culture, identity and values.* Deaf Studies V: Towards Diversity and Unity. April 17–20, 1997. Washington, DC: College for Continuing Education, Gallaudet University.

Plue, C. (1998–99). *Deaf Asian/Pacific Island students: How can we enlarge their visions and dreams?* The Deaf American Monograph Series. Silver Spring, MD: National Association of the Deaf.

Plue, C. (1999a). A history of Deaf Asians/Pacific Islanders in America. *Deaf Studies VI: Making the Connection Conference Proceedings,* April 8–11, 1999. Washington, DC: College for Continuing Education, Gallaudet University.

Plue, C. (1999b). *A descriptive study of achievement, social identity, and cultural influences of Asian/Pacific Island American Deaf students in California and Hawaii.* Unpublished doctoral dissertation, Lamar University, Beaumont, Texas.

Shamshudin, A. (1994). Deaf culture in Pakistan. In C. J. Ertling, R. C. Johnson, D. L. Smith, & B. D. Snider (Eds.), *The Deaf way: Perspectives from the international conference on Deaf culture* (pp. 75–77). Washington, DC: Gallaudet University Press.

Stokoe, W. (1960). *Sign language structure: An outline of the visual communication systems of the American Deaf* (Occasional Papers 8). Buffalo, NY: University of Buffalo.

Strassler, B. (1997, November 30). *Deaf digest*. Message posted to the Deaf Digest Gold Edition listserv.

Sue, D. W., and D. Sue. 1990. *Counseling the culturally diverse*. New York: John Wiley & Sons.

Suwanarat, M. (1994). Deaf Thai culture in Siam: The land of smiles. In C. J. Ertling, R. C. Johnson, D. L. Smith, & B. D. Snider (Eds.), *The Deaf way: Perspectives from the international conference on Deaf culture* (pp. 61–64). Washington, DC: Gallaudet University Press.

Tsuchiya, M. (1994). The Deaf Japanese and their self-identity. In C. J. Ertling, R. C. Johnson, D. L. Smith, & B. D. Snider (Eds.), *The Deaf way: Perspectives from the international conference on Deaf culture* (pp. 65–68). Washington, DC: Gallaudet University Press.

Vasishta, M., & Sethna, M. (1994). Clubs for Deaf people in India. In C. J. Ertling, R. C. Johnson, D. L. Smith, & B. D. Snider (Eds.), *The Deaf way: Perspectives from the international conference on Deaf culture* (pp. 464–469). Washington, DC: Gallaudet University Press.

Wong, H. Z. (1980). Asian and Pacific Americans. In L. R. Snowden (Ed.), *Reaching the underserved: Mental health needs of neglected populations*. Beverly Hills, CA: Sage.

Wu, C., & Grant, N. (1997). Asian, American, and Deaf: A framework for professionals. *American Annals of the Deaf*, 142(2), 85–89.

Academic Writing of Deaf Students in Higher Education: Processing and Improving

KRISTER SCHÖNSTRÖM

In this essay, I discuss some experience from my work with deaf students in Swedish as a Second Language for the Deaf, at the Department of Scandinavian Languages, Stockholm University, particularly processing academic writing and improving their writing skills. Our goals and methods for improving deaf students' writing skills is described and discussed.

Background

Since 1981, courses in Swedish as a Second Language for the Deaf have been given at the Department of Scandinavian Languages, Stockholm University. In these courses, deaf students can learn their second language on their own rules. Because of their deafness, the students have to learn the language of the community in its written form and not as a spoken language (see Svartholm 1993 for further discussion). The subject was founded by Professor Kristina Svartholm in the beginning of the 1980s and has successively developed to become an academic subject at the department with courses up to the master's level and doctoral level in the subject. In 1998, it was established as a full academic subject with a professorship of its own.

In this subject area, students may study different courses including practical writing, the grammar of Swedish, text analysis, theory and practice of translation between Swedish and Swedish Sign Language, and bilingualism. Currently three people are working at the department with the subject, of whom one is hearing and two are deaf. In addition to teaching, research in the second language of the deaf is conducted as well as developmental work of different kinds.

Description of the Course(s)

There are four different levels of the subject: basic, immediate, advanced, and specialized. If studying all the courses, it takes two years of full-time studies to complete. In the basic course, there are four different course units: "Proficiency in Swedish Writing," "Structures of Swedish," "Deaf Bilingualism," and "Text Analysis and Text

Production." The basic course aims to give students knowledge of modern Swedish written language and to develop their reading ability and writing proficiency. They will also gain basic knowledge of bilingualism of the deaf. In the following, I focus on the course unit called "Proficiency in Swedish Writing."

Through practice, "Proficiency in Swedish Writing" aims to teach students to express themselves in writing as well as in analyze text composition and norm deviation. By practicing this course in parallel to another course unit named "Structures of Swedish," which is based on studying the grammar of Swedish, students learn grammar rules in Swedish and learn how to use the new knowledge in writing. In this way deaf students are trained to use their new knowledge in grammar when practicing writing and also for analyzing and discussing the texts with each other.

The Students

The students come from all around Sweden and are deaf or, in some cases, hard of hearing. They may have different kinds of background; for example, they may have attended different schools earlier in life. However, most of them have studied at one of the five schools for deaf students in Sweden. During the past few years, the number of students with a bilingual childhood has increased. In contrast, a few of the students may have attended schools for hard of hearing or hearing students. However, in principle all of them use sign language. If students with low-level skills in sign language attend the course, they will have difficulties keeping up with the other students, especially understanding the contrastive analysis and translation discussions of sign language versus Swedish. Most of them usually do not pass the course.

The students' skills in Swedish may differ as a result of their different school background. It may sometimes be a problem, especially for those who have lower level skills, and normally these will not pass the course. If any student has a lack of knowledge, he or she will have to work more outside class by practicing writing or understanding the grammar of Swedish, and often this works well. However, it is important to note that students must have reached a good level in the Swedish language before entering the courses. The entrance qualifications are the same as for hearing students at any other university course.

Teaching and Course Contents

Deaf and hearing teachers with a bilingual approach give all lessons in Swedish Sign Language. Lessons include lectures, group discussions, and student presentations but focus on group discussions. In the course unit "Structures of Swedish," teaching is based upon lectures and different practices that students discuss in the lessons. Different grammar rules at different language levels, such as morphological, syntactical, and discourse level, are practiced and discussed. The teacher takes advantage of questions from the students and explains in sign language; if possible, the teacher compares the grammar of Swedish with the grammar of Swedish Sign Language. The focus remains on the written form of Swedish. The written language is the representation of Swedish that deaf students meet daily in the Swedish community, and the teacher takes this exposure into account.

In "Proficiency in Swedish Writing," the lessons are mostly scheduled as group discussions that include discussions based on homework. The course is built up on the students' home exercises. The teacher presents different home exercises to the students every week including different exercises in academic writing. Examples of exercises are pieces of informative writing, descriptive and narrative writing, and different kinds of texts such as letters, informative papers, stories, descriptions, book reviews. The exercises are primarily given by the teachers, but sometimes the students are allowed to choose a free exercise that meet criteria defined by the teachers (for example, that the exercise should be an informative text that would be possible to print in a Swedish morning paper). The students also have to adapt their writing to different target groups such as people in general, the authorities, and friends. In this way, the students become better prepared to write different texts to different target groups, and their self-criticism and consciousness of writing improve. We believe that this is more important than correctly writing every grammatical detail. Furthermore, we think that the role of correct grammar should be subordinated to the role of developing writing strategies and awareness about the writing process as such.

Every week the students exchange their exercise texts with each other in the same small group, which often consists of approximately four students. They are expected to analyze each other's texts at home, looking for failures and successes in different areas: the exercise goals, language structure on all levels, and grammatical rules. Although Swedish is their second language, they have to build analytical ability in Swedish, critical thinking, and so on. When home analysis is over, the students meet again in the lessons for group discussions. Here they get a chance to criticize and discuss each other's texts. They have to use real grammar arguments with references to the grammar books used in the other course unit, "Structures in Swedish." To argue based on their own feelings is not enough; even if they are correct, the other student can still rebut the argument. Thus the students have to use some language rule from the literature that can explain the grammatical error and argue from that reference.

One of the course books about writing that is used is Strömqvist's 1994 text. This book is a key reference in which the students can seek tips and learn about steps in the writing process. The book also shows good examples of different kinds of texts. There is a lot of valuable information that is necessary to consider before starting to write and arrange texts.

As mentioned earlier, the courses "Proficiency in Swedish Writing" and "Structures of Swedish" are taught in parallel during one semester. The students' knowledge improves after one semester, but they should still continue their writing by themselves after the courses to improve their awareness of their new skills. The courses only act as a starter for increasing the students' consciousness of writing and self-analysis of texts rather than transforming them into perfect writers overnight. Language development takes time, and a first step—the most important one—is to improve their awareness of process writing and the purposes of writing found within the real community.

Once they pass the course unit, they can take another course unit called "Text Analysis and Text Production." In it, they learn how to analyze different texts on a higher level by analyzing different text styles to see what components of language differ from one style to another. Here the demands on their analyzing ability are higher, and the students thus get a deeper knowledge of their second language and the function of written texts.

Conclusion

The students' expectations are very positive when they begin their studies. They expect themselves to become better writers and to improve their skills in Swedish generally. Interestingly, most of them expect to improve their grammar in writing rather than improve their writing strategies (a short discussion about this is found in Andersson 1991). It can be explained by the fact that traditional teaching methods in the schools for deaf students in Sweden (and in other schools) have focused on writing correct forms and on drill exercises on lower-order units rather than on improving the deaf learner's skills by analyzing and discussing strategies and targets of writing in higher-order units.

Svartholm (1994) claims that explanations in courses for second languages for deaf students should be given in a contrastive perspective, in which sign language and written language are explicitly compared. It is important to use sign language as a tool both for communication and for comparisons between the two languages when teaching deaf students to write. Teaching the students to use both top-down and bottom-up strategies as interactive ways to process the rules when writing texts is also important. Once deaf students gain awareness of written Swedish (or another second language), they can work on improving their skills themselves.

The response from the students has been positive; they feel that they get a deeper consciousness of written Swedish and how to write academic texts of different kinds. I see by my experiences that deaf students have no problems in learning the rules of writing and processing writing if those rules have been explained to them. I think the problem is that those rules have not been explained to deaf students until now.

References

Andersson, R. 1991. *I arbete med sakprosetexter med döva elever*. Institutionen för nordiska språk: Stockholms universitet.
Strömqvist, S. 1994. *Skrivboken—skrivprocess, skrivråd och skrivstrategier*. Andra Upplagan: Gleerups.
Svartholm, K. 1993. Bilingual education for the Deaf in Sweden. *Sign Language Studies* 81: 291–332.
———. 1994. Second language learning in the Deaf. In *Bilingualism in deaf education: International studies on sign language and communication of the deaf 27*, ed. I. Ahlgren and K. Hyltenstam, 61–70. Hamburg: Signum Press.

PART FOUR

Family

Deaf Couples and Adoption

RUNE ANDA

Some people have asked me how a deaf couple can qualify to adopt children. In some countries, deaf people are forbidden to adopt, so we feel lucky. I begin by discussing our experience with the adoption process in the Norwegian system. Each county has a different adoption system. First, we applied through the adoption authorities in our country, and then their representative came to evaluate us in our home. Among other things, they checked our age (we could not be too old), our health, our disabilities (deaf), and our financial status. They also learned that we had been married for several years and that we had a good and stable relationship. They also asked questions about our family and the rest of our family, including the grandparents, to determine whether we all had positive attitudes toward adoption. Our application and related papers were then sent to the country of origin, in this case, China. The officials in China needed to evaluate our papers, and they had the final decision. It was possible that they would not approve our request to adopt because we were deaf. We were fortunate with both adoptions, after expressing our persuasive arguments to the authorities. We argued that deaf children need homes where they can communicate easily with their parents; in our case, we would teach our children Norwegian Sign Language.

We first adopted my son, Marius, as a small boy at age six. One day we were reading the newspaper in Norway, and there was an article with a picture of a child from Ecuador. The article said that he was deaf and that no one wanted to adopt him. So my wife and I both looked at each other and quite soon agreed that we wanted to contact the adoption authorities and find out how we could become adoptive parents. We sent in our application for this child in Ecuador. We went through the home study, and the authorities checked our health, age, relationship, and so forth. We waited and finally got a telephone call telling us that this deaf boy had disappeared and that no one knew where he went. We were quite disappointed, but we decided to keep our application with the authorities anyway because we still wanted to adopt a deaf child from somewhere. In our country, Norway, there were three adoption agencies. All three of them started searching for a deaf child, using their connections all over the world. Soon the reply came that there was a deaf boy six years of age in a children's home in China. It only took a week for us to get confirmation that Marius was indeed in that children's home and was available for adoption. We said that yes, we would like to bring him into our home. Within three months, we had Marius at home in

Norway. It happened quickly, because the authorities *knew* about him. They may have known about him for three years, without putting him on a so-called adoption list, possibly because he was deaf. It is possible that the authorities, both in Norway and China, were surprised that anybody at all *wanted deaf children*.

We traveled to China to bring Marius home and learned a little about his past. We learned that he was found on the streets in Nanjing, wandering around alone when he was three years old. The people who found him left him in a children's home, and he stayed there for three years. He turned four, then five, and then six years old, waiting to be adopted. There were three hundred children in the orphanage—from babies to young teens thirteen or fourteen years of age—and he was the only deaf child there. I am told that it is common to have deaf children isolated in various orphanages. Marius saw his playmates disappear one by one as families came to adopt them. My guess is that he was considered unadoptable because he was deaf. He did not have any language and used only gestures, but he took our hand and wanted to leave the orphanage with us right away. We actually had to hold him back and said, "Wait, wait." He was *telling* us to take him out of the orphanage, *now*. He just wanted to get out of there with us. When my wife and I traveled to China to adopt Marius, we met with different officials, including the police and adoption authorities. One official that met with us became quite shocked after realizing that we were deaf. Perhaps this alone would be enough for us to not be allowed to adopt children, let alone deaf children. He was visibly concerned and, through an interpreter, we explained about how deaf children in Norway learn in deaf schools, their job opportunities, and the quality of life they have. We had to do a lot of convincing, but luckily it ended all right because after awhile he became relieved and very pleased to have this information. Thus we were allowed to adopt Marius, after making a promise to this official that we would bring him up properly. We also had to pledge to tell him that he was from China and that we would give him information about Chinese culture and history. We both agreed to that and feel it is important for children adopted internationally to understand the culture in which they were born.

Teaching Marius how to communicate was very interesting and exciting, but this period was also frustrating at times. We had to start from scratch because he basically had no language until he came to our home at age six. We started out with very simple gestures in international sign language and then slowly converted into Norwegian Sign Language. If he had been adopted by a hearing family that did not use signs, he would have had a much harder time.

When Marius was about seven years old, after a year with us learning language, he made some drawings. He wanted to do these drawings about the orphanage in China. There were beds in a row with a woman standing near them with a stick. I asked him about the stick, and he said that sometimes the woman would beat the children and it hurt. I asked him why; he said probably they had not done what she had told them to do. He said, "I thought that maybe since I was deaf I wouldn't understand what she had told me to do." He must have suffered some pain as well as emotional trauma through that.

Two years later the adoption agency contacted us and told us that they found another deaf boy in China and asked us if we wanted him; we said, "Yes, please!" We went through the whole application process again, and the social worker came to visit us and check our family, as before. Then we got a phone message telling us that the authorities in China had found this boy's parents and returned him to the parents, so we could not have him. We kept our application in anyway, because we wanted to adopt another child from China. So, we waited. And we waited. They searched for a deaf child. China is such a big country; it has 1.3 billion people. There should be lots of deaf children in orphanages there. We started wondering whether there is something wrong with the search process. We waited a full year. Finally they found a deaf girl who was two years old. After that, only a little more than a month passed before we traveled to China and brought Lena home with us.

Lena was found on the streets in Wuhan when she was only a small baby. She was taken to the children's home there and stayed there until she was two years old. We flew to China in 1994 to adopt her. Lena had a close tie to a particular woman who worked at the orphanage. When she was given to us through the adoption agency, she cried and cried; she did not want to go with us. She cried very loudly for two days, and then two days later, she smiled. Finally!

Now Lena is ten years old, and she goes to an elementary school for deaf children in Norway. Marius is seventeen years old, and he goes to a vocational school for deaf students in Norway.

I often wonder about my children's early history and why they were abandoned. China has a one-child policy, and often girls are abandoned because families in China prefer boys to carry on the family line. Perhaps Lena was abandoned because she was a girl (she was too young for anyone to know she was deaf). Marius, on the other hand, was three years old when he was abandoned, and his deafness was probably noticed. His parents may have abandoned him because the parents did not wish to have a deaf child as the *only* child. I am only speculating here, and it is possible the parents were too young or too poor to raise them.

Chinese culture has not caught up with Western culture in terms of accepting people with disabilities. Giving birth to a child with any disability is often a source of shame. In Norway in the period from 1991 to 1995, there were one hundred children adopted from China through the adoption organization that we used. Out of those, ninety-seven were girls and only three were boys. Interestingly, all three boys had some kind of disability. One had a heart failure. Marius was deaf; that was his disability. The third had another kind of disability.

There are lots of orphanages in the world and lots of orphaned children. There are many different reasons why children are abandoned by their biological parents, from country to country—poverty, war, stigma, age, illegitimacy, and increasingly, the children orphaned by parents with AIDS.

All children have a right to grow up in a family. It is certain that there are many orphaned *deaf* children in children's homes in the world, but the authorities are not keeping data on them. When we first applied, we got Marius quite quickly because the authorities knew about him. The next time we had to wait quite a while. I think the authorities and people who work with adoption make lists of the children that are in the orphanages, but they write down that the children in their care are *deaf* children. Maybe they think that *nobody* wants to adopt them. When we applied and said that we wanted a deaf child, the authorities were quite surprised.

Now and then the adoptive organizations all over the world receive messages about orphaned deaf children. How can we connect deaf children quickly enough to get placed in the homes where they can thrive in a language-rich environment, using sign language? Will they keep lingering in children's homes? Unfortunately, the adoption authorities do not know about the rich resource that the deaf community all over the world can provide to deaf children who need families. Maybe these authorities have already placed many deaf children into new homes with hearing parents who do not use sign language or did not know anything about raising deaf children? We need to influence our governments to make stronger policies on behalf of deaf children and insist that they have a right to a culturally appropriate home where sign language is used to help them grow socially and intellectually.

We are proud to be deaf role models and help hearing parents nurture their deaf children. My wife and I recently attended a meeting with some hearing parents who had deaf children of preschool age. A psychologist at the meeting with knowledge about deaf people explained to the hearing parents that they will experience a time of grief because their child is deaf. They may feel the world collapsing. The psychologist then pointed at the two of us and said: "They *wanted* to adopt a child, a deaf child. They felt happiness afterwards because they realized they were able to provide a deaf child with a better family life."

I think about all the deaf children in the world. We have got to do something about this. Something has to be done for them to share in the same opportunities as their peers. I think that if there is a deaf child needing a family, that deaf parents should be considered first as adoptive parents. There are many deaf couples facing infertility who should be given a chance at adoption. However, if hearing parents adopt them, they should be fluent in sign language and the culture of deaf people. This is the same concern that the authorities had when we pledged to teach Marius about his Chinese culture and history. Parents of deaf children need to do the same; teach their deaf child to be proud of who they are and cherish their deaf culture.

Hearing people who do not know about deaf people and sign language would not be able to understand how important sign language is. Unfortunately, many of them would often be told, or be led to believe, that sign language destroys the ability to learn speech and affects language development. Such thinking has made it very difficult to get the adoptive authorities to accept the idea that deaf couples ought to be allowed to adopt deaf children. There is too much incorrect information about deaf people and their ability to raise deaf—or even hearing—children. We must work to change our society's image of deaf people through public relations and education.

In 1995, I went to the World Congress of the World Federation of the Deaf (WFD) in Vienna, Austria. I gave a paper on this same subject. But before that, I sent out a questionnaire to about one hundred countries all over the world and asked them what the options were for deaf adoption in their country. I suspect that even if deaf people were allowed to adopt, there were few of them who got the opportunity to adopt deaf children. Thus, the questionnaire also asked whether deaf people in their country had adopted a deaf child. I got twenty-three responses, with only seven countries providing approximate numbers of adopted children. The United States had most, with around forty deaf couples who had adopted children, mostly deaf children. Norway was number two. Most of other countries had about one to five couples with adopted children.

I was able to connect with Dr. Barbara White of Gallaudet University, who hosted me and my family in 1996 at her home in Maryland. Barbara and her husband, Bruce, adopted a daughter, Allison, who is thirteen now. Barbara did interesting research for her doctoral degree in social work at the Catholic University of America. She studied fifty-five deaf parents who adopted deaf children. She learned through a survey and through interviews that deaf parents have a strong sense of entitlement to their deaf children, meaning that these parents feel positive about their right to parent their deaf child and raise them as their own. She also found that these families function well in spite of not having formal support services after the adoption. (Her dissertation is titled "The Effects of Perceptions of Social Support and Perceptions of Entitlement on Family Functioning in Deaf-Parented Adoptive Families." The dissertation, published in 1999, can be ordered through University Microfilms International, no. 9925899).

There is a lot of useful information in Barbara's research. I also hope that these findings on the strengths of deaf-parented adoptive families will be accessible to the whole world and particularly to the adoptive authorities, both to "knock down prejudices" and to convince them that deaf children will get a safe and good future in families where sign language is used.

In 1994, Jamie Burke, also an American, established a Web page listing deaf children who wait for permanent homes. It is called Deaf Adoption News Service (DANS), and its Web address is http://users.erols.com/berke/deafchildren.html. The Web page provides information about deaf children, with their name, a picture, whom to contact if you want to apply to adopt a particular child, but the Web site is not an adoption agency. Today there are about fifty deaf or hard of hearing children on this list. From 1994 until now more than forty deaf children have been adopted as a result of this Web site. The most recent development is the discussion forum online where parents who have adopted deaf children, or who want to adopt them, can get support and discuss their concerns. To subscribe to the discussion forum you can e-mail deaf-adoption-subscribe@yahoogroups.com.

Many people agreed that there ought to be some form of affiliation between DANS and the WFD, so we started working on that. DANS became a special interest group of the WFD in 1997. Through the WFD, we can more effectively inform authorities in different countries—both countries of origin and the receiving countries—about adoption of deaf children.

Since that time, we received financial support in Norway to print and distribute an informational booklet written by Barbara White and Susan Knolls, one of her students. This was an information sheet about beginning the adoption process. We have an English version and a Spanish version that have been widely distributed. We sent letters and booklets out to adoptive authorities in different countries containing general information about deaf people and about sign language, although we do not know whether some cultures might have a negative attitude toward sign language. We did not ask them to reply directly; we just sent this information out. Then we got a letter back from India that thanked us for the booklets and indicated that they had spread them through India. That was really nice to have that kind of response.

We also sent letters and information booklets to the deaf associations all over the world. We asked them to put information in their magazines. I do not know whether they have put the information in the magazines, but they were asked to. Four months ago a psychologist in Europe contacted me because he had been contacted by a deaf couple that wanted to adopt. The psychologist was quite skeptical, so he asked me, can deaf people really adopt? I said, yes, they could. He asked me about how a deaf person could bring up a child. There are some strange attitudes out there. I hope the deaf couple that he was in contact with got through the system and successfully adopted.

I hope the DANS Web site continues in spite of the fact that confidentiality is a concern when putting children's pictures online. There are only a few people I know of working on this issue, and we welcome anyone to get more involved. All it takes is a letter or a call to authorities and adoption agencies to find out if there are any deaf children in orphanages who are waiting for parents. Please tell the authorities that there are deaf people who would like to raise deaf children. If you live in receiving countries, you can contact the adoption authorities and ask them if deaf people can apply for adoption. If they say no, then work with them and ask them why. Your advocacy can pay off, even if it is only educating others and correcting their misconceptions about deaf people. You can tell deaf magazines in your countries about DANS; have them write an article about DANS and spread the information about how to go through the adoption process and how to apply for adoption. There are many useful tips on the Internet now about applying for adoption, but we must end discrimination against deaf adopters so that many more deaf couples will be able to adopt deaf children who need permanent and loving homes.

The Psychological Support Offered to "New Parents" of Deaf and Hard of Hearing Children in Cyprus

KIKA HADJIKAKOU

All families with deaf or hard of hearing children will require, at one time or another, relevant information on hearing loss and guidance for their children's educational, communicative, and/or career options, which should be accurate and practical. Most parents will also need some form of psychological support (Cunningham & Davis, 1995). This study examined the psychological support and counseling program offered to "new" parents of deaf and hard of hearing children in Cyprus. To obtain relevant information, two focus group meetings were organized. Participants in the first group were five parents of deaf or hard of hearing children (with different sex and ages, different degrees of hearing loss, different ages at detection, and different types of school and communication). Participants in the second group were two teachers of the deaf, one audiologist, one ear, nose, and throat (ENT) doctor, and one pediatrician.

A qualitative data analysis software was used to analyze all interview data. The results indicated that parents' experiences and professionals' opinions of the counseling process and the psychological support offered were as follows: (1) the counseling services are not well organized and there is no coordination, (2) parents did not receive any support once the hearing impairment of their children was detected or the results were communicated to them, and (3) the guidance program offered by the school for Deaf student to new parents is inadequate in supporting, training, and educating the parents of deaf or hard of hearing children, especially those with profound hearing loss. They also made recommendations that could form the basis for improved support and guidance services for families with children with permanent hearing impairment in Cyprus.

Background

Family system theory suggests that all the parts of the family are inextricably interrelated. One part of the system cannot be altered without every other part being affected (Jones, 1993). Luterman (1987, p. 100) states that "the discovery of deafness in a child is a very powerful extrafamiliar stress on the family system."

However, it appears that the process of grieving "may go more quickly and smoothly when parents are provided a linguistic—rather than pathological—framework for viewing their child's interactions, education, and future" (Mahshie, 1995, p. 66). Mahshie also stresses that "support for hearing parents of young Deaf children has traditionally come from family and friends who have little information about the real possibilities. Often it comes in the form of sympathy, reinforcing the idea that the child's deafness is a tragedy" (66).

Families faced with a child with special needs will require relevant information and guidance that is accurate and practical, so that they may become independent in their efforts to meet their own emotional needs and the needs of their children (Cunningham & Davis, 1995). Parents' increased knowledge about their children's hearing loss leads to more acceptance and sensitivity to the restrictions that their children may encounter. Programs that provide parent education and tutoring yield significant gains in the children's future academic achievement (Luterman, 1987). It is well known that parents' initial contacts with support and guidance services may determine the subsequent nature of relationships between parents and professionals (Beazley & Moore, 1995).

In Cyprus, the School for the Deaf offers a parent guidance program. During this program, the director of the school, the educational audiologist, and a senior member of the staff run guidance sessions for parents of preschool deaf or hard of hearing children (from detection until the children are three years old). These guidance sessions are held in the school. The guidance program "provides information about the pathology of deafness, hearing aid use, language and speech development, education provision and social and emotional adjustment" (Markides, 1990, p. 14). This study examined the psychological support and counseling (guidance) program offered to new parents of deaf or hard of hearing children in Cyprus.

Methodology

Two focus group meetings were organized at the School for the Deaf in Nicosia. Convenience sampling, which is the most common method for selecting participants in focus groups, was applied in our study (Stewart & Shamdasani, 1990). Consequently, a number of individuals who were known to the researcher and also thought to be representative of the larger population of interest were invited. These were divided into two groups: the first group consisted of five parents of deaf or hard of hearing children (with different ages, different degrees of hearing loss, and different types of school), and the second group consisted of five professionals (two teachers of the deaf, one audiologist, one ENT doctor, and one pediatrician).

The invitees were seated in a manner that provided maximum opportunity for eye contact with both the moderator and the group members. At the beginning, the moderator (the researcher) attempted to create an atmosphere of trust, and the invitees were assured of anonymity. Group members were introduced to build a sense of group identity. After that, the moderator introduced the topics, and the discussion started.

During the meeting, all respondents were encouraged to participate. Generally, the moderator used an interviewing style somewhere between the detective and nondetective approaches. Observers took notes at the focus group meetings, and the session was recorded on audiotape. The meeting lasted approximately two hours.

A computer-assisted approach (ETHNOGRAPH) was applied to facilitate the analysis of the qualitative data. ETHNOGRAPH is organized into three groups of procedures (data procedures, preparation of data, and selection of the file's line numbering).

Results

All participants had the opportunity to share their experiences and knowledge and to give important information concerning the communication of the results, the guidance program, and the overall psychological support.

The communication of the results was the most painful memory of the overall identification process for most of the parents:

- ❖ "The doctor communicated the results. He told me, 'Your child has a problem with his/her hearing. Take your child and leave. You will suffer a lot from now on, since your child can probably hear almost nothing.'"
- ❖ "Cyprus ENTs' way of announcing the results is awful. There is no support."
- ❖ "The Institute [of Neurology and Genetics] mailed the results in English. They did not explain anything to us and there was no support."

However, the experiences of parents who were given the results abroad was quite different:

"Doctors in Israel told us about our child's hearing loss. They were very good and they told us that our child could learn many things. They showed understanding, they supported and encouraged us."

On the other hand, professionals said of the communication of the results to the parents: "The hardest part is when I communicate the results to the parents. I'm trying to be gentle and stress the things that the child will be able to do despite his hearing impairment. The first reaction of the parents is that there is something wrong with the diagnosis. I always encourage them to ask for a second opinion. I may tell then some things about the hearing loss. It always depends on the case. I also prepare them for the hearing aids and when asked if the hearing loss can be cured, I tell them 'no.'"

The next step after the announcement of the results is the counseling process and the overall psychological support. The professionals admitted that the current guidance program in Cyprus is not well organized and not always good for all children:

- ❖ "Once the results are announced, the counseling program starts. There is a counseling program in the School for the Deaf in Nicosia and a teacher of the Deaf supports (psychologically) and educates the parents. The aim of the program is to enable the parents to help their children to obtain language, speech. This program lasts till the child's entrance into established educational provision (three years of age). . . . The counseling program is

good for children with severe hearing loss. However, there are some problems with the program for children with profound hearing losses."
- ❖ "It is a fact that there isn't a well-organized service (including teachers of the Deaf, audiologists) for the psychological support and counseling of the parents in Cyprus. Parents need not only counseling so as to help their children to obtain language, speech, and to achieve communication. Parents not only need counseling, but training as well."
- ❖ "The services are not well organized. There is no coordination."
- ❖ "Pediatric implantation has become a widespread procedure for seriously and profoundly deaf or hard of hearing children in Cyprus. Half of the children in the guidance programme in Cyprus have had a cochlear implantation in the private sector (since there is not a government cochlear program in Cyprus). Parents make the decision for a cochlear implantation, being consulted by people (mainly doctors) in the private sector. The teachers are not involved in this decision. Initial tuning and regular reprogramming takes place in Greece or in the private sector in Cyprus. There is not a complete pediatric cochlear implant team in Cyprus and only one or two people are involved in cochlear implantation. Thus, educators in the counseling program are not trained in cochlear implantation and they consequently assume that the activities used with hearing-aided children are suitable for those with cochlear implants."
- ❖ "The audiologist involved in the guidance programme does not participate in the tuning session or in the reprogramming of the implant system. He/she only detects faults in the functioning of external parts."

As with counseling, the psychological support provided by teachers of the Deaf is not satisfactory. The professionals stated the following:

- ❖ "The psychological support is provided by teachers of the deaf, who are not, of course, psychologists themselves."
- ❖ "If there was a specialist psychologist for the Deaf, he/she could help. However, any other psychologist wouldn't be such a good idea."

Likewise, parents were not very satisfied with the counseling program and with the support received:

- ❖ "I went with my child to the School for the Deaf for counseling. The child was satisfied since he/she could play with the teacher. However, I was not satisfied."
- ❖ "There is no counseling, no support."
- ❖ "There is no parents' support in Cyprus. Once your child's hearing loss is identified, you're alone."
- ❖ "A teacher of the Deaf supported us (psychologically) in the private sector. My experiences during the first year were very bad. Counseling and support are vital."

The habilitation process, as described, is not very satisfactory. Hence, both parents and professionals agreed that there is room for improvement. Concerning the counseling and ongoing support, the professionals stated:

- ❖ "A lot of work and a valuation of the attempts need to be done in this area [counseling]. In most of the cases, the mother is the person who gets involved. However, the rest of the family should be involved."
- ❖ "Parents are not all the same. Even children with the same degree of hearing loss are different. Therefore, there will probably be a need to see one child every day, and another not."

Parents similarly stressed the following:

- ❖ "Counseling should be offered to parents. There should be home visits by a teacher of the Deaf and a counselor, at least for [the first] three years."
- ❖ "The family needs support as well."
- ❖ "Ongoing support is insufficient. Teachers of the Deaf and speech therapists should be trained."

Overall, the results indicated that the parents' experiences and the professionals' opinions of the counseling process and the psychological support offered were mostly negative:

- ❖ The counseling services are not well organized, and there is no coordination.
- ❖ Parents did not receive any support once the hearing impairment of their children was detected and the results had been communicated to them.
- ❖ The guidance program offered by the School for the Deaf to new parents is inadequate in supporting, training, and educating the parents of deaf or hard of hearing children, especially those with profound hearing loss.

Recommendations

Our focus groups revealed the need for early counseling and ongoing support. The NDCS (1994, p. 4) also suggests that "parents should receive sensitive counseling and guidance about the test results and be given clear information about the planned follow-up." Markides (1990, p. 58) stresses that "the discovery of deafness should be revealed to the parents immediately following diagnosis but with extreme care and sensitivity." Markides also suggests that parents of deaf or hard of hearing children will "have special needs and they will require guidance and skilled support to understand, adjust to and accept the disability of their child and to develop modes of behavior and attitudes most conductive to their child's growth" (57).

The guidance program in the School for the Deaf is in need of improvement, and educational services should evaluate and improve the counseling program offering to the deaf or hard of hearing children and to their families:

- Psychological support should be provided by psychologists, who are specialists in deafness, to all family members soon after the detection, in order to come into terms with deafness (Warner, 1994). Ongoing psychological support is also vital for all family members at all stages of the deaf children's lives.
- Deaf adults should be involved in the family support program. Parents, who see their children interacting with Deaf adults from an early age, recognize the particular skills that are being demonstrated and value the contribution that Deaf adults can make to their family (Pickersgill, 1998).
- New parents should meet and interact with other parents of deaf children (Gregory & Knight, 1998).
- Establishing a route to communication between the family and the deaf child should be considered a pressing matter (Pickersgill, 1998). There is no evidence to support that early sign language acquisition interferes with the acquisition of speech in Greek; on the contrary, research data support the beneficial results of bilingual education for deaf children (Mahshie, 1995; Pickersgill, 1998). Thus, sign language should be introduced in the early years and should not be regarded as the last resort for deaf children who cannot acquire speech.
- The process of cochlear implantation followed in other countries, which is divided into four areas—assessment, surgery and initial tuning, rehabilitation, and maintenance (Archbold, 1997)—should be applied in Cyprus as well; cochlear implantation and rehabilitation in Cyprus should be considered from a complete pediatric cochlear implant team's job (including parents, doctors, teachers of deaf students, audiologists, psychologists, speech therapists, and members of the Deaf community).

References

Archbold, S. (1997). Cochlear implants. In W. McCracken & S. Laoide-Kemp (Eds.). *Audiology in education* (pp. 239–266). London: David Fulton Publishers.

Beazley, S., & Moore, M. (1995). *Deaf children, their families, and professionals dismantling barriers.* London: David Fulton Publishers.

Cunningham, C., & Davis, H. (1995). *Working with parents: Frameworks for collaboration.* Milton Keynes, U.K.: Open University Press.

Gregory, S., & Knight, P. (1998). Social development and family life. In S. Gregory, P. Knight, W. McCracken, S. Powers, & L. Watson (Eds.), *Issues in deaf education* (pp. 3–11). London: David Fulton Publishers.

Jones, E. (1993). *Family systems therapy: Developments in the Milan-systematic therapies.* Chichester, UK: John Wiley & Sons.

Luterman, D. (1987). *Deafness in the family.* San Diego, CA: Hill Press.

Mahshie, S. N. (1995). *Educating deaf children bilingually.* Washington, DC: Gallaudet University.

Markides, A. (1990). *Special educational needs of hearing-impaired children and young adults in Cyprus* (Report submitted to the Minister of Education of the Republic of Cyprus). Manchester, UK: University of Manchester.

NDCS. (1994). *Quality standards in paediatric audiology, Vol. 1: Guidelines for the early identification of hearing impairment in children.* London: National Deaf Children's Society.

Pickersgill, M. (1998). Bilingualism—current policy and practice. In S. Gregory, K. Knight, W. McCracken, S. Powers, & L. Watson (Eds.), *Issues in deaf education* (pp. 88–97). London: David Fulton Publishers.

Stewart, D. W., & Shamdasani, P. N. (1990). *Focus groups: Theory and practice.* London: Sage Publications.

Warner, B. (1994). Family therapy systems with deaf people and their families. *Deafness and well being* (pp. 42–43). Paris: Editions Charles Leopold Mayer.

The Missing Link in Literacy Development—A Parent's Perspective

NAYANTRA KANAYE

Because of the nature of Deafness and its implications, Deaf children are often severely hampered in their acquisition of literacy skills. There are a number of factors that inhibit language development in Deaf children. The most important are late diagnosis of a hearing disorder, inability of parents to accept to accept the Deafness and thereby provide the necessary stimulation, a lack of early educational programs catering to the specific needs of Deaf infants, and uncertainty of the best method of communication. Davis and Silverman (1978) reinforce the concept of an early intervention program for Deaf babies as a way of ensuring that the development of literacy skills starts as early as possible.

How the Diagnosis Is Presented to Parents

Our experience as parents at the time of diagnosis mirrors exactly what Davis and Silverman (1978), Moores (1987) and Lane, Hoffmeister, and Bahan (1996) report in their findings with parents: shock and disbelief at the diagnosis, denial, guilt at perhaps in some way being the cause, being totally at a loss as to what the future implications might be for our child, and wanting to ignore the diagnosis and to hope for a miracle. We did not want to accept the diagnosis and visited one doctor after another hoping that the last one had made a mistake. Our idea of Deafness at that time included the notion that our child would be, to some degree, retarded. Of course, I now realize that this is an absolutely nonsensical idea, given the fact that both she and her brother (also Deaf) have graduated with bachelor of science degrees (her degree achieved magna cum laude) in the finance and accounting field from the Gallaudet University in Washington, D.C. It is for this reason that I would like parents to understand that all is not lost when they receive news that their child is Deaf; a lot can be achieved provided appropriate intervention takes place as soon as possible and adequate educational support is provided.

Parents need to be handled with understanding at this delicate stage. My experience endorses the findings of researchers that not enough training is provided to physicians and other health professionals, who find it difficult to deal with the unpleasantness of facing families in pain and therefore resort to simply presenting the diagnosis in a clinical manner. Because of their discomfort, too, they may fail to provide necessary factual information and a balanced view of what steps to take (Lane et al., 1996). I have never gotten over the insensitivity of the doctor who presented the diagnosis to me with the words, "This child is stone Deaf," and I still have extremely negative feelings about him. I regarded him as the person who shattered my dreams and knew that I would never consult him again regardless of how good he might be in his field.

Emotional State of Parents: The Need for Counseling

This extremely upsetting news is further aggravated when the parents have little or no understanding about the disability concerned. Parents always look forward to a baby with a lot of dreams and aspirations for the child's future, and the possibility that the child may have a disability is usually never considered. When my daughter was diagnosed as Deaf just before she turned two years old, I felt as if the whole world had come crashing down around me. These dreams for our daughter did not include therapeutic intervention, which I realized would have to make up the bulk of our days. To say that this news shattered our dreams is to put it very mildly. We were devastated. I felt that I had suffered a loss so severe that I despaired of ever recovering from that loss, and I can only liken this intense pain that I felt, this immense feeling of sadness and helplessness, to that which one may experience at the death of a loved one.

During the crucial months after the diagnosis is made, it is important that parents are given the chance to work through these intense, conflicting emotions by receiving counseling and support. If these emotions are not appropriately dealt with, they will continue to fester beneath the surface, inhibiting adjustment to the Deafness as well as appropriate and timely intervention. I did not receive any help in this area and had to work through these emotions on my own over a long period by reading extensively on the subject and pursuing studies in this field. I realize now how helpful it would have been for me if I had an understanding professional to talk to at that time, someone who was objective, allowed me space to be just a parent, understood what I was experiencing, and would not judge me or coerce me into accepting a particular approach that they assumed was best for my child.

My children are profoundly Deaf, and the advice I was given was that I should fit them with hearing aids and start speech therapy. I was told that the success of my children depended entirely on me and whether I would commit to providing this intensive training needed to enable my children to lipread, to speak, and thus to be able to fit into "normal society." The burden that this placed on me was so great that when we did start sign language with our children, I could not shake off the guilt that I had failed them in the worst possible way. These feelings of guilt only changed for me when I had the opportunity to meet a Deaf adult, Alan Jones, who did not have good oral skills but was successfully employed as a computer analyst and, best of all, communicated through sign language.

Grappling with Different Issues

Parents and close relatives, especially in the community from which I come (the South African Indian community), often overprotect their Deaf children, shielding them from the outside world and contact with other children, treating them as if they are incapable of doing anything by doing everything for them, absolving them of any responsibilities or chores that other siblings may be required to do and also often not reprimanding them for misbehavior and wrongdoing. They are thus unable to distinguish between right and wrong, thereby denying them opportunities for normal development, and as a result education is often delayed. This is not confined to South African communities alone. Lane (1994), in describing the American situation, states that because Deaf people are judged as physically defective, people assume that this gives rise to undesirable character traits such as impulsive behavior and lack of abstract thought.

Parents also need to be made aware that hearing aids do not automatically restore hearing in the same way that a pair of spectacles corrects vision. This would avoid the frustration that sets in when progress is limited. I remember how difficult and frustrating it was during those endless hours of speech training that I did with my children, assuming that the hearing aids served a similar purpose to a pair of spectacles. This was because they are classified as profoundly Deaf, and in hindsight, it is obvious that the oral approach was not the appropriate route for them.

The controversy about the use of sign language versus the oral means of communication continues, and this often causes a dilemma in the minds of parents. Parents have often never met Deaf people before and may perhaps be ignorant of the concept of Deaf culture, as has been my own experience. It is therefore not surprising that they often choose the oral route, assuming it to be the best possible way for their child, because professionals whom the parents encounter at this stage, such as doctors; ear, nose, and throat (ENT) specialists; and audiologists, often recommend this. However, as Moores (1987) explains, a prelingually Deaf child will develop little or no speech without specific training and stimulation, and because professionals often advise parents that it is imperative to start this process as early as possible, parents fear that if they do not comply they may be doing their child a disservice. In most instances, such as my own, parents are not told that speech competency depends on the degree of hearing loss. Parents often equate speech competency with language competency and only realize their error in judgment years later when the Deaf child does not develop adequate speech, is language delayed, and is now advised to use sign language.

When sign language is recommended at a much later stage, almost as a last resort, parents get the impression that it is not the optimal recommendation but rather that it is only to be used with those children who fail in speech therapy to develop adequate lipreading and vocal skills. This initial oral approach, which is often recommended by professionals, is what Lane (1994) and Lane, Hoffmeister, and Bahan (1996) refer to as the medical or infirmity model, a model that is described as attempting to make Deaf people poor imitations of hearing people, as opposed to a cultural model, which concedes that sign language is indeed a language which Deaf people are entitled to use freely and which forms the basis of their cultural identity.

The frustration that Deaf children undergo at being unable to communicate freely because of the unwillingness of hearing professionals to acknowledge that there is another language, although not a spoken one, which Deaf children can be exposed to and be allowed to develop, can only be imagined. Exposing our children to sign language was not an option that we would even consider at that time, because then we would be sentencing them to becoming low-functioning Deaf people; that was the idea that was subtly conveyed by all whom we came into contact at that stage. Successful Deaf people were oral Deaf people! Thus, if the "experts" are advocating a particular route, how do emotionally weak parents who are still reeling from the shock of the diagnosis choose otherwise?

Acculturation into the Deaf Community: The Parent Factor

Despite the route parents may take, there eventually comes a time when Deaf children become immersed in the Deaf community and acquire sign language. I have often heard parents say that their Deaf children are happiest when they are with other Deaf people and that when they reach their late teens, parents lose them to the Deaf community. The relationship between Deaf children and their parents must not be merely a biological one, and Deaf children need not become divorced from their parents to become part of the Deaf community. Parents of Deaf children need to embrace Deaf culture as a crucial part of their children's lives to ensure that their children are not isolated from them. The relationship between parents and the Deaf community has to be a symbiotic one in order to create an environment of warmth and acceptance for their Deaf children. During my studies in the United States when I met, studied, and socialized with many Deaf adults, I realized how important it is for parents to be able to do this because it provided many insights for me about the significance of Deaf culture and what it means for Deaf people.

Parents also need to meet and interact with adult Deaf role models on an ongoing basis. This is an excellent way of enabling parents to come to terms with the Deafness and of making acceptance easier, giving parents an indication of what the future may be like for their child and allowing them to see the positive consequences of accepting sign language as a communication mode for their child. Being able to meet adult Deaf role models was one of the most positive influencing factors in my life. When I visited Gallaudet University and the National Technical Institute for the Deaf, both of which are in the United States, and saw the large numbers of college graduates, it changed my view of sign language and opened the way for a brighter future for my children.

However, a disturbing factor that is often encountered in our community is Deaf people who have adopted the negative attitudes of hearing people toward sign language and who regard themselves as superior if they have acquired some vocal skills. This often creates feelings of ambiguity toward the language in Deaf people themselves, thus making the choice for parents even more difficult. In fact, schools also continue to display their oral successes without explaining that these are the minority, and parents are given to understand that this is true for all Deaf children who go through the program, regardless of the degree of hearing loss. Therefore, it is important that parents have opportunities to develop a positive attitude toward Deafness in order to develop in their children a sense of pride and acceptance of their language and culture.

Points to Consider in Ensuring Deaf Children Develop Literacy Skills

Faced with all of this, how do we ensure that parents participate fully in the intellectual development of their Deaf children? How do we ensure that Deaf children develop the literacy skills so necessary for success in their educational careers?

First and foremost is the introduction of sign language as soon as diagnosis is made. The different degrees of hearing loss and the wide range of losses that one finds among Deaf children means that some children may benefit from oral intervention, and it is certainly not my intention to completely discredit the oral route. Developing vocal skills is commendable if it benefits the child; after all, they do have to live and function in a hearing world. However, for the large majority of Deaf children who are classified profoundly Deaf, this is not possible, and encouraging parents to follow a route that has minimal success is deceptive, in my opinion. Blame for failure often falls on the shoulders of the parents, who have to pick up the pieces later after precious time is lost, a factor acknowledged by Lane, Hoffmeister, and Bahan (1996) in their book *A Journey into the Deaf-World*. Deaf children are then condemned to a lifelong struggle to acquire literacy skills, eventually leaving school with insufficient skills to cope in the real world, and having to suffer the indignity of being stuck in low-paying jobs. In my opinion, it would be more appropriate to follow a combined approach: introduce the child to sign language and at the same time follow a program to develop their oral skills. This will give emotionally charged parents who may be having ambiguous feelings some respite from having to make a crucial decision and, at the same time, valuable time is not being lost.

The United States, Sweden, and Denmark have large numbers of Deaf college graduates, bearing testimony to the importance of sign language in the development of the whole child. A program to emulate is the bilingual and bicultural program instituted by Sweden in 1981 as the official policy in their schools for Deaf students (Lane et al., 1996). To forge bilingual education, block mainstreaming, and ensure that Deaf children are not deprived of sign language, Swedish Sign Language is used to teach Swedish, which is taught as a second language. Deaf people are widely respected for their knowledge concerning their language and culture and play an important role in additional services such as Swedish Sign Language classes, parents' meetings hosted by Deaf clubs, special preschools, Deaf home visitors, and short-term live-in arrangements as a way of bringing Deaf adults into the homes of hearing families with Deaf children.

In South Africa, even though sign language is now recognized as a language of instruction in schools for Deaf students, in reality, schools continue to have large numbers of personnel who are either not fluent in sign language or have very minimal signing skills. Students still have to pass two languages to qualify for university entrance, and sign language is not one of them. Bilingualism for Deaf people as described by Grosjean (1982), involving sign language and the use of written English, must be encouraged in schools for Deaf students and, in fact, in all educational programs in South Africa. Sign and written English bilingualism is very rare among South African Deaf people. At present one in three Deaf adults in South Africa is functionally illiterate, and the average Deaf school dropout has a written language comprehension ability equivalent to that of an average eight-year-old hearing child (DEAFSA, 1997).

Higher Education for Deaf Students

There is very little access to tertiary education for Deaf people in South Africa. Universities such as University of the Witwatersrand (Center for Deaf Studies Unit) that have units for students with disabilities also have entrance requirements as described previously, which make it virtually impossible for the average Deaf student. The South African College of Open Learning (previously Springfield College of Education) started a teacher-training program for Deaf students in 1998 but has not taken new students since 2000. The program catering to Deaf students at the Durban Institute of Technology has now grown to include approximately thirty students, all studying toward the Diploma in Information Technology. Two interpreters and a coordinator of the Deaf Program were employed in an attempt to meet some of the needs of the Deaf students. However, for many of these students this diploma is not necessarily their preferred field of study but they take the coursework simply because there is some support in place, as limited as it might be. Very little or no support structures are in place, at present, in South African colleges and universities to meet the needs of Deaf students desiring to continue with further education.

The mere provision of interpreters for Deaf students in a tertiary institution is not enough to meet their needs for success in studies. Education at schools for Deaf students in South Africa and at mainstream schools is vastly different, and Deaf students face an ongoing problem regarding inadequate literacy skills. To address this inadequacy, it is important for tertiary institutions that accept Deaf students to make adequate provision for their specific needs, such as the availability of tutors and tutorial centers, note takers, and a bridging module designed to offer intensive training in developing literacy and numeracy skills.

Conclusion

Parents have to play a critical role in the lives of their Deaf children if they want to enable their children to take their rightful place in society: that of a citizen of the country with the same rights as any other for a fair and equitable education with all the support necessary to be able to succeed in their studies without unceasing effort. We parents need to have support groups and parent lobbyist groups to make our voices heard loud and clear to all concerned: professionals, educational professionals, and the government alike.

Historically, the ancient Hebrew and Roman laws classed Deaf people with those who were mentally challenged and with children by assuming that they were not able to take normal adult responsibility and therefore gave them no legal rights (Bender, 1981). This kind of attitude continues to prevail in many countries throughout the world. For example, Lane, Hoffmeister, and Bahan (1996) report that in developing countries such as Burundi there is no provision for the education of Deaf children.

According to a report titled "Special Education in the Developing Countries of the (British) Commonwealth," "Deaf children cannot think in words, so their mental growth is severely retarded." Thus, it can be seen that we all need to work together to rid the world of these archaic ideas and replace them with more progressive ways of thinking.

References

Bender, R. E. (1981). *The conquest of deafness: A history of the long struggle to make possible normal living to those handicapped by lack of normal hearing.* Cleveland: Interstate Printers and Publishers.

Davis, H., and Silverman, R. (1978). *Hearing and deafness.* New York: Holt, Rinehart, and Winston.

Deaf Federation of South Africa (DEAFSA). (1996). *South African Sign Language: Curriculum for level 1, 2, 3.* Johannesburg, South Africa: Author.

Grosjean, F. (1982). *Life with two languages.* Cambridge, MA: Harvard University Press.

Lane, H. (1994). *The mask of benevolence: Disabling the Deaf community.* New York: Alfred A. Knopf.

Lane, H., Hoffmeister, R., and Bahan, B. (1996). *A journey into the Deaf-world.* California: DawnSign Press.

Moores, D. F. (1987). *Educating the Deaf.* Boston: Houghton Mifflin Company.

The Silent Garden: Reaching Out to Your Deaf Children

PAUL W. OGDEN

Hearing parents of a newborn deaf child—indeed, hearing people generally—are unaware of the diversity within the deaf and hard of hearing population, including the amount of hearing loss a deaf or hard of hearing person has, the age at which the loss occurred, and the type of hearing loss, whether conductive (damage to the parts of the ear that conduct sound to the inner ear), sensorineural (damage to the hair cells and neurons that transmit the sound to the brain), or mixed (a little of each of the previous two). The causes of hearing loss also vary, extending from accidents and infections to genetics.

For the family of a deaf newborn, these considerations are interesting but academic. Hearing parents, in particular, are sometimes quite thrown by the birth of a deaf child and react emotionally when the diagnosis is formally made. They sense a feeling of loss themselves, loss of their expectations and dreams, and the growing knowledge that their private world has been shaken to its core. Some parents of deaf children feel overwhelmed as they look ahead to the obstacles they know they will have to confront as they struggle to make the right choices for their children, guiding them through their early years into adolescence and adulthood in a society filled with negative stereotypes and practical obstacles to achieving "the good life" parents want for their children.

When a child is diagnosed with a hearing loss, parents and family members enter a grieving process that entails moving through predictable stages of shock and denial, anger, guilt, depression, and anxiety. Understanding the process and going through it is the first step to coping with their new reality and learning how to recover their lost feelings of anticipation and joy.

Throughout the grieving phases, it is important for parents and family members to confide in each other and to express their true feelings, even the unacceptable ones of guilt and anger. Some parents think they are responsible for their child being deaf; some cultures see it as a punishment for wrongdoing, even when they cannot pinpoint the nature of the wrongdoing. Just as guilt recedes, depression and anxiety, too, will give way to feelings of renewed confidence as parents begin to reevaluate their competency and discover in themselves the resources they need to create a full life for their child.

Coping begins when parents are able to reassess what they view as "normal" and to *contain the loss*, that is, to recognize that the ramifications of raising a deaf child are not as ominous as they feared. One of the unanticipated rewards of moving through the grieving process is to find that the scope of one's world is enlarged. Rather than dwell on comparisons of deaf versus hearing where the latter always comes out ahead, they begin to appreciate their child's individual accomplishments and assets over the days and years.

Other coping strategies for families, besides sharing fully with each other, is to reach out to find people going through similar experiences, to allow themselves time to recover—everyone is different in this regard, to recognize that grief for the fantasy child will not last forever, to avoid isolation, to hold on to a sense of humor, and to take care of *themselves* as much as their child. A parent who is anxious and tired is not only of little use to a child but can transmit those fears and concerns to the child. Whether in a deaf or hearing environment, the family is the first to provide them with opportunities to grow and learn, and it is the family that is responsible for their child feeling supported and cared for and developing a strong sense of self. Perhaps most important for parents to remember is that they *will* make mistakes and that parenting under any circumstances involves a lot of trial and error. Being gentle with themselves and not giving in to the temptation to criticize themselves constantly is vital if they are to come to terms with their new reality.

Once parents have "come out the other side," they need to begin focusing on communicating with their child. Regardless of how parents choose to communicate (with sign language, speech, or speechreading, for example), the child needs to have full access to language and all the conversations his brothers and sisters are privy to. In fact, because deaf and hard of hearing children will pick up less incidental information because of their hearing loss, parents must plan to go out of their way to explain things and to teach their deaf or hard of hearing child the myriad things that hearing children pick up on their own on a daily basis.

Communicating with a deaf child can be demanding. Parents and siblings need to be patient and to persevere. These early years are critical, and the home environment means everything now. Trust develops between mother and infant as she responds to cries and comforts the child through touch and facial expression. For the deaf child, parents need to focus on tactile and visual equivalents to talking, establishing and maintaining eye contact and using facial expressions to communicate. Exposing the child to purposeful gestures and signs, whether formal or "home grown," and paying strict attention to keeping the child in the loop is critical. The foundations of conversation, in fact, are laid at this stage. When parents give in to feelings of frustration and helplessness and stop communicating with their deaf child, the effect on the child—on any child, in fact—is to withdraw into a private world and become isolated.

Recognizing the different ways a deaf or hard of hearing child communicates should help parents strike a balance between fostering independence and being attentive to the very real frustrations their child is experiencing in its struggle to be acknowledged and understood. When the child learns he or she can forge solid relationships through communication, the family and child become more healthy and robust.

Like hearing children, deaf children should be exposed to books early. Stories can be read to infants and toddlers. For all children, early language exposure is extremely important to the child's cognitive development. Studies show that children who are read to and see parents and other family members reading do well in school and show measurable results in their future academic success, and the deaf child is no exception. As in all families, perhaps the most enjoyable thing parents can do is play with their child. The whole family can participate and take a break from the stresses of everyday life as they bond over a game of charades or baking a batch of cookies. The family can be considered a mosaic, each member representing a thing of beauty in itself and commanding attention both for its individual contributions and its participation in the whole.

As the deaf child matures, he or she needs to be fully integrated into the family. Two specific steps parents can take to ensure that their child has the foundation for becoming a productive, well-adjusted, successful adult are to equip the child, as soon as he or she seems ready, to deal with her "differentness" from the hearing world, or, as appropriate, from siblings, and to provide the child with deaf adult role models. Beyond this, parents need to be explicit when interacting with their child, never leaving him or her out of a conversation as if they are not present. Next, they need to be direct in their praise and in their criticism or constructive feedback. The most serious odds deaf children face are the consequences of being left out of the communication process within the family. At all costs, the deaf child must be discouraged from using his or her deafness as an excuse to slack off or to withdraw.

To enter the outside world, children need to know what the values and morals of the family are and to know how they are expected to behave around others. Deaf and hard of hearing children, like hearing children, need to learn independence; and parents should allow them to make mistakes and take responsibility for their actions. Parents are likely to find themselves acting as ambassadors for their child and for deaf children in general as they proceed on their journey of learning.

Having a deaf brother and sister can be a strain for siblings. After all, seeing their parents preoccupied with the deaf child, they may feel left out and worry about what the new family situation means for them. Parents need to reassure them that the deafness of their brother or sister is not the end of their family life and although deafness means the child cannot hear, everything else with the child is fine. At the same time, parents would be wise to sense when the siblings have had enough explaining, educating, and defending. Siblings should not be forced to be the interpreter for their deaf brother or sister all the time, and the responsibility for the deaf child should not be allowed to limit the hearing child's development and love of life. For the health of the family, it is important that parents commit to creating an environment that is conducive to open communication and, further, that they stay alert to whether they might unwittingly be unfairly shifting burdens on the hearing children.

If parents pay special attention to setting aside time for each of their children individually, being honest about deafness within their family and with other people, educating their children about deafness, reinforcing positive interactions between siblings, insisting on a lack of favoritism in the immediate and extended family, and focusing on the importance of the family as a whole, they can offset or eliminate the disruption that can otherwise burden the entire family. Ultimately, family members will come to appreciate the uniqueness of their children and what each brings to the family. Yes, the journey demands much of both parents and siblings, but the insights learned about family dynamics and the importance of inclusion and open and honest communication yield many unexpected rewards for the parents of a deaf child.

References

Ogden, P. W. (1996). *The silent garden: Raising your deaf child*. Washington, DC: Gallaudet University Press.

Ogden, P. W. (2002). *El jardin silencioso: Criando a su hijo sordo*. Hillsboro, OR: Butte Publications (Spanish translation of *The silent garden*).

Deaf Parents with Teenage Children

PAUL PRESTON

A few years ago, I did a four-year national study on people like myself: adult hearing children of deaf parents throughout the United States. Increasingly, in the United States as well as several other countries, we are often referred to as "codas." Data for that study included life histories and interviews with 150 men and women—all of whom were hearing and who were raised by profoundly deaf parents. This study resulted in a book I wrote, *Mother Father Deaf,* published by Harvard University Press.

Now I will describe a new national research project I am working on, which focuses on deaf parents with teenage children.

First, however, I want to emphasize that this project concerns deaf parents in the United States. Although we are here at Deaf Way as a testimony to the global Deaf community, we need to recognize that there are also differences among our Deaf communities—at the local, regional, and national levels. Over the years, we have tried very hard to get hearing people to recognize Deaf culture, and often the main emphasis has been to concentrate on the sign languages of the world. However, culture does not involve only language, and we need to start recognizing that we have paid very little attention to other kinds of cultural differences among Deaf people—how they think, how they behave, how they interact with the hearing people of their country, how they live their lives. *Culture* is a slippery concept to define: we know it, we feel it, but it is often hard to put into words exactly what it is. To me, as an anthropologist, culture includes four components: (1) a system of shared ideas and behaviors, (2) which are distinct, (3) which are learned, and (4) which provide a template for personal and social interaction.

So, why are we even talking about deaf parents and their families? Let us not be naive. When we talk about only certain kinds of families, when we focus on deaf parents and their children, what are we really saying? That there is something wrong with them? There is good reason to be cautious, to be suspicious. A lot has been written about deaf parents, about their children, and about our families that is harmful. Many people still see us as broken people who can produce only broken children, but they are wrong.

Many deaf parents have raised their families successfully, and they are inappropriately stigmatized because of misguided presumptions about their parenting capabilities. However, some deaf-parented families are vulnerable to dysfunction, even child abuse or neglect because of risk factors comparable to those within hearing families. These risk factors include low economic status, lack of social supports, lack of parenting knowledge, and the child's problematic behavior. For those deaf parents who need information or services, resources are virtually nonexistent. Without appropriate information or intervention, in the most extreme situations deaf parents are at risk of losing custody of their children because of presumed negligence or maltreatment. In less extreme cases, a number of barriers may seriously impede adequate parenting and increase the risk of family dysfunction or dissolution.

A National Study of Deaf Parents with Teenagers

Research for a new study, the first National Study of Deaf Parents with Teenagers, is being conducted by an agency I codirect in Berkeley, California: Through the Looking Glass. Through the Looking Glass is a national resource center for parents with disabilities. Our research project on deaf parents go on for another year, so there is still a lot more data and more analysis that needs to happen before we can really discuss the final results. In the meantime, I can describe what the project is and what we have learned so far.

Who Is Involved?

Our study of deaf parents with teenagers is part of a large national study concerning parents with disabilities and deaf parents, all of whom have teenage children. Our study includes families that have parents with physical disabilities, parents with cognitive disabilities, blind parents, parents with multiple sclerosis, and deaf parents. A recent study estimates that there are at least 8.1 million American families with children in which one or both parents are deaf or have a disability, approximately 10.9 percent of all American families. Although this national research also studies other parents with teenagers, I discuss our research project with deaf parents and their teenagers.

The deaf parent portion of our research project targets two populations: (1) deaf and hard of hearing parents who have at least one teenaged child eleven to seventeen years old living at home with them and (2) any hearing or deaf teenagers (aged eleven to seventeen) who live with at least one deaf or hard of hearing parent. These parents and teenagers can live anywhere in the United States. Also, please note that in our study, all of the "deaf" parents who are participating so far are both functionally deaf as well as culturally Deaf, but we would also include parents who have a hearing loss but who are not necessarily culturally Deaf.

Why Study Families with Teenagers?

Research has paid almost no attention to deaf parents with teenagers. Why bother to study these particular families? As children reach adolescence they may take on increased responsibilities in the family—including those related to their parent's deafness. How is a teenager's natural progression toward greater independence and separation from their family influenced by a parent's deafness? As most of us realize—from our own experience as teenagers (or if you have teenagers of your own)—becoming a teenager usually means wanting to be more private, more separate from parents and the rest of the family. Adolescence is marked by strong interaction with and allegiance to peers. Teenagers' sensitivity to their teenage peers may increase their embarrassment about their parents. At the same time, many teens with deaf parents may feel strong cultural ties to their Deaf families. They may feel conflicted about their responsibilities at home and their desire for independence. What kind of roles do teens with deaf parents take on, and how are they different from the roles of teens with hearing parents? Adolescence is a time for a readjustment of the parent-child relationship. It is especially important for deaf parents and members of the Deaf community to address how our families navigate our children's developmental transition to independence during the adolescent period.

One of the strengths of the Deaf community is its peer support. Deaf people have traditionally been the main source of information and support for other deaf people. This is an especially important resource for deaf parents. However, peer resources are not always available. In some situations, access is limited because of geographic distance. In other cases, a deaf individual may not have strong ties to the local Deaf community because of differences in ethnicity or socioeconomic status compared to the larger group. Still other deaf adults are minimally connected to the local Deaf community because of poorly developed sign language skills or because they have not had long-term ties to the Deaf community; this is particularly true in the case of recent deaf immigrants in the United States.

Deaf parents and their adolescents currently grapple too often with family issues in isolation from one another. There is a profound need for materials and networking that alleviate their isolation. For the most stressed families in the community, there is also a need for intervention that is informed by a Deaf community perspective as well as state-of-the-art research. There is very little available practical material to guide deaf parents in parenting teenagers or to inform teenagers in these families. There are no materials focused on adolescence written from the point of view of the Deaf community, drawing on the experiences of parents and adolescents.

Research Questions

Here are some of the key research questions that we are hoping to answer when we finish this project:

1. How many deaf and hard of hearing parents with teenagers are there in the United States? How many families are there in which both parents are deaf? How many families have one hearing and one deaf parent? How many children are usually in the family? Do families live in certain parts of the country? Are there more in cities or in rural areas?
2. What themes and issues are common to families of deaf parents and teens? How do these compare with themes in families with hearing parents? Blind parents? Physically disabled parents?
3. What is the difference between families who feel they are basically happy and

those families who are not happy? What kinds of information or support might make a difference in promoting positive family functioning and happiness?

4. Are there any particular issues or events that are easier or more difficult for families with deaf parents and their teens (for example, entering middle or high school, separation, risk taking)? Does it make any difference if the teenager is hearing or deaf?
5. What kinds of tasks do teenagers of deaf parents do around the house? How do these compare to teenagers with hearing parents or teenagers of parents with disabilities?
6. What makes the difference in deciding who does what around the family? Is it the gender of the teenager? The birth order of the teenager? Whether both parents are deaf, or one is deaf and one is hearing? How many other children are in the house?

Research Methods

To answer these questions, our research project on deaf parents and teenagers has four phases.

Phase 1: Existing Data from the U.S. Census and the National Health Interview Survey

The main objectives in Phase 1 are to estimate how many families there are in the United States with deaf parents who have teenagers and also to describe the characteristics of these families. We also draw data from a national study I was involved in a few years ago, the first National Survey of Parents with Disabilities.

Phase 2: Focus Groups

Phase 2 was designed to gather initial feedback from deaf parents and their teenagers. I conducted focus groups of deaf parents with teenagers in Orlando, Florida; Monterey, California; Rochester, New York; and Cincinnati, Ohio. I also conducted focus groups with teenagers of deaf parents.

Phase 3: National Survey

Phase 3 is a national survey of deaf parents and their teenage children. We are surveying both parents and teenagers. There are separate questions for the parents and for the teens. One of the things we are hoping to do is to compare the parents and the teens' perspectives. Do the parents think their teenagers help a lot around the house? What do the teenagers think? Do the teenagers think they can or cannot do some things because their parents are deaf? What do their parents think? What are the positive aspects of having deaf parents?

In developing this national survey, we are trying out several different approaches: (1) a printed survey that is mailed to deaf parents and their teens all over the United States; (2) an online version of the printed survey, and (3) in-person interviews with deaf parents. These interviews will include all the questions from the print survey but will allow parents to discuss their responses at greater length as well as additional issues not included in the survey. Deaf parents are being interviewed in the following areas: Seattle, Washington; Rochester, New York; Santa Fe, New Mexico; Topeka, Kansas; and San Francisco, California.

You might wonder why we bother with printed surveys because it is possible that most deaf people would prefer to be interviewed in person. Well, one reason is that it is a lot cheaper to mail several surveys to deaf parents all over the United States than it is to have an interviewer travel and meet with each deaf parent. Unfortunately, the U.S. Department of Education—which sponsored this research—did not give us much money to travel all over the United States conducting interviews. Also, maybe some deaf parents would prefer to fill out a survey—they do not ever have to use their names, so no one would know who they are. We are trying to compromise. We will do as many printed surveys as we can, and also do as many face-to-face interviews as we can. Another result of using these different approaches will be that we will be able to compare how deaf parents responded to these three different approaches: print survey, online survey, and in-person interview.

Phase 4: In-Depth Exploration

We will also be gathering information from the families we work with locally in the San Francisco Bay Area, providing in-home support services. Most of these families are experiencing considerable difficulties and crises—ranging from premature babies, babies and young children with medical problems, to parents with abuse or violence histories. It is important to keep in mind that these families are not typical families with deaf parents. However, they can help us understand some of the difficulties that some families experience and also help us understand what works best to help these families.

What Have We Learned So Far?

Even though we still are not finished with our research, here is a summary of what deaf parents and their teens have talked about most so far.

One thing they all talked a lot about was communication. One Deaf mom said: "My hearing children would talk with their friends and talk on the phone and talk all the time. And I don't know what they were talking about. They would leave us out. I would say, What did you say? They would say, Oh, nothing. How do you control that? I would say, Come on, I want to know what you're talking about. And they would say, Nothing!"

But, communication issues were not present only if there were hearing teens. For example, one Deaf dad with two deaf teens said: "My biggest challenge with two deaf teens? They complain that I know too much about them. Because I have a lot of networking with deaf parents and teachers and all that kind of thing. So, I know what is going on in their lives, and they don't like that. I think they don't like that I can understand everything they're talking about because we all sign."

Another issue? Feeling stigmatized. Feeling different from others. Sometimes hearing people criticized or had negative ideas about Deaf people. One teen talked about how her family felt different than other hearing families. "I'm always being teased a lot. Some kids make fun of how my Mom and Dad talk. I just get embarrassed about it. Sometimes my friends are being nice and they want to ask me a million questions about sign language and deafness and all that. But sometimes I just don't want to deal with being so different."

A Deaf mom gave her perspectives on this: "My daughter and I go out in public and we don't sign. I talk to her. Maybe because my voice is different, she'll say, Be quiet, don't talk! I remember when I was at the school, I didn't want my mother to fingerspell to me. Mom, put your hand down, I don't want people staring at me."

Another Deaf mom described similar feelings: "Sometimes, my daughter will be walking and I'll be talking. And she can hear negative comments from people around me. My gosh, look at that! There's a deaf person!"

What else did teens talk about? Especially the hearing teens? I think it might be something that you would expect: interpreting. So, what did teens say about interpreting? You might think they complained a lot. Well, yes, some did complain, but many teens said they really enjoyed interpreting; many loved to interpret. Sometimes they were a little mischievous and did not always interpret exactly what was going on. A few teens I interviewed were angry about having to interpret too much. Some said they felt too much responsibility, but there seems to be some differences of opinion about this. Many of the deaf parents I talked with said their teens often think they are more responsible for things than they really are. This kind of thing is also showing up among other families in our study: the teens of disabled parents say they do more chores around the house than the parents say they do. This is even true among nondisabled families: teens say they do more chores around the house than their parents say they do.

Several deaf parents discussed how current technology and more available resources affect their families and their children. Teens often said they felt that technology gave them greater flexibility and more options about how much they needed to help their parents out. Most deaf parents felt that newer technologies had made communication much easier but that there were still significant problems, for example, poor captioning, equipment that does not always work or work as well as it is described. Some noted that not all deaf people had or used all these technologies, so they could not contact all their deaf friends. Almost every deaf parent said they still preferred face-to-face interaction. Many also said that although they were less dependent on their children to interpret or assist in some situations, there were still many occasions when the equipment would not work, was not available, was too expensive, or was not as good as promised. Regarding using outside interpreters, almost all these parents agreed there were times when they would not want to use an outside interpreter because of privacy issues or funding issues: who is going to pay for it?

This underscores one area of need that was identified by a broad range of deaf parents with hearing children. Deaf parents with hearing teens repeatedly described how they are excluded from active participation in their hearing child's education. Deaf parents reported that their hearing child's school system almost never provides interpreters for routine parent-teacher meetings or other school functions. School administrators remain uncertain of their legal obligations to provide communication access to deaf parents.

A deaf mom felt that the lack of available interpreters often interfered with her ability to be part of her children's lives: "I feel that for me, probably the toughest thing for me was to get through to the school to get to talk to the teacher or to be part of my children's school life. Really, I have to admit that it came to the point where I gave up. I would show up to my kid's activities but I was not a part of the school. I never felt welcomed. The barriers were too great there."

Additionally, teachers of hearing children of deaf parents often have misconceptions about deaf parents and their hearing children. For example, some teachers presume all young codas need speech therapy or special education classes. The rich cultural and linguistic heritage of hearing children of deaf parents is often unrecognized and underappreciated. Sometimes deaf parents ended up being cultural brokers for their children, as this one mom explained: "When my son was growing up, when I had to go to school, I would try to explain to the teachers that my son comes from a deaf family and we sign. My son signs and he is very animated with his face. A lot of people think he's aping them or doesn't agree with the teacher. The teachers write him up and make him go to detention. That's part of our culture. And they say, What's your culture? Many times the teachers just don't understand. He's from a deaf family and they just nod at me. It's really tough."

Policies underlying services and programs for deaf parents and their children rarely consider how deaf-parented families function positively—without intervention. Nor do such policies take into account that Deaf-parented families are often scrutinized according to cultural standards no more appropriate than if applied to other ethnic or racial minorities. Such biases can have devastating effects on whether some families remain intact. As one dad explained: "What do deaf parents need the most? How to be assertive, I think. We actually have to make the inroads and we have to be the ones to be part of our child's hearing world. We have to get more involved. And it's not easy."

Our national resource center at Through the Looking Glass has found a critical need for education of the family courts and of medical and social service professionals working with families in which one or both parents are Deaf. The lack of Deaf awareness and Deaf-appropriate services throughout these systems—whether using children as interpreters in custody hearings or excluding deaf parents from active participation in their hearing children's education—jeopardizes positive outcomes for many of these families.

I am looking forward to completing our interviews, analyzing the data and sharing our results.

Deaf Parents with Hearing Children: A CODA Symposium

THOMAS H. BULL, ELIZABETH BELDON, AND BERT PICKELL

CODA Identity and Deaf Parental Empowerment

In the United States in the 1960s and 1970s, we were called HCDPs, hearing children with deaf parents. In 1983, Millie Brother of Santa Barbara, California, distributed the first newsletter of the new organization CODA International (Children of Deaf Adults). Our annual international conferences began in 1986 and have drawn participants from seventeen countries. Our largest conference so far was in 1998 with 285 attendees from seven countries.

The first CODA conference held outside of the United States was in 1999 in Brisbane, Australia, after the World Federation of the Deaf (WFD) Congress there. CODA conferences were held in tandem with Deaf Way I and II and will be held around the time of the WFD Congresses in Toronto (2003) and Spain (2007). There is a growing international interest about CODAs.

At the 1999 WFD Congress in Australia, there was an emphasis on family in the program. It was good to see that four of the six speakers were codas, who discussed our experiences and concerns. At that time, Millie Brother was on a panel and said, "We are the children of the [Deaf World] and you can't separate us" from you. In the same spirit, this year at Deaf Way II, we are presenting on this topic as a part of the "family" strand.

In the United States, 90–95 percent of deaf children are born to hearing parents. A great deal has been written about how to bridge the language, educational, and cultural differences that become apparent in this hearing-parent-with-deaf-child family. Also in the United States, 90–95 percent of the children born to Deaf parents have normal hearing. Within the Deaf community, little attention has been paid to the special challenges present in this bilingual and bicultural family system.

KODA is an organization begun in 1991 in Rockville, Maryland. A group of deaf parents with hearing children wanted to meet to learn from each other, and they also wanted their hearing young children to have opportunities for activities with other children like them. There are now groups providing activities for KODA children and their parents in Australia, Canada, Finland, Sweden, and various states in the United States.

The experience of being deaf is a unique one that unites more than ten thousand deaf people from 108 countries here at Deaf Way II. Deaf people are people of the eye and use the language of the hands. In the same way, when we hearing codas get together, even though our countries, socioeconomic status, histories, languages, life experiences, and cultures are different, we all share a very unique experience of being hearing in the Deaf world. We feel very close to each other because we spend half our lives explaining deaf people to hearing people and the other half of our lives explaining hearing people to the Deaf community.

Deaf people have struggled for their social identity and personal freedom against such demeaning terms and stigma perpetuated by such terms as "deaf mute," "deaf and dumb," and "hearing impaired." Today, in the Deaf world, there is pride in saying I am Deaf or hard of hearing.

Many of us hearing codas, raised in Deaf culture, also struggle with our Deaf and hearing identities. We grow up feeling different. We are children of the people of the eye. We are your children who use the language of the hands, but we can also hear. As a result, we can feel confused, different, and alone growing up hearing in the Deaf world. Often we grow up extremely aware of our difference in society and of our difference within our own families. I was a bilingual and bicultural person who needed eye contact. I had internalized Deaf cultural values, but growing up, I had little understanding of what this meant.

This identity conflict has been described in the following ways: "I'm caught in between deaf and hearing." "I'm neither one nor the other." "I felt like I visited two homes but had no place for myself." We are hearing but with "mother father deaf."

Just as deaf people find their identity and are empowered in so many ways here at DW II and other gatherings, I found my identity as hearing *and* deaf at a gathering. It was a CODA conference. When I attended my first CODA conference, I was forty-two years old. That is when I finally found my home, my people, those who were like me. I was changed forever! I became one person: hearing and deaf and CODA. That is my identity: a bilingual and bicultural person.

A dream of mine is that Deaf parents rearing hearing children will share their experiences with the next generation of Deaf parents, but in the past, Deaf parents have not done that. For example, in the United States, there are *no books* written by Deaf parents about parenting hearing children. There are at least twenty books written by hearing parents who have Deaf children.

In the past thirty years in England and America, to my knowledge there are only nine articles written by Deaf parents for a total of about twenty-five pages. In contrast, there are hundreds of articles written by hearing parents who have raised deaf and hard of hearing children, where they share with other hearing parents the benefit of their experiences, be they negative or positive. Also, since 1980, only a handful of children's stories written for KODA children have Deaf or hard of hearing parents in them. Of the eighty-one doctoral and master's studies listed in *On the Edge of Deaf Culture*, only one is a study by a Deaf parent who has hearing children (Mary Weiner).

All parents, whether Deaf, hard of hearing, or hearing, need help as parents. Of the three programs available for Deaf parents with hearing children, all are thirteen to eighteen years old and have not been revised.

In the United States in 1988, the world saw deaf students protest the selection of a hearing woman as president of Gallaudet University, which became the historic Deaf President Now revolution. In my opinion, we need another DPN, this time a Deaf Parents Now movement whereby seasoned Deaf parents (who have hearing children) and who are empowered can share their experiences through writing, film and video, workshops (as Elizabeth Beldon has given), research (as Tammy Weiner has conducted), and other ways. In that way, the benefit of their expertise will be passed along to the next generation of Deaf parents.

Let me share an e-mail received from a Deaf mother who describes an incident with her hearing KODA daughter about her identity:

> A few weeks ago, my daughter and I were having a conversation. I had just found out that I was pregnant. My daughter was asking me why it happened and all sorts of 5-year-old questions. I am not a religious person, but I thought talking about God would help her put things in perspective. I said 'You know, I'm deaf and God chose for me to be deaf . . . same thing with your daddy.' Then I said: 'God chose for you to be hearing and your brother to be hearing.' She said: 'No, I am not hearing. . . . I am hearing and deaf!' Stunned, I asked her who told her this. She said: 'God told me.' She said this with a little sweet smile.

This mother goes on to say: "It was the most beautiful thing that happened. It really said something to me about her identity . . . that she has been exploring it herself and this is obviously how she feels. I think it's wonderful."

I also think it is wonderful, but as an empowered and enlightened Deaf mother today, my hope is that she will now say, "Yes, you are deaf and hearing *and* a KODA."

Through the Eyes of an American Deaf Mother with Hearing Children

Elizabeth Beldon

Each passing generation has a distinct culture that invariably helps to determine the parenting styles of its adults. This statement is just as true for Deaf parents.

I am Deaf and was born to Deaf parents. Because deafness is a hereditary trait in my family, I have a long line of Deaf relatives. One could also label my family as hillbillies, a stereotype I have accepted. I am a proud mother of one Deaf son and two hearing daughters. I also have nine grandchildren (four Deaf and five hearing) so you can see why, as a grandmother, I continue to be actively involved in my grandchildren's lives.

Unlike the typical twentieth-century family dynamic of hearing parents responding to their deaf children with an overriding paternalist coddling, leaving the children with a sense of inferiority, my hearing relatives often possessed so little that they did not exhibit an attitude of superiority over their Deaf relatives. In fact, many of my relatives, like my grandmother, were disadvantaged, lacking an education and other basic life skills. In contrast, it was the Deaf family members who were the advantaged, having received an education from state-funded institutions. They often found themselves educating the hearing family members. This unusual environment enabled me to possess a confidence and a general awareness about life unlike that of my Deaf peers raised by hearing parents.

My interest in the relational dynamics of Deaf parents and their hearing children was spawned during my graduate studies in family counseling. Between the years

1984–2001, I began a period of interviewing and public speaking that elicited an extensive collection of empirical and anecdotal information. My greatest fear is that this rich historical experience shared by my generation and the generations before will be lost to a new generation. Today's generation of hearing children of Deaf parents is living a different life. This collective experience is our culture's history and must be preserved.

Many historical milestones have led to this disparate experience between my generation and the current one:

1. The validation of ASL as a true language and the subsequent public interest in teaching ASL to hearing people.
2. The recognition of our culture and increased respect for its members.
3. The advantages gained by the exponential advancement of technology that surpass those of my day.

As part of my research into this diachronic study of Deaf parents and their hearing children, I conducted two surveys. The first survey was given to a group of Deaf adults who reared hearing children between the 1950s and 1980s. The focus question was "What are your greatest concerns in raising hearing children?" The top six concerns were the following (ranked):

1. Selecting the child's name and knowing the correct pronunciation.
2. Knowing when the infant was crying.
3. Assessing the appropriateness of TV programs, music, or other auditory media for content as well as sound level.
4. Exposing the child to English or sign language.
5. Using the telephone as an effective means of communication.
6. Getting the hearing child's attention for dinner, bedtime, and so forth.

These concerns forced Deaf parents to systematize behaviors that hearing parents do without much thought.

The second survey posed the same question but shifted the time frame from the 1980s to the present. Not surprisingly, the concerns about the children's names and getting the child's attention for dinner remained the same.

However, there were other concerns not found in the first survey. One of these is the role of a hearing child within a changing Deaf community. One example of such a change is the role of the Deaf club. The Deaf club used to be one of the primary social outlets and vehicles for acculturation for Deaf people as well as their hearing children. Prior to the 1980s, hearing children were so involved with the Deaf community that during their early years they were often oblivious to the fact that they were different than Deaf people: they could hear.

Today's Deaf community has less dependence on congregating at the clubs for interaction and information sharing. Because of technological advances in communications such as e-mail, fax, and even video phones, Deaf people are getting their social needs met in a variety of ways. Therefore, parents are more likely to direct their energies toward meeting the hearing child's social needs rather than their own. Thus, hearing children's lives become aligned with mainstream society earlier.

Another concern that appeared in the second survey but not in the first was the successful transmission of Deaf culture to hearing children of Deaf parents. Prior to the 1980s, acculturation was a natural consequence of being a hearing child, but as more Deaf adults tiptoe about mainstream society, their hearing children are encouraged more toward a blended or perhaps even a completely mainstream experience. The issue is redefining a hearing child's cultural identity. Is the child bilingual, bicultural, or both? If the child's maturation is primarily within the mainstream experience, can he or she claim any affiliation to the Deaf community?

Now I want to touch on another interesting aspect of this discussion. During my public speaking, information I shared brought about new insights for many Deaf parents. One idea that came up was the misunderstanding brought on by a hearing child's search for identity and his or her response to the parents' deafness. For example, during puberty a child may not want his parents to sign in public when the child is present. The parents might believe this means he or she is embarrassed by them when in fact this behavior is a normal reflection of a child's developmental stages.

Another insight for Deaf parents was the physiological changes experienced by boys as they mature, in particular, the change in voice during puberty. Many parents were shocked to realize boys' voices changed, and some were saddened by the fact that they missed this developmental milestone.

Again, another insight was about the language parents taught their hearing children. During the 1950s–80s, Total Communication was popular. Deaf parents felt because their children were hearing they should use an English-based signing system with them. My question was whether this was the right decision. Did their child miss out on acquiring a rich sign language, American Sign Language? At the time parents did not realize that they could teach their hearing children ASL *and* English. They did not realize their children could be part of both the Deaf and the hearing communities at the same time.

In sum, the generation of Deaf parents raising hearing children prior to the twenty-first century had a unique life. Our lives required the use of ingenuity unheard of today. What a shame it would be to lose this history! To date, no one has preserved these aspects of the lives of hearing children of Deaf parents. Just as George Veditz's *The Preservation of the Sign Language* has given us a glimpse into an earlier time, we need to encourage an international effort to archive this fascinating part of our history so that future generations can be inspired to chronicle their stories as well.

Deaf Parents, Hearing Children: What We Have Learned from KODA Camp

Bert Pickell

It has been my good fortune to be the director of a KODA Camp program for the past four years at Camp Mark 7 in Old Forge, New York. We have developed a program to work with KODA kids ages nine to sixteen there. The program's main objective is to provide an opportunity for KODA kids to gain an understanding of their identity as bicultural individuals and to further explore this individually. We have had an overwhelming response to this program, and more than 85 percent of our attendees return for the next summer. Clearly this means there is a need for this type of program from the perspective of the kids as well as the parents. KODA kids benefit from this experience because the opportunities to understand and to see themselves reflected in other people who have a similar background are so rare. The fact is that most of the world does not recognize them as bicultural.

We attempt to accomplish our goals through three types of activities that assist the kids in starting to understand themselves better. First, we recognize that American Sign Language (ASL) is the language of the Deaf community in America. Few have had the opportunity to study and truly understand their native language. Most study English in school and their sign language becomes very English based. We provide a workshop on and activities that allow them to explore some of this. Ultimately there is a talent show where the campers can perform for their parents in sign language, and we work with them to improve their ASL skills. We do respect parents' choices in what language system they use with their kids. Many kids do not sign very well or even at all. Still, it is important to expose them to the language so they can make choices as to how much they want to be able to communicate with other deaf people.

The second way we support their growth in understanding themselves is by having a workshop on Deaf culture and hearing culture. Again, it is important to remember that only people involved with the Deaf community even talk about "hearing culture." Few parents are really knowledgeable enough to discuss the differences between the two cultures and help their kids figure out how to navigate through both of them. This is not unique to Deaf people; people of all cultures would find it difficult to explain their own culture and compare it to others. The kids are given an opportunity to talk about this and to put it into words to explain it better. This is a big part of the KODA experience because they are often the mediators between these two cultures.

The third activity is to have a chance to share our KODA stories. It is so nice to have a place where we can share the experiences of growing up without having to spend time explaining everything to other people. Other KODAs just understand. This helps them to see that their experiences are not so limited; many others share them.

The kids then spend time getting to know each other and share more experiences with each other. This builds their concept of a group identity. They now feel as though they belong to a bigger group and do not feel so alone. Many KODAs share a feeling of isolation or not fitting in, and the camp experience helps them to not feel that way. Many of the kids refer to camp as their second home or the one place that they feel like they fit in with everyone else. Some people feel that things that may have been issues for KODAs in the past are no longer relevant and so things should be easier. For example, there are televisions with captions now, and kids do not stand next to the television and interpret anymore. Telephone relay services are available now so kids do not have to make as many phone calls.

The kids today have shown me that much of their experience is the same today as it has been in the past. This is important in understanding the true nature of the KODA experience. It comes down to this idea: KODAs are bicultural individuals who are not recognized as such by the rest of the world. They have little opportunity to understand themselves in order to develop a healthy sense of identity. I am blessed to have had the opportunity to continue my own growth and understanding of myself through running this camp program and sharing that growth and understanding with the kids and the families who attend.

References (Beldon)

American Academy of Pediatrics. (2002). *Puberty: Information for boys and girls.* Retrieved June 2002 from http://www.aap.org/family/puberty.htm.

Beldon, Elizabeth. (1984–2001). The hidden treasures of Deaf parents raising hearing children and A behind the scenes look at Deaf parenting of hearing children, six workshops.

Walker, Lou Ann. (1987). *A loss for words.* New York: Harper Collins.

Veditz, George W. (1913). *The preservation of the sign language.* Washington, D.C.: National Association of the Deaf.

References (Bull)

Bull, T. H. (Ed.). (1998). *On the edge of Deaf culture: Hearing children/Deaf parents annotated bibliography.* Alexandria, VA: Deaf Family Research Press.

Filer, R. D., & Filer, P. A. (2000, Winter). Practical considerations for counselors working with hearing children of deaf parents. *Journal of Counseling and Development, 78* (1), 38–43.

Paris, V. (2001, Spring). Wall of sound: Silence, music, and raising an abled child. *Brain child: The magazine for thinking mothers, 2* (2), 12–13.

Preston, P. M. (1994). *Mother father Deaf: Living between sound and silence.* Cambridge, MA: Harvard University Press.

Prickett, D. (2000, Fall). The CODA connection: Do your parents know Braille? *Gallaudet Today, 31* (1), 26–35.

Sanford, R. (2000, December). Kids of deaf adults (KODA): Are you the Deaf parent/parents of a hearing child/children? Read on! *Vibes, 27* (4), 24.

Shultz-Myers, S., Myers, R. R., & Marcus, A. L. (1999). Hearing children of Deaf parents: Issues and interventions within a bicultural context. In I. W. Leigh (Ed.), *Psychotherapy with Deaf clients from diverse groups* (pp. 121–148). Washington, DC: Gallaudet University Press.

Singleton, J. (2002, Summer). Hearing children of deaf parents bridging two languages and two cultures. *CSD Spectrum, 2* (2), 26–28. Retrieved from http://www.c-s-d.org/pdfs/spectrum/2002_Summer.pdf.

Singleton, J. L., & Tittle, M. D. (2000, Summer). Deaf parents and their hearing children. *Journal of Deaf Studies and Deaf Education, 5* (3), 221–236.

Weiner, M. T. (1997, December). Raising bicultural and bilingual children: Deaf parents' perceptions. *Dissertation Abstracts International.*

Parent Education Program

Neubacher, M. (1987). *Pathways for parenting, parents guide: Our baby is hearing.* Detroit, MI: Lutheran Social Services of Michigan.

Neubacher, M. (1987). *Pathways for parenting, parents guide: Our child—two worlds.* Detroit, MI: Lutheran Social Services of Michigan.

Neubacher, M. (1987). *Pathways for parenting, parents guide: Adolescence to grown-up.* Detroit, MI: Lutheran Social Services of Michigan.

Parenting: Bringing two worlds together [VHS Videotapes]. (1992). Fairfax, VA: Northern Virginia Resource Center for Deaf and Hard of Hearing Persons.

Parenting skills: Bringing together two worlds, one home, two cultures. (1992). Fairfax, VA: Northern Virginia Resource Center for Deaf and Hard of Hearing Persons.

Pathways for parenting video: A video program for deaf parents with hearing children [Videotapes]. (1987). Detroit, MI: Lutheran Social Services of Michigan, Family Counseling and Education.

Tebelman, L. (1989a). *Pathways for parenting video: Facilitator's guide.* Detroit, MI: Lutheran Social Services of Michigan.

Tebelman, L. (1989b). *Pathways for parenting video: Parent's guide.* Detroit, MI: Lutheran Social Services of Michigan, Detroit.

CODA Autobiographies

Abrams, C. (1996). *The silents*. Washington, DC: Gallaudet University Press.
Allan, J. (2002). *Because I love you: The silent shadow of child sexual abuse*. Charlottesville, VA: Virginia Foundation for the Humanities Press.
Barash, H. L., & Barash-Dicker, E. (1991). *Our father Abe: The story of a Deaf shoe repairman*. Madison, WI: Abar Press.
Blake, M. F. (1993). *Lon Chaney: The man behind the thousand faces*. Lanham, MD: Vestal Press.
Chism, S.C. (2002). *A search for identity: The unfolding of an unknown past*. Philadelphia: Xlibris Corporation.
Clark, G. (2000). *Sounds from silence: Graeme Clark and the bionic ear story*. St. Leonards, Australia: Allen & Unwin.
Corfmat, P. (1990). *"Please sign here": The world of the Deaf*. Worthing, U.K.: Churchman Publishing.
Crowe, D. I. (1993). *Dummy's little girl*. New York: Carlton Press.
Davis, L. J. (2000). *My sense of silence: Memoirs of a childhood with deafness*. Urbana: University of Illinois Press.
Miller-Hall, M. (1994). *Deaf, dumb and black: An account of an actual life of a family*. New York: Carlton Press.
Perez, J. E. (1985). *A sign of love*. Glenn, CA: Janet Enos Perez.
Sidransky, R. (1990). *In silence: Growing up hearing in a Deaf world*. New York: St. Martin's Press.
Slocombe, A. (1996). *My parents' voice*. Surrey, U.K.: A. Slocombe.
Vivo, P. (1991/1996). *Turn right at the next corner*. Granville, OH: Trudy Knox.
Walker, L. A. (1986). *A loss for words*. New York: Harper and Row.
Worzel-Miller, L. (2000). *The best of both worlds (a-not-so-silent life)*. San Jose, CA: Writers Club Press.

CODA Fiction

Glickfeld, C. L. (1989). *Useful gifts*. Athens: University of Georgia Press.
Greenberg, J. (1970). *In this sign*. New York: Holt, Rinehart and Winston.
Jeffers, A. (1995/1998). *Safe as houses*. London: Gay Men's Press.

CODA Videotapes

Davie, Cameron. (1992). *Passport without a country* [VHS videotape]. Queensland, Australia: Centre for Deafness Study and Research, Griffith University.
Kraft, Bonnie. (1997). *Tomorrow Dad will still be deaf and other stories* [VHS videotape]. San Diego, CA: DawnSignPress.

World Wide Web Resources

Camp Mark Seven in New York. http://www.campmark7.org
CODA—Children of Deaf Adults International. P.O. Box 30715, Santa Barbara, CA 93130-0715. http://www.coda-international.org/
KODA—Kids of Deaf Adults. http://www.mmkoda.org/ and http://www.kodainfo.com/index.htm

Mailing lists:

- deafparenting-subscribe@yahoogroups.com
- Mother_Father_Deaf-subscribe@yahoogroups.com (or contact Art Smith at Smith_ASLI@comcast.net)

PART FIVE

Health and Mental Health

Mental Health and Deafness Go Global

BARBARA BRAUER

The United States is the first country in the world to make mental health services available to its deaf population. Most deafness professionals would agree that the New York State Psychiatric Institute in New York City, with its Mental Health Project for the Deaf, was the very first provider of mental health services to deaf people during the late 1950s. This program was also the first one to do research on deaf patients. It provided training for psychiatric students. It was the first to publish its research findings. All of that pioneering work was made possible by a grant from the U.S. Rehabilitation Services Administration. From my two years of experience as an assistant research scientist with this program, I can tell you that the professionals in this New York program were first-class researchers and first-class mental health professionals. Unfortunately, they knew and understood very little or nothing about deafness, deaf people, deaf culture, or sign language. As a result, the deaf residents of New York City underutilized this program. The so-called experts of that program had a lot to learn. Nonetheless, the important point to make here is that, even if they knew very little or nothing, they were willing and interested enough to learn and to participate in something that would make history and something that would get things started.

After New York, other programs providing mental health services to deaf individuals were established across the country. Most notable were the ones in Washington, D.C. (Saint Elizabeth's Hospital), Chicago (Michael Reese Hospital), Minneapolis (St. Paul-Ramsey Hospital), and San Francisco (University of California Center on Deafness). As with the New York project, most of the administrators of these other programs were also first-class hearing mental health professionals who, however, also knew and understood very little or nothing about the deaf people they served. The deaf residents of these different cities also underutilized these programs. It took quite some time before those professionals began to learn more about deafness and deaf people. However, they continued to view deafness from the medical model, to view deafness as a pathological condition, and to view deaf people in negative ways. They believed that deaf people, because of their deafness, were more vulnerable or predisposed to emotional disturbances and mental illness. It was not until the numbers of mental health professionals who are deaf themselves grew that the field became more educated about deafness, deaf people, and so forth.

During the late 1980s in Europe, mental health professionals from several countries organized themselves to establish the European Society on Mental Health and Deafness (ESMHD). Countries involved with that organization included France, Germany, England, Spain, Italy, Holland, Belgium, Austria, Denmark, Sweden, Norway. and Finland. That such an organization could be possible with members who spoke different languages, had different cultures, and yet were able to come together and share their knowledge with each other made a big impression on me. The first ESMHD Congress took place in 1988 in Rotterdam, Holland. Congresses met every three years, and venues have included Namur, Belgium; Paris, France; Manchester, England; and Copenhagen, Denmark. The Sixth Congress will take place next year in Austria.

I had the good fortune to be able to attend the Paris and Manchester Congresses, where I became acquainted with several ESMHD officials and inquired about their possible interest in a world conference. They expressed much interest, and the First World Conference on Mental Health and Deafness took place in 1998 at Gallaudet University. It was a huge success with participants representing many different countries throughout the world. The Second World Conference took place in 2000 in Copenhagen. That happened simultaneously with the Fifth ESMHD Congress. I had the pleasure of co-chairing that with Lars von der Lieth, professor at the University of Copenhagen. That was also a huge success. At this time, no decision has been made as to how frequently we should have a world conference. During the international advisory meeting in Copenhagen, two things had happened.

The first was that two psychiatrists from South Africa made their bid for the nomination of South Africa as a proposed venue for the next world conference. They reported that considerable support has developed in South Africa for hosting the Third World Conference on Mental Health and Deafness. This will take place in the year 2005 in Cape Town. Obviously, these world conferences are meeting a worldwide need.

The second important thing that took place was a request made by officials at this international advisory meeting for someone to develop a mental health and Deafness international Web site. Links from the Web sites of other mental health service, training, and research programs can be placed on this international Web site to allow any of us to keep track of what is happening in our field worldwide. The address for this Web site is http://mhdeafintl.gallaudet.edu/directory.html.

Yes, the United States took the lead in establishing the first programs of mental health service delivery to deaf individuals, the first research in this area, and the first training programs at Gallaudet University in counseling, psychology, and social work. However, European member nations of ESMHD took the lead in getting themselves organized for the international cooperation and sharing of knowledge, findings, and insights with each other. My opinion is that we in the United States need to do better than what we are doing now within the American Deafness and Rehabilitation Association (ADARA)—we need to work something out with ADARA to give our field more legitimacy and recognition within the Americas as well as throughout the world. Moreover, we need to emphasize the wellness model. We need to depathologize deafness. We need to destigmatize psychological disorders and mental illnesses.

In conclusion, here are some random thoughts based on my thirty-six years in the field. You may or may not agree with me. These are just my thoughts from the perspective of a deaf female clinical psychologist.

1. There are hearing mental health professionals who say that they have deaf spouses, as if marrying a deaf person qualifies them as Deafness professionals. Nothing could be further from the truth! To be qualified, more emphasis has to be placed on training.
2. A psychiatrist from Norway coined the word *surdophrenia* to describe deaf people as having a mentality different from the hearing and who, among other things, function badly socially. The reason I bring this up is to alert you to this diagnosis. That is, when you come across this so-called diagnosis in psychiatric or psychological assessment reports, this must become a red flag to you that the psychiatrist or psychologist simply was not fluent or intuitive enough for communication with the deaf patient, inmate, or client. During my long tenure in this field, I have never come across a deaf patient, inmate, or client who could not communicate something. There is a deaf female mental health professional from the Netherlands who would agree with me—she coined the word *surdophobia* to describe hearing professionals who have a phobia or aversion to working with deaf individuals.
3. This is a random thought that is not particularly germane to mental health and Deafness, but this is a point about which I feel strongly should be mentioned. There are interpreters who will "voice" for deaf mental health professionals, even if and when these deaf professionals are speaking for themselves. This is rude and unprofessional and must be stopped. Arrangements about this issue must be made with the deaf speaker beforehand.
4. Fortunately, there are increasing numbers of mental health professionals who are deaf, many more in the field now than previously. However, there remains very little solidarity and too much backstabbing among themselves. Competition for clients, for recognition, for grants, and for awards is fine, but the behaviors need to become more professional.
5. Recent articles published about the history of mental health and deafness often mention hearing mental health professionals as pioneers in the field but seldom mention deaf pioneers. These hearing pioneers may have started programs of service, training, and research, but the deaf pioneers had to teach them about deafness, deaf people, deaf culture, and deaf sign language. The truth is that mental health services began to improve with the advent of deaf mental health professionals. As mentioned earlier, a happy development is that there are more deaf mental health professionals in countries all over the world today. Mental health services have improved considerably because more deaf mental health professionals are training both deaf and hearing students who will be future mental health professionals serving deaf individuals. This training is now taking place in colleges and universities worldwide, at conferences and workshops, in continuing education and training institutes, and so forth. The past fifty years saw amazing increases in opportunities for graduate and professional training for people who are deaf. This has been of benefit to people who are hearing and wish to work with deaf individuals. Yet, in spite of this progress, we still have a long way to go.

Next year, on May 5, 2003, in Bad Ischl, Austria, we shall have the next ESMHD Congress. It will be held in the northern region of Austria.

Mental Health Services in the Philippines: A Deaf Perspective

MARIA TANYA L. DE GUZMAN

My beloved country, the Philippines, is a third world or developing country in Asia. It has approximately 7,107 islands. There are three major islands: Luzon, Visaya, and Mindanao. It is the third-largest English-speaking country in the world. It has a rich history that combines Asian, European, and American influences. The population is 78.4 million, with more than one hundred thousand Deaf and hard of hearing people. (See map.)

History of Counseling for Deaf People in the Philippines

In 1907, the first Insular School for the Deaf and Blind, presently known as the Philippine School for the Deaf, was created in Manila. The Philippine Association of the Deaf (PAD) opened its own school, the second oldest in the Philippines. Both schools currently have guidance counselors for the Deaf pupils.

In 1975, PAD, a private school, had a hearing guidance counselor, who assisted and responded to the students' needs and who also provided facts and resources on deafness.

This made me curious: are there any research studies on mental health issues that apply to Deaf Filipino culture?

Presently, there are very few services in the Manila area or elsewhere in the Philippines. Fortunately, there are two places that have ample counseling services for the Deaf population, including mental health counseling. First, the Catholic Ministry to Deaf People, Inc. (CMDP), a nonprofit organization, provides personal safety classes, which provide individual and family counseling and therapy for Deaf survivors from sexual abuse. Second, De La Salle-College of Saint Benilde's (DLS-CSB's) Counseling Resource Unit for Deaf Esteem and Formation, under the School of Deaf Education and Applied Studies, offers guidance and individual and group counseling services to Deaf students including guidance workshops, seminars, and other activities that focus on their esteem, self-awareness, and identity.

There is a classic case of an unschooled Deaf woman who worked as a house helper. Her employer's husband was stabbed to death, and she was accused of this

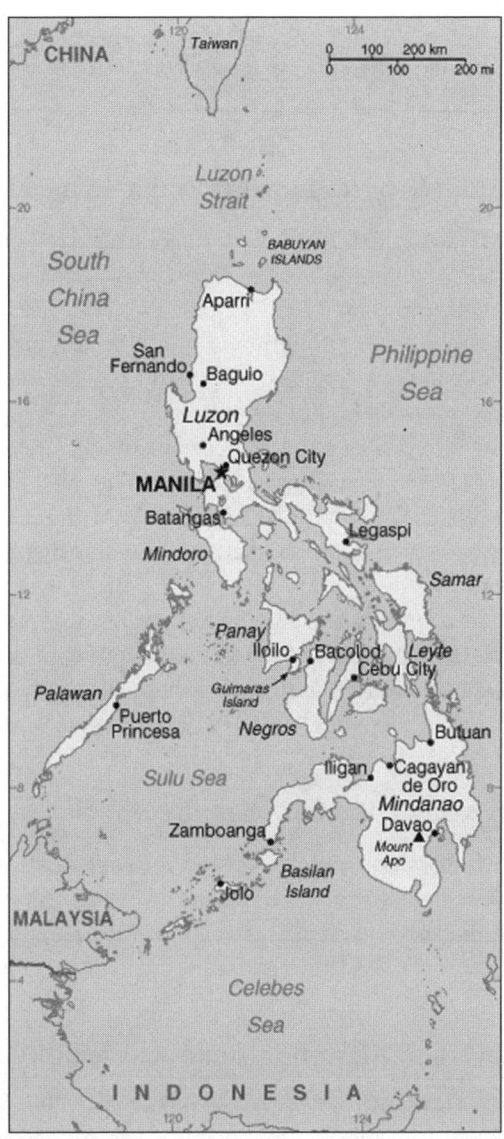

crime. The court was not able to understand the Deaf woman because of her gestures and nonstandard signs. Even her lawyer tried to communicate with her but failed to get the full details, and so the court ordered a Deaf person with communication skills to be the intermediary. Eventually, a Deaf man was found. He tried to communicate with the Deaf woman by using gestures and sketching on paper to get details of the incident. He was able to get through to her, and she began to express in her own words how she had been a victim for a long time from sexual harassment, abuse, and rape by her employer's husband. She was able to communicate on paper through the patient help of the Deaf man. In the end, the Deaf woman won the case. However, the court did not know how to help the Deaf woman and where to refer her for mental health services. This illustrates the lack of accessibility to mental health services for the Deaf.

Lack of Mental Health Services for Deaf People in the Philippines

The Philippine Mental Health Association is a major organization in Manila that provides crisis intervention and counseling for acute mental health situations, as well as other related services. Unfortunately, it has no services for Deaf people because the association does not know how to communicate in sign language. Another problem is that Deaf people have the responsibility to get and pay for interpreters, and this is a very difficult situation for Deaf Filipinos.

The Deaf minority is in dire need of intensive mental health services to overcome the weakening effects of their own internal problems, as well as external pressures. The mental health needs of the Filipino Deaf people remain unaddressed because of the existing language barrier. In addition, there are very few mental health professionals available to provide this service.

However, I have a vision that one day the Philippines will establish the first mental health organization, unit, or agency for deaf people and the rest of CMDP and DLS-CSB will offer a well-structured and comprehensive guidance and counseling program. This will support the overall needs of Deaf people in the Philippines.

Lack of Full Resources for Mental Health Issues

The reality is that Deaf Filipinos are way behind in terms of knowledge about mental health issues because they do not have enough resources, data, or research on Deaf mental health issues. We also need to determine how hearing and Deaf Filipino counselors can be trained to work with Deaf clients.

Lack of Strong Advocacy, Networking, and Accessibility

There is clearly a lack of advocacy, networking, and accessibility in the Philippines for Deaf needs. Very few organizations for Deaf people in Manila have taken responsibility for developing these services. For instance, the Philippine Federation of the Deaf (PFD) does advocacy work to the hearing society on Deaf awareness. The PFD disseminates information on Deaf culture and Filipino Sign Language. It is important for the hearing public to know the needs of the Deaf so that they may be able to assist and respond to the Deaf community's needs. Guidance counselors should know that language use is important for Deaf people, because it plays a crucial role in the counseling process. It serves as a therapeutic intervention and a tool in transmitting knowledge, beliefs, and traditions. It is also closely linked to the history and culture of the individual.

Lack of Awareness about Deaf Culture and Linguistics

Our present problems are accentuated because of the communication differences between Deaf and hearing worlds. There is a big need for recognition about the effective use of sign language and communication, coupled with increased awareness of aspects of deafness. The PFD and the Philippine Deaf Resource Center worked hard to identify the true natural sign language and culture of Deaf Filipinos.

Common Attitudes of Hearing People toward Deaf People, which Lead to Mental Health Problems

Deaf people suffer various emotions such as hurt, anger, depression, embarrassment, and frustration from their experiences with hearing people. This sometimes makes them suspicious of hearing people. Here are some commonly seen attitudes of hearing people toward Deaf people in the Philippines.

Discrimination

Most Deaf people do not have equal opportunity for hiring, promotion, compensation, and accommodation in employment. Access to quality education, vocational rehabilitation services, telecommunication systems, and mass media is lacking. The hearing society sometimes thinks that Deaf Filipinos do not have higher education, and they tend to think Deaf people cannot do everything that hearing people can do because of communication barriers. Hearing Filipinos themselves are not aware of Deaf Filipinos' abilities and the differences between the hearing and Deaf worlds.

Laughing at Deaf People

Here is an example of a true incident in Manila. Some young Deaf people rode in a jeepney (Philippine mini-bus), and they were conversing in sign language. Hearing passengers could not stop watching them and laughed at them because they thought that sign language looked very funny, like monkeys communicating to each other. Such behavior offends Deaf people and causes them to become suspicious when hearing people laugh. Sometimes, Deaf people become passive and refuse to sign in public places.

Disbelief

Hearing people sometimes do not believe that deaf people can do many things, such as writing and reading. Of course, some hard of hearing people can speak and use the telephone, which confuses hearing people who do not understand the Deaf world and hard of hearing culture. Some hearing people are shocked when they see the abilities of Deaf people.

Rudeness

Sometimes Deaf people receive rude looks from hearing people when they try to communicate with them. For instance, most hearing sales clerks become annoyed when the Deaf customers ask them to get pen and paper so that they can communicate. Other times, hearing sales clerks are impatient when communicating by writing with the Deaf customers.

Bad Words

Some hearing Filipinos say, "Pip! Pipi!" (in Tagalog, a Filipino native language: "Mute! Mute!") when they see Deaf people signing. Deaf people can guess what hearing people say because they notice the obvious oral speech of hearing people with their facial expression and laughing or showing disgust. This does not make Deaf people feel good at all.

No Support

Many Deaf people feel frustrated and disappointed when they receive no support or encouragement from their hearing families, schoolteachers, and so forth. Sometimes, hearing people pay little attention to Deaf people's needs. Hearing people have difficulty in communicating with Deaf people because of lack of patience and the attitude that Deaf people are not important. Communication barriers are very common.

Critical Need for Mental Health Professionals Trained to Work with Deaf People

There is obviously a great need for trained professionals to help Deaf people deal with these attitudes and oppression in the Philippines. Of course it would be ideal to have more Deaf professionals because Deaf professionals can identify with their clients. They share similar experiences and feelings about their deafness.

We have legislation, the Magna Carta for Disabled Persons enacted in the Philippines in 1992, which is similar to the Americans with Disabilities Act in that it mandates access for disabled people. However, it has not been implemented appropriately for Deaf people. This is the major reason I chose to become a mental health professional.

Becoming a Professional Counselor

When I was a religious and moral values teacher in Manila, many deaf students came to ask me for help solving their problems. Many Deaf students were victims of physical and sexual abuse, experienced communication barriers, struggled to accept their real identity, and had other issues. I discovered Deaf students suffered even more because they were not satisfied or comfortable with their hearing counselors because of communication problems, different views, or difficulty in getting an interpreter. This motivated me to become a professional counselor so I could provide services for those Deaf Filipinos who badly needed someone who could work with them. I began my master's studies in school counseling in the Philippines but later decided to transfer to Gallaudet University to study mental health counseling instead. I came to Gallaudet because I wanted to learn more about the needs of the Deaf community and to focus on how to apply counseling to Deaf people and our culture.

At Gallaudet, I am climbing a tough mountain to become an effective mental health counselor. I am learning many new things not offered in the Philippines and feel that my study for a master's degree is very challenging. Gallaudet is a wonderful school, and I find this to be like my home because I feel that I am part of the Deaf world here. I feel empowered and more competent. I do not want to be the only Deaf Filipino working in the field of mental health, but as far as I know, I am the only Deaf Filipino who has received this advanced training. Someday I plan to go to the Philippines to contribute the following services:

- guidance and counseling training for professionals and paraprofessionals;
- guidance workshops for Deaf individuals and their hearing families;
- workshops and seminars on prevention and education (e.g., depression, suicide, prevention of sex abuse, etc.); and
- counseling resources for deaf people.

In conclusion, there are three major needs in the Philippines that need to be resolved. First, we need more Deaf and hearing counselors who are proficient in Filipino Sign Language, who are knowledgeable about Deaf culture, and who have positive attitudes. Second, we need more research studies on the mental health status of Deaf people so that we can respond better to their needs. Third, we need to establish professional training programs for counselors. I hope to see these services and training programs develop by creating a partnership between the Deaf and hearing communities.

For instance, information sharing should be encouraged during and after Deaf Way II to ensure that deaf people are involved and consulted during the process of development. This is vital for the benefit of the Filipino Deaf community.

Cancer Awareness Project: Deaf Cancer Wise

CARLY MUNRO

Deaf Connections is a charity based in Glasgow, Scotland, that provides a diverse range of services for Deaf people living in the west of Scotland. "Deaf Cancer Wise," a cancer awareness project for Deaf people, is one of the projects run by Deaf Connections, and I discuss how the project began, its aims, and the progress made so far. This project has been running for a year now, with two years remaining. I also discuss a model that encourages Deaf people to change lifestyles.

The health care system in Scotland consists of fifteen health boards responsible for health services and patients in their region. Deaf Cancer Wise works with two health boards in the west of Scotland. Consultations between the boards and Deaf people indicated that health services had not met Deaf people's needs, caused by poor or no accessibility to health services and information. A selection of examples of such problems and barriers are as follows:

- ❖ At a General Practicioner surgery or hospital, Deaf people detest waiting for their name to be called, because they often find themselves constantly watching the receptionist in case they miss their name. In cases when the receptionist has been asked to notify the Deaf person directly, the Deaf person remains "forgotten," especially during busy periods.
- ❖ Many health workers are unaware of the importance of clear communication with Deaf people. They do not realize that a majority of Deaf people prefer to use British Sign Language (BSL), a separate language from English.
- ❖ Similar problems arise with medical jargon: a lot of medical terms are not understood by Deaf people. Doctors do not spend enough time with Deaf patients, often preferring to give a synopsis of information instead of the full explanation that they would give to their hearing patients.
- ❖ In Glasgow, a free communication support service is available for Deaf people attending medical appointments. Many health workers do not know how to work effectively with communication support workers, consequently leading to further communication problems for Deaf people. Cases of Deaf people attending appointments without communication support or

having to reschedule appointments are common because of the acute shortage of communication support in Scotland. Communication support cannot be booked for immediate appointments.

Some Deaf people bring family members—siblings or parents—to act as "communicators" when they either are unable to book communication support or are skeptical of the ability of communication support workers to maintain confidentiality. This means that the family member would know what is wrong with the person before the Deaf person.

From time to time, Deaf patients are notified during medical appointments that "somebody here knows sign language," that is, that one of their colleagues can act as a signer. This worker frequently has very basic sign language skills and is not able to understand the Deaf person.

Health information sent out from health services, such as leaflets, are usually inaccessible to Deaf people because they tend to be written in complicated text with little visual information. Information available in other media formats, such as television advertisements, seldom includes subtitles. These access barriers to information cause Deaf people to be concerned that they are missing essential health information such as prevention techniques for certain illnesses, such as cancer.

Cases have arisen where communication support workers overstepped their ethical boundaries during interpreting appointments by expressing their opinions, for example, by advising Deaf patients what they should do about their own health.

Two cancer screening services are available for women in Scotland: breast and cervical screenings. Because of lack of access to information and communication, many Deaf women, as a result of ignorance, do not attend screening appointments and are unaware of the benefits.

A variety of support groups for people with certain types of cancer are problematic for Deaf people, again because of the shortage of communication support. Only two qualified counselors are available in the whole of Scotland to work with Deaf people, and neither specializes in cancer-related illnesses, which consequently leads to greater frustration for Deaf people seeking support.

These examples are only some of the difficulties Deaf people face when accessing health services in Scotland, which are unacceptable because Deaf patients have the right to receive as much information as possible to make informed decisions about their health. They cause Deaf people to put off visiting their doctor until they are really ill. For some who may have cancer and certain other illnesses, it may be too late for successful treatment.

Deaf Cancer Wise takes all this into account and aims to remove, or at least reduce, these to improve access to cancer-related health and information services for Deaf people.

Cancer is a major illness in Scotland. In a country with a population of around 5.5 million people,

- ❖ 26,000 Scots are diagnosed as having cancer every year,
- ❖ 15,000 die from it every year, and
- ❖ 14,740 died in 1999.

It should be noted that those 15,000 are not necessarily from the 26,000 that are diagnosed that year; they might have been diagnosed previously. These figures are high in terms of the percentage of the whole Scottish population.

"Cancer in Scotland: Action for Change," a research article from the *Scottish Executive* (July 2001), indicates that many Scottish people do not reach their life expectancy. Cancer is a leading cause of premature deaths for roughly one in three men and one in four women by the time they reach the age of seventy-four. The article forecasts that if the current trend continues, an average of one in two deaths will be from cancer within the next decade.

In the Deaf community, as with many diverse communities, incorrect rumors run wildly about cancer, such as that cancer can be caused by bumping into something hard or that cancer is passed from person to person. This creates a great deal of concern and anxiety among Deaf people who are uncertain of the truth of these rumors, though they are aware of an increasing incidence of cancer in Scotland.

In response to this serious concern about inaccessible health information, four organizations—Deaf Connections, St. Vincent's Centre for Deaf People, Greater Glasgow National Health Service (NHS) Board, and Lanarkshire NHS Board—partnered together to produce a pilot video project called "Breast Screening: A User's Guide," which has information presented in BSL by Deaf people. The video was accompanied by a visual pamphlet on breast awareness. The aim was to educate Deaf women about the main purposes of breast screening, including an explanation of the procedure of a typical appointment. The Deaf community responded positively, indicating that their information needs had been addressed with information provided in this language format. This was then used as evidence that health information should be provided in BSL to the Deaf community to ensure full access.

The pilot video project enabled Deaf Connections to obtain funding for three years from the New Opportunities Fund, which is part of the British National Lottery Scheme. Deaf Cancer Wise was consequently set up in September 2001.

The aim of Deaf Cancer Wise was not postdiagnosis care but cancer prevention. Research shows that unhealthy lifestyles increase the incidence of cancer; 80 percent of cancer is believed to be caused by unhealthy lifestyle factors such as poor diet, smoking, high body mass, high alcohol consumption, too much exposure to the sun, and low physical exercise levels.

It is commonly said that prevention is better than cure. The project aims to provide accessible information to the Deaf community on healthy lifestyles, along with information on certain cancers, to reduce risk of developing cancer.

The project does not focus only on delivering information to Deaf people but also on delivering Deaf awareness training for cancer-related health professionals and volunteers, to promote deaf-friendly and accessible environments within these services.

Initial plans for Deaf Cancer Wise included various aims, such as the establishment of a drop-in resource center where Deaf people may ask for clarification or ask questions about cancer-related issues. Further video packages and visual resources with explanations of cancer-related jargon were planned, along with a Web site produced specifically for Deaf people on cancer issues. Counseling services were to be examined to see how these services could be adapted to serve the needs of Deaf people who have cancer.

Deaf Cancer Wise has one employee, which is myself, and it has not been possible for me to work with every Deaf person who needs support or information on cancer. To overcome this, four lay health workers, or "sessional workers," were recruited, which enabled the project to perform its aims more effectively within the Deaf community. The workers, all Deaf themselves, were provided with some basic training on cancer issues and lifestyles. The project focused on two lifestyle factors during the first year—smoking and healthy eating.

In Scotland, the most common cause of cancer is smoking, which causes 90 percent of lung cancers and 30 percent of other types of cancers. Further, the most common cancer-related deaths are those with lung cancer. Smoking is considered the main cause for 20 percent of all deaths.

Practically, approximately one-third of the Scottish population aged between sixteen and seventy-four (34 percent of men and 32 percent of women) smoke. In terms of reducing cancer deaths, this situation is by far easiest to change—by stopping smoking.

Deaf Cancer Wise has worked with Smoking Concerns, a mainstream smoking-cessation group within the Greater Glasgow NHS Board, to ensure that their information is deaf-friendly because many Deaf people are frustrated with the lack of access to information on smoking cessation. Deaf people, when asked, showed ignorance of various support therapies available for people who want to stop smoking. Their doctors tended, instead, to provide them with nicotine patches without instructions on how to use them and without explaining about other therapies such as nicotine chewing gums, sprays, and lozenges. Also, in Scotland, people can see their pharmacist to discuss problems, withdrawal symptoms they may have, or seek reassurance. Deaf people do not have this type of access, and this is where Deaf Cancer Wise comes in to provide a similar service in their own language, BSL. Deaf people have an opportunity to come in to see us every week for 10 minutes to discuss these issues or concerns.

A theoretical model to assist people in successfully changing their lifestyle or habits has been adopted by Smoking Concerns to help people stop smoking. The stages of change model (Prochaska et al., 1988) has already been identified as a success with hearing people, and it was agreed that this model would be tried with Deaf people.

The model consists of a pie chart with seven segments of stages, which people go through during change. The model can be used to help create successful strategies for any lifestyle change, not just on smoking cessation. One-to-one consultations are generally more appropriate so that individual needs can be identified and met. The seven stages of the circle are as follows:

1. not interested,
2. thinking,
3. preparing,
4. trying to change,
5. maintaining change,
6. remaining stable, and
7. relapsing.

The model is used initially to assist in judging whether an individual is ready to make a lifestyle change. People in stage 1 may not be interested in making a lifestyle change, because they are quite happy continuing with the behavior. Once accessible information is provided to the individuals on the benefits of changing behavior, a seed of doubt may be planted between stages 1 and 2. From stage 2, thinking, people then move to stage 3, in which they take time to prepare for the change, because immediate action often leads to failure. Once people decide how to prepare for the change, they move to stage 4 and make the actual change. At stage 5, the individuals have to maintain that changed behavior to prevent relapse. If all things are going well, they move to stage 6, where they are stable and do not fall back into the undesired previous behavior, although there remains the risk of relapsing. If this occurs, this is not seen as a failure, and the individuals have the choice to go through the cycle again. The good thing about this model is that after failure people can reflect on the reason(s) for the relapse to prevent these from happening again.

In terms of smoking cessation, people may be quite happy to continue smoking (stage 1). They may be asked why they wish to continue smoking, and after receiving information on the dangers of smoking, they might start contemplating and weighing the positives and negatives of smoking (stage 2). They may then decide to stop smoking but require preparation before stopping (stage 3). Preparation includes consideration on appropriate times to stop; for example, people may already have weekend plans with friends, which may increase the likelihood of failure. Instead of stopping before the weekend, a date of stopping may be set for the following Monday (stage 4). The individuals actually stop smoking (stage 5) and remain committed, achieving stability as a nonsmoker (stage 6), unless they have a relapse (stage 7). If this happens, the individuals have the opportunity to look back at the model and see what has gone wrong, which reduces risk of relapse if they wish to attempt it again.

This has been a useful model for Deaf people. Following this service, we hope to see a reduction in the number of Deaf people who smoke. This will be reviewed in two years time when the project funding ends to see the overall impact.

The second area that the project has focused on is nutrition. Poor diets in the west of Scotland are believed to cause up to 30 percent of cancer cases. In Scotland, stomach cancer is the sixth most common form of cancer. Here, a poor diet means food with too much fat, salt, and sugar, not enough fruits and vegetables, and not enough carbohydrates and fiber.

Deaf Cancer Wise aims to provide information on healthy eating to Deaf people, but it is also important to consider other factors, such as not having enough money to buy healthy food, which is normally more expensive. Relapse is likely a result of people not being able to afford healthy food. The model assists people during preparation so they can prevent relapse before making changes to their diets.

The project works in partnership with the Nutrition Department of the Greater Glasgow NHS Board. Their nutritional information needed to be adapted to make it accessible to Deaf people. Workshops and group sessions were held about how to actually buy healthy food cheaply and how to prepare for changing their diets. Cooking classes teaching basic healthy cooking skills were also offered. We forecast that the project will later produce videos in BSL about buying and cooking healthy food.

The stages of change model assists people in changing their lifestyles, but it is also important to remember that people cannot be forced to change. If this happens, people tend to become defensive and refuse to change. The best way to plant the seed is by providing as much accessible information as possible to these people and let them decide what they wish to do.

In Scotland, although more people are diagnosed as having cancer, an increasing number of people are surviving after being diagnosed. This indicates that information is reaching people and encouraging them to check out any doubts early with their doctors, which makes diagnosis and treatment easier. If the information is life saving, we have to examine whether Deaf people have access to the information. Quite often they are disenfranchised, do not have access, and so may not necessarily be positively affected by that. It is important to build partnerships with mainstream health and voluntary organizations, such as Breast Cancer Care and Cancer BACUP, remind them of the existence and needs of Deaf people, and make sure that the information they have is accessible to Deaf people. Hearing people are not out there alone suffering from cancer, but Deaf people as well.

The main goal of my presentation was to notify other countries about what has been happening in the west of Scotland with the hope that a similar kind of project could be set up elsewhere, because the project appears to be a success with the Deaf population, who are desperate for health-related information and support. There is a high incidence of cancer in the rest of the United Kingdom, but there is no other project like Deaf Cancer Wise there.

I hope that at the end of the three-year project, if it proves to be successful, additional funding will be obtained to cover a larger area including the whole of Scotland and perhaps England and Northern Ireland as well.

Reference

Prochaska, J. O., Velicer, W. F., DiClemente, C. C., & Fava, J. L. (1988). Measuring processes of change: Applications to the cessation of smoking. *Journal of Consulting and Clinical Psychology, 56*, 520–528.

AIDS and Deaf People: Health Service Delivery and Prevention for Deaf People by Deaf People

JULIE ELAINE ROY AND MICHEL TURGEON

The purpose of this essay is to share with other Deaf people how we came to create a community health information and prevention center for Deaf people, managed by Deaf people, with a special interest in HIV, AIDS, and other venereal diseases.

Following an important meeting of Deaf people in Montreal organized by the Association des Bonnes Gens Sourds (ABGS) and the Comite Sida Aide Montreal (CSAM) to inform Deaf people about venereal diseases and AIDS, it became obvious that a permanent association was needed to provide the Deaf population with information on HIV and AIDS issues. The meeting also made abundantly clear that Deaf people with HIV and AIDS needed help and assistance and that a volunteer service of some sort had to be established. Michel Turgeon, who is deaf himself, came up with the idea to set up a special organization to serve the Deaf community. One of the key reasons for creating a health education center for Deaf people was the realization that unless something was done to break the circle of ignorance, there was a real risk that the Deaf community in Quebec could disappear.

Coalition Sida des Sourds du Quebec (CSSQ), the Quebec Deaf AIDS Coalition, was founded in April 1992 and incorporated in July of the same year. Michel Turgeon is the executive director of the center. Membership on the Board of Directors is subject to two conditions, namely that members must be deaf and at least two members must be HIV positive or have full-blown AIDS. In addition, the eastern and western part of the province must also be represented on the board.

The coalition is supported financially by two levels of governments: federal (Canada) and provincial (Quebec). Corporate and other donors are also invited to support our organization. The coalition organizes various other events, activities, and functions to raise funds, provide information on HIV and AIDS, and reach out to the Deaf and hearing communities.

The coalition is accessible to French- and English-speaking Deaf and hard of hearing individuals, regardless of sexual orientation, because the disease affects us all.

I must point out, at this time, that the coalition is run and operated for Deaf people by Deaf people. Deaf people seek out other Deaf people for help, and the communication barriers that Deaf people meet when seeking information are removed when that information is communicated by another Deaf person. This said, we also seek out partnerships with other AIDS organizations in Quebec and in Canada to make sure we are on top of the latest information on this deadly disease.

Deaf people are a group often labeled the forgotten ones regarding information about HIV and AIDS. Research in France and in the United States has shown that the rate of infection in the Deaf community is double that of the hearing communities, and that it is mostly Deaf heterosexuals who are infected. Most Deaf people think AIDS is a gay disease or, worse yet, that it affects only hearing people.

We now know that the epidemic trends of HIV infection identify hard drug users, especially intravenous ones, as the people most at risk. We are now working on a new program to reach out to that subgroup, so that Deaf drug users know the risk of contracting HIV and ways to avoid it without having to stop their drug habit.

Here are some of the many services offered by the coalition:

- ❖ AIDS and HIV prevention among Deaf people is one of our primary goals. On a regular basis, we visit different organizations and schools for Deaf students across the province with videotapes, flyers, and general information packages on HIV/AIDS education and prevention. We offer workshops on HIV, AIDS, and safe sex. Obviously, the workshops are all given in sign language by a Deaf person. We also have an awareness and outreach program. An infected Deaf person goes out in the community, as a spokesperson and a living example of the terrible impact of this disease on one's life. We also distribute condoms at all major events and functions held in the Deaf community, and this has been very successful.
- ❖ We run a support and assistance program for Deaf patients, whether they are infected with HIV and AIDS or not. Services include psychological counseling, group therapy, spiritual support, social support, and rest and recuperation in a country setting. There is also a program operated by Deaf volunteers to help ill people with different chores, including accompanying them to medical appointments, house cleaning, and grocery shopping. There are also programs aimed at improving the quality of life of infected patients by taking them out to a restaurant or other social events.
- ❖ The coalition provides financial support to patients who do not have the money to pay for their medication through a special money-for-medication program. We teach infected persons how to take their medication, especially with new treatments such as tritherapy (combining fixed doses of antiretrovirals, involving three medicinal drugs of two different classes in the same tablet).
- ❖ We established an information hotline with a 1-800 number and TTY answering service for Deaf people who have HIV or AIDS or others who simply have questions about HIV and AIDS.
- ❖ We seek out partnerships with other associations who serve the AIDS and HIV community. We share knowledge and experience and search together

for solutions in difficult situations. We also try to forge partnerships with government agencies that deal specifically with the Deaf population. The Raymond-Dewar Institute in Montreal is a case in point. This agency supports the work of the coalition by making a psychologist and social worker available. There are times when professional help for Deaf patients who are infected with HIV or AIDS is essential.

- We have produced and adapted a lot of material that was developed for and by Deaf people. Our goal is to ensure that every Deaf person has the same information on HIV and AIDS as hearing people do. We adapted reading material by simplifying the vocabulary and by adding lots of drawings, graphics, and illustrations.
- With funds from Health Canada, we produced a videotape in Quebec Sign Language (LSQ) captioned with French subtitles. This videotape, which is half fiction and half documentary, explains the reality of HIV and AIDS to Deaf people in Quebec.
- We also cover the cost of having a member of each of the Deaf clubs in Quebec Province to travel to Montreal for a two-day workshop on AIDS and HIV education and prevention. Consequently, we wrote a new training handbook that enables those who received the training in Montreal to pass on their new knowledge to other Deaf people back home.
- Through workshops, we are regularly training Deaf people to become volunteers to support Deaf people with HIV or AIDS.
- We also encourage sign-language interpreters to participate in our training program so they will be ready to accompany Deaf patients to their medical appointments.
- We created a glossary of signs related to AIDS and HIV in areas such as health sciences, sexuality, sexually transmitted diseases, medication, and so forth.

In conclusion, given the growth of the HIV/AIDS epidemic, especially in the Deaf community, the establishment of a special-purpose health center for the Deaf community, managed and operated by Deaf people, became imperative. The very survival of the Deaf community in Quebec was at risk. Yet, the coalition's continued existence is not assured. Finding creative and ingenious means of raising awareness and funds remains one of our primary functions, and we continue to rely heavily on the support of the Deaf community as well of hearing volunteers.

Reference

Peinkofer, James R. 1994. HIV education for the Deaf, a vulnerable minority. *Public Health Reports* 109, no. 3: 390–96.

Reconstructing Deafness: A Solution-Focused Approach to Mental Health

SUE E. OUELLETTE

Traditional psychotherapy with deaf and hard of hearing people has been hampered by adherence to two basic assumptions. First, many therapists believe that deafness represents a pathology that predisposes persons who are deaf or hard of hearing to various mental and emotional disorders. Such a premise underlies much of the literature on deafness and mental health. There have been various iterations of this assumption, ranging from a belief that deafness itself yields mental illness to theories that blame the deaf person's family, school, or community for failures that eventually emerge as mental health problems. This model also views deafness in and of itself as a pathological condition to be placed on Axis III of *The Diagnostic and Statistical Manual of Mental Disorders* (fourth edition text revision, 2000), along with other indicators that explain and describe the patient's symptoms.

Second, practitioners in the field of deafness have shared with the larger field of mental health an assumption that problems are improved by a better understanding of the nature of the problem. This assumption then defines the process of therapy as a problem-solving process. The well-known stages of problem solving include definition of the problem (diagnosis), intervention guided by assessment, and evaluation of the intervention (De Jong and Berg, 1996).

An alternative model for therapy is presented in the work of Steve de Shazer and Insoo Kim Berg, who have developed solution-focused therapy. This model fits within the philosophy of social constructionism, which holds that human beings attribute meaning to their experiences through the interactions they have with others. The experience of deafness, for example, has been construed by the hearing community as involving concepts of disability, deviation, and limitations. Many deaf and hard of hearing individuals grow into adulthood subscribing to this view imposed by the dominant hearing culture. The deaf community, on the other hand, has construed the experience of deafness quite differently, that is, as a cultural variant rather than a disability. Both of these very different constructions of deafness are arrived at through interaction with different groups of people (the hearing community versus the deaf community). The attribution that deaf or hard of hearing people hold concerning their physical difference will greatly influence how they think, feel, and act.

As such, it makes sense to approach the treatment of mental health issues with deaf and hard of hearing people from a constructivist perspective. Because the experience of many deaf people has unfortunately been focused on what they cannot do and on the problems and limitations they experience, it is therapeutically useful to focus on the many strengths and abilities that deaf individuals have been able to bring to bear on surviving in an environment that is not optimally supportive.

Solution-focused therapy provides a framework for deconstructing the myths of deafness as problem saturated and focused on limitations and, instead, constructing with the client a view of capability, resourcefulness, and success. The model is briefly outlined next.

The Model

Solution-focused therapy began approximately thirty years ago with the work of Steve de Shazer and Insoo Kim Berg at the Brief Family Therapy Center in Milwaukee, Wisconsin. Their approach was purely inductive in nature in that they and their team intently observed large numbers of clients in an effort to determine what worked for them therapeutically. The model that resulted from these efforts has gained immense popularity and acceptance in the United States, Europe, and Asia. De Shazer and Berg have been joined in their exploration of this model by a number of scholars, researchers, and clinicians who focus their effort on this model. As a result, the model has evolved with various different emphases and understanding. Notable among those who are developing versions of this model are O'Hanlon, Walter, Peller, Miller, Dolan, Lipchick, and Weiner-Davis.

An understanding of the assumptions of the solution-focused model is key to understanding the model. Walter and Peller (1992) detail a number of assumptions of the model:

1. Advantages of a positive focus. *Assumption: Focusing on the positive, the solution, and the future facilitates change in the desired direction. Therefore, focus on solution-oriented talk rather than problem-oriented talk.*
2. Exceptions suggest solutions. *Assumption: Exceptions to every problem can be created by the therapist and client, which can be used to build solutions.*
3. Nothing is always the same. *Assumption: Change is occurring all the time.*
4. Small change is generative. *Assumption: Small changing leads to larger changing.*
5. Cooperation is inevitable. *Assumption: Clients are always cooperating. They are showing us how they think change takes place. As we understand their thinking and act accordingly, cooperation is inevitable (de Shazer, 1982, 1984, 1985).*
6. People are resourceful. *Assumption: People have all they need to solve their problems.*
7. Meaning and experience are interactionally constructed. *Assumption: Meaning is in the word or medium in which we live. We inform meaning into our experience, and it is our experience at the same time. Meaning is not imposed from without or determined from outside of ourselves. We inform our world through interaction.*
8. Recursiveness. *Assumption: Actions and descriptions are circular.*

9. *Meaning is in the response. Assumption: The meaning of the message is in the response you receive.*
10. *The client is the expert. Assumption: Therapy is a goal- or solution-focused endeavor with the client as the expert.*
11. *Unity. Assumption: Any change in how clients describe a goal (solution) and/or what they do affects future interactions with all involved.*
12. *Treatment group membership. Assumption: The members in a treatment group are those who share a goal and state their desire to do something about making it happen.*

The actual process of solution-focused therapy involves inviting clients to explore and define two things: (1) what they want to be different in their lives and (2) what strengths, resources, and abilities they have to bring to bear on getting whatever it is that they want (De Jong and Berg, 1996): "The practitioner affirms and amplifies client definition of goals, past successes, strengths, and resources as they emerge through conversation. Consequently, these conversations focus more on building solutions than on solving problems" (p. 377).

De Jong and Berg (1996) note the following stages of solution-focused therapy.

Description of the Problem

Arrived at by asking the client (s), "How can I be useful to you?"

Development of Well-Formed Goals

Distinctive to this approach is the use of a miracle question that assists the therapist in constructing with the client a sense of what the client wants. This is accomplished by inviting the client to construct "a vision of an alternative future that *concretely identifies what will be present in a more satisfying future*" and that focuses on what clients might do differently to make that future happen (De Jong and Berg, 1996, p. 381). The miracle question might be phrased as such, "Imagine that we finish here tonight and you go home and have dinner, maybe watch a little television. Then you finally go to bed and fall asleep and, while you are sleeping, a miracle occurs and the problem that brought you here today is completely solved. Because you are sleeping, though, you don't know that this miracle has occurred. When you wake up tomorrow, what will be the first sign to you that something has happened, that the problem is gone? How will other people know that something has happened to you?" de Shazer (1994) refers to the miracle question as "a way to begin constructing a bridge between client and therapist built around the [future] success of therapy (p. 95).

The therapist seeks to construct goals with the client that are

1. small rather than large;
2. salient to clients;
3. described in specific, concrete behavioral terms;
4. achievable within the practical context of clients' lives;
5. perceived by the clients as involving their "hard work";
6. described as the "start of something" and not the "end of something"; and

7. treated as involving new behavior(s) rather than the absence or cessation of existing behavior(s) (de Shazer, 1991).

This process is accomplished through the use of the miracle question and constructing with the client what he or she will be doing differently when the problem is solved.

Exploring Exceptions

The next task of the solution-focused therapist is to look for times when the problem is not happening or is less severe. These are exceptions to the problem and represent times when the client is already exhibiting the kind of behavior or thinking associated with an absence of the problem. The therapist strives to identify times when the problem does not occur or when the client is already doing some of what he or she wants to do. The therapist then seeks to contrast the contextual differences by soliciting information regarding what is different during these times of exception. Exceptions are always elicited that are within the client's frame of reference and have to do with what he or she is doing or thinking differently. Questions may also seek to identify what other people would perceive as being different about the client were they to observe the client during one of these times of exception. When the client is unable to identify exceptions that have already occurred, the therapist can move to a future orientation by asking the client to identify times when just a small amount of the miracle may have already occurred in his or her life.

End of Session Feedback

A central feature of this model is the use of a consultation break. The model was originally developed in a setting that employed a team model. The consultation break provided an opportunity for the therapist to leave the therapy room, go behind the one-way mirror, and consult with team members who assisted the therapist in identifying things the client was doing that represented exceptions or were good for the client and should be continued. De Shazer and Berg continue to use consultation breaks even in the absence of a formal team; in fact, the use of a consultation break is considered to be a core component of the model. The break allows the therapist to identify compliments and clues. Compliments affirm the client's strengths and resources whereas clues suggest ways in which these can be brought to bear on solving the presenting problem. Compliments and clues both flow from a thorough investigation of exceptions.

Evaluation of Client Progress

Solution-focused therapists regularly ask clients, "On a scale of one to ten with ten being the day after the miracle when the problem is solved and one being as bad as the problem has ever been, where is the problem now on the scale?" This question allows the client to reevaluate the severity of the presenting problem at the end of the session after solutions have been explored. It is not uncommon for a client to state a number followed by an explanation that "if you had asked me that question at the beginning of this session, I would have said the problem was a *one* (or a *minus ten* or some other negative number). Now, though, I realize that I have been able to fix some parts of the problem so I'd probably say it's more like a *five*." This scaling question allows the therapist to measure progress from session to session. It also allows the therapist to ask the client what would be a small sign that he or she was moving closer to a *six*, which is useful in emphasizing future change.

A second scaling question asks the client how confident he or she is that the problem can be kept at the number it has been scaled at. The therapist might ask, "How confident are you that the problem will stay a 5 this coming week?"

Subsequent Sessions

Subsequent sessions are often begun with the simple question, "What's better since the last time I saw you?" The goal of the therapist in second or subsequent sessions is to determine what is better, what the client did to make things better, and whether or not it is better enough.

Applications to Working with Deaf and Hard of Hearing Clients

Torres (1995) presents a cogent argument for adopting a constructivist perspective in the provision of mental health services to deaf and hard of hearing individuals. She uses the work of Hinkle (1994) to note the necessity of therapists resisting any temptation to impose their own worldviews on their clients. She concludes, correctly, that the worldview of a hearing therapist will differ significantly from that of a deaf client and that only through an awareness of this difference can the problem of disparate worldviews be solved. She also notes that a social constructivist paradigm fits well with the way deaf people are currently constructing the experience of deafness as one that embodies self-determination and empowerment. She concludes that this congruence between the changing social construction of deafness and the therapeutic approach creates an environment in which therapy is more likely to be collaborative and productive.

Solution-focused therapy provides a framework for deconstructing the myths of deafness as problem-saturated and focused on limitations and, instead, constructing with the client a view of capability, resourcefulness, and success. This is done by focusing on the positive, the future, and on times when the problem does not occur rather than perseverating the problem. In so doing, the client and therapist reconstruct the problem as capable of being solved and the client as capable of taking action to solve the problem. Further, the client identifies strategies he or she has already used successfully that can be brought to bear on the presenting. Finally, scaling offers a way to reinforce the newly constructed description.

References

American Psychiatric Association. (2000). *Diagnostic and statistical manual of mental disorders* (4th rev. ed.). Washington, DC: Author.

De Jong, P., & Berg, I. (1996). *Interviewing for solutions.* Pacific Grove, CA: Brooks/Cole.
de Shazer, S. (1982). *Patterns of brief family therapy.* New York: Guilford.
de Shazer, S. (1984). The death of resistance. *Family Process, 23*(1), 11–21.
de Shazer, S. (1985). *Keys to solutions in brief therapy.* New York: W. W. Norton.
de Shazer, S. (1991). *Putting differences to work.* New York: W. W. Norton.
de Shazer, S. (1994). *Words were originally magic.* New York: W. W. Norton
Hinkle, J. (1994). Ecosystems and mental health counseling: Reactions to Becvar and Becvar. *Journal of Mental Health Counseling, 16,* 33–36.
Torres, M. (1995). A postmodern perspective on the issue of deafness as culture versus pathology. *JADARA, 29*(2), 1–7.
Walter, J., & Peller, J. (1992). *Becoming solution-focused in therapy.* New York: Brunner/Mazel.

PART SIX

History

Russian Deaf Towns

ELENA SILIANOVA

I describe a unique phenomenon that still determines the life of many Deaf Russians. I call it "unique" because I and my colleagues do not know whether things like it exist somewhere else. I know that there are similar places in Bulgaria, for example. The phenomenon is the following: in some big Russian cities or in their suburbs, there are areas or districts that are inhabited mainly by Deaf people. The center or the core of these settlements is a factory or a workshop where the majority of the workers are Deaf. Usually there are few apartment blocks near the factory (there can be one or two or sometimes four big blocks of apartments) where mainly people from the factory live. There is usually a Deaf club with a gym where Deaf people can do different sports. There can be a store or a kiosk, sometimes a post office, and people who work there use some sort of signing. It is an important fact that those people who live or work in the "Deaf area" can sign.

Let us go back to the past. Traditional historic literature about the foundation of the All Russian Federation (Society) of the Deaf describes the first Deaf workshops as appearing only after the Communist Revolution of 1917. However, I found some archives proving that the first workshop for deaf people was founded at the end of the nineteenth century (1898). That year the Russian Empress Maria Fedorovna (the wife of the Russian Emperor Alexandre the Third, the daughter of the Danish King Christian the Ninth) set up a charity with the aim of helping Deaf people in education, vocational training, employment, and culture. The head of the charity, Ivan Karlovich Moerder, started the construction of a big brick building for the college in August 1900 on the plot of land donated by Count Apraksin. It was on the bank of the Neva River in the St. Petersburg suburbs. At the same time, a school-farm opened where the girls were taught literacy and farming skills and had speech therapy classes. There were a big kitchen garden, an orchard, a cattle farm, and a poultry farm. Besides ordinary classes, special workshops for boys were opened where they had some professional training in areas such as shoe making, carpentry, and so forth.

In 1899, Ivan Moerder set up school-farms in Sestroretsk (near St. Petersburg) and near Narva (now Estonia). The charity issued a special document about Deaf workshops describing in detail the life of Deaf workers there. They spent all their life there—they ate, lived, slept, had classes, and, of course, worked.

To tell you the truth, in my opinion, these workshops strongly reminded me of an army or a prison with guards and supervisors. However, the workshops were usually the only employment choice for Deaf people then. They worked either in workshops attached to the schools for Deaf students, meaning that the school graduates stayed there after finishing the academic courses, or they were taken to these "sheltered homes" (caring houses) at different ages and were given mainly professional training. At the beginning of the century, the charity organized thirty-eight settlements for 1,100 Deaf people, but the arrangement could provide "bread and bed" to only 5 percent of the Deaf Russians.

After the revolution of 1917, the charity ceased to exist and the governmental committees on employment and social security began to organize labor communes for Deaf people (called houses of labor) and the education of the deaf-mutes. The first house was opened in 1919 to teach shoe making, joinery, and sewing. The profit from the workshops went to food, clothes, and rent. One of the first workshops was opened in Moscow to manufacture socks, stockings, and knitted clothes. It was the first union of Deaf workers, which became the prototype for later workshops and factories. At that time there also existed a few other cooperatives for Deaf people. The All-Russian Society of the Deaf was founded in 1926 (the Russian abbreviation is VOG). Its first chairman, Pavel Saveliev, was very active in opening factories and workshops: full employment of the Deaf population was the goal. At that time there were twenty-four workshops for 399 people. If we look at the figures from the beginning of the century, 1,100 employed Deaf people, it is a regress, but we must keep in mind general unemployment, starvation, and decline after the revolution of 1917.) In 1929, the Soviet government issued a special decree on the employment of Deaf people, and by 1932, there were 1,002 Deaf workers. In 1937, the VOG owned seventy-three workshops and factories; some of them were rather big, such as a boat engine factory in Moscow, mechanic workshops in Saratov and Kostroma, and numerous sewing factories. Most of the factories were very profitable; the income went both to the VOG Central Board and to the federal budget. Either educated Deaf people or hearing professionals organized evening classes for illiterate Deaf workers. Approximately 9,500 Deaf people received professional training. Factories started hiring sign language interpreters. The VOG began building hostels for Deaf trainees and workers. Hostels attracted many people from rural areas to big towns. Before World War II, 3,000 Deaf people lived in hostels owned by the VOG.

Because Deaf people were not recruited by the army, they worked very hard at VOG workshops and factories. They specialized in different goods for the army, including hospital linen, clothes, and boots. During the war there were opened groups of Deaf workers with interpreters within ordinary factories: Deaf people produced tanks, armament, and airplanes. Of course, some factory buildings, clubs, and hostels were destroyed during the war, but the Soviet government provided enough funds to restore them, and in 1945 the VOG had sixty-seven factories and workshops. The postwar time was the period when VOG paid much more attention to the development of other facilities around workshops; more hostels, apartment blocks, clubs, evening schools, stadiums, and gyms appeared. Pavel Sutyagin, chairman of VOG for twenty-one years (1950–71), was the initiator and the heart of the process. In 1954, VOG became a self-financed organization, meaning that the government budget did not give any money for its social, cultural, sport, or economic activities. Pavel Sutyagin was the author of the idea of Deaf towns. Deaf towns, or VOGograds, developed and flourished at that time.

All workshops were turned into big factories; the smallest counted fifty workers, the biggest factories up to four hundred Deaf workers. Evening schools (usually four evenings a week) gave secondary education and vocational training. Usually young Deaf workers lived in hostels near the factory but when they got married they were given free flats. "Good" Deaf people often had free holidays on the Black Sea coast in one of the rest homes owned by VOG and had a special food supply. Of course many Deaf people of the older generation and middle-age people are nostalgic. Many of them dream of getting this "wonderful" time back. Before I comment, here are a few more dry figures of the current situation.

Though the economic situation in Russia is really very difficult and complicated, the special training-industrial enterprises managed to survive even though many of them do not give much or any profit at all. It is hard for them to compete within the market economy. Some sixty-eight factories are doing better, some not. In general, there are fewer Deaf workers in the factories then used to be before; in some of them fewer than 51 percent of employees are Deaf. A young face is a rarity; the majority consists of old qualified workers. The younger generation is looking for better-paying jobs. Some factory managers prefer to employ hearing workers. VOG used to own eighty-two apartment blocks, but now it tries to get rid of them because they are too expensive to keep (heating, electricity, plumbing), and some of the buildings were transferred to the jurisdiction of local municipal authorities. Many clubs are either closed or rented out—local VOG branches receive profit from the rent, but some of the clubs are dark and cold. Deaf sports culture is trying hard not to die, but only recently the government has started financing national sports teams.

Three more examples to illustrate the current situation: There are two factories in Moscow: one on the north, the other one is in the east. The northern one was founded as early as in 1929, and in its better times employed 500 Deaf workers. There are 65 employees now, and they mainly produce shoes, boots, some badges, and tin covers for jars. Many rooms at the factory, including a Deaf meeting room and gym, are let out to other businesses. Not far there is a block of flats for the workers. The eastern factory is a little better off: of 167 employees 142 are Deaf, and they produce various plastic goods and some filters. There are two blocks of flats for both Deaf factory workers and for Deaf actors from the Theatre of Mime and Gesture.

In the town of Smolensk, which is about five hundred kilometers from Moscow, there are only 300 Deaf people, 53 of whom make linen at the local industrial enterprise. The workers' salary depends on the orders. If there are no orders at all, no one works and they each get about $20 a month. (The subsistence wage in Moscow per person is $300 a month.) Near the Smolensk factory, there are two blocks of flats for mainly Deaf inhabitants. The neighbors meet each other at the courtyard, where women usually chat and gossip and men share a bottle of vodka. There is a shop nearby with a signing shop assistant.

The most striking example of a Deaf town is the place called Silikatnava, forty kilometers from Moscow. The factory was founded after World War II. Of course, it has seen better days, but now it is also trying hard to survive by manufacturing lamps, folding beds, and plastic goods such as combs or hair clips. Though only 143 Deaf people work at the factory, there are 300 Deaf people in town altogether. They live in four apartment blocks each of one hundred flats. Three-quarters of the area's population is Deaf. Deaf people who do not work at the factory are either pensioners or commute to better-paying jobs in Moscow. There used to be two hostels but now only one is left; it is in bad condition, and only seven young families live there (there are no free flats for them now). The other hostel is closed, and the evening school does not function either. The Deaf club is in a separate big building attached to the factory. It works, but events do not occur often—people go to the library or sometimes in the evenings an interpreter interprets soap operas on television. Virtually fifty meters from the factory, there are summer cabins with little plots of land where Deaf people grow vegetables and spend their summer weekends. Only one shop out of two is open. Most hearing people use some form of signing. I was really surprised that very few Silikatnaya inhabitants go to Moscow and Moscow Deaf clubs, where the life is totally different. Most of the people only think about "wonderful past" and complain. No one does anything to change the situation.

These Russian Deaf towns will probably soon disappear. Now there are still people who remember the past. Further research is needed; otherwise it will be too late to save the towns and document the past.

Iranian Deaf Culture

ABBAS ALI BEHMANESH

In the Islamic Republic of Iran, the officially announced literacy rate is 48 percent to 52 percent of the population. There are fifty deaf institutions, and twenty-six deaf institutions are in the capital, Tehran. There are only three high schools for deaf students in Iran, and they are in Tehran and Mashhad. There are sixty-nine languages listed for Iran. Of those, sixty-eight are living languages, such as Farsi otherwise known as Persian.

Deaf Education

According to a prominent, well-respected teacher and one of the best-known lecturers in deaf education in Iran, Samineh Baghcheban, deaf education was established in Iran in 1926, or 1305 in the Iranian calendar. The founder of deaf education in Iran was Jabar Baghcheban, Samineh's father. Originally named Jabar Asgaerzadeh, he was born in Irvan, in the country of Armenia, formerly of Russia. He was a reporter for several newspapers. During the Russian Revolutionary War, he wandered from place to place and returned to Tabriz, northwest of Iran.

In 1924 (1303), Baghcheban founded a public school with the assistance of a friend who worked in the Department of Education. He also established a class for three deaf students in 1926 (1305). Prior to establishing this class for the deaf students, the mother of one of the deaf students came to the public school and complained to Baghcheban. She was frustrated because the school was of the opinion that her son could not be educated. Baghcheban thought of teaching deaf students. After Baghcheban established the class for the deaf students, he invented a sign language method, now called Total Communication. After a while, Baghchaban intended to demonstrate his method of teaching the three deaf students in his class. To his surprise, many people wanted to witness his program. People expressed disbelief when they saw that his deaf students were able to read and write. Baghcheban acted as a pioneer in Iranian deaf education. He did not study deaf education previously but invented his own methods at the time.

In 1927 (1306), the Iranian government cut off financial assistance for the deaf program. Baghcheban was persuaded to move to another city, Shiraz, south of Iran in 1928 (1307). He established a deaf school with a kindergarten program there in Shiraz. Kindergarten was unheard of in Iran. During the course of his career in teaching, he decided to move to the capital city, Tehran. In 1933 (1312), Baghcheban established another deaf school in the Yousef Abad, a locality in Tehran, which was later relocated across the street and renamed the National School for the Deaf.

During his teaching tenure, he was chosen by the government to supervise the Persian language curriculum of all the public schools in Iran. The official objective was to reduce the illiteracy rate in Iran. To my knowledge, Baghcheban's pedagogy is one of the best teaching methods in Iran so far. After Baghcheban's death at eighty-two years of age in 1966 (1345), his daughter, Samineh Baghchaban-Pirnazar, assumed his teaching responsibilities and also became principal of the deaf school.

Samineh was born in 1927 (1306) in Tabriz, Iran. Samineh followed her father's steps. She was familiar with her father's teaching methods because she had attended her father's schools as a child. As a result, Samineh received early training in deaf education. She has devoted many years of her life to helping Iranian deaf people and has lectured in many places about deaf people's needs.

Samineh received a bachelor's degree in education from the Teachers College of the University of Tehran and a master's degree in Deaf Education in the United States from Smith College in Northampton. She received additional training at the oral Clarke School for the Deaf and returned to Iran in 1950. After returning from the United States, Samineh became involved in many organizations, such as the National Rehabilitation Center for the Deaf, where she held the position of director general in 1971; the Iranian National Association for Welfare of the Deaf Organization (Sazman Meli Refah Nashenavayan Iran), where she held the position of president in 1973; and the World Federation for the Deaf, where she held the positions of director and fourth regional secretariat in 1977. She retired from these positions during the 1979 revolution in Iran when the fundamentalists overthrew the Shah. She rejoined her family in the United States. Today, she still works in the field of foreign language studies, for example, teaching Persian to Iranian American children and non-Iranian people.

Samineh also established resources for training hearing people who wanted to become teachers of deaf students. With assistance from Farah Pahlavi, the Shah's wife and the queen of Iran, four hearing teachers from Syria came to Iran to learn how to teach deaf students in 1977. Afterward, four men from Africa attended this program. Samineh's departure from Iran was a devastating blow dealt to the Iranian Deaf community. Samineh was one of the greatest leaders in deaf education.

From 1977 until the revolution, Farah Pahlavi sponsored deaf education and strived to improve the situation for deaf people by providing impoverished deaf children with clothes, essential supplies, and financial assistance for vocational school. With her assistance, the Iranian government sponsored the first convention celebrating fifty years of deaf education in 1977. This resulted in expanded resources, for example, the creation of tools to educate hearing people about the abilities of deaf people. American, European, and African scholars attended the convention in Tehran, including Fredrick Schrieber, the president of the National Association for the Deaf (NAD) at that time. The most important outcome of this convention in Tehran was the establishment of a regional center for training teachers of deaf students. The World Federation for the Deaf also recognized the achievements of this convention.

The Deaf Community after the 1979 Revolution

After the 1979 revolution, many skilled people in deaf education left Iran for the West. This situation placed the Iranian deaf people in a difficult predicament and caused a "Dark Age" for them. Today, the schools are all conducted orally, and many Iranian deaf people do not understand what the teachers say. Fortunately, the Department of Health employs some literate deaf people.

Deaf Schools

Deaf children throughout Iran are shocked when they visit the deaf schools. The environment is different than what they are used to. For all students, there is compulsory religious instruction at school. Girls are taught that learning to be a good mother is more important than pursuing careers. Iranian women are discouraged from leaving their homes. The government proscribes the intermingling of men and women in public places. A dress code is mandatory for all Iranians as well. Unlike girls, boys are expected to pursue higher educational or vocational training.

Deaf Women

Prior to the 1979 revolution, women were able to freely associate with men. However, after the 1979 revolution, this was no longer true. In particular, Deaf Iranian women had difficulty in adjusting to the societal changes caused by the 1979 revolution. For example, courtship was considerably more difficult for deaf Iranian women. During the reign of the Shah, educational and judicial reforms were put into place that lessened the influence of the religious classes and laid the basis of a modern state. Women were freed from the *hijab* and *chador*. (The *hijab* and *chador* are Farsi terms meaning clothing that cover the hair and bodies of women.) Divorce laws were modified in women's favor.

The most common form of recreation in Iran for deaf people is visiting friends and relatives, most often two or three times a week. Deaf Iranians develop very close relationships with each other. Often, a great deal of social life centers on the clubs and sport places where deaf people gather to play and pass the time with guests and visitors. Chatting, card games, and backgammon are also very popular pastimes.

Because deaf children put in long hours doing homework, and deaf girls often help with household duties, they have little time for recreation during the school year. Deaf clubhouses and sport clubs tend to be at full capacity during the weekends, when the forbidden American movies are shown. Club patrons also watch soccer to fill their long days of summer. Today, however, deaf unmarried women are forbidden by cultural conventions from patronizing the clubhouses or sport clubs unless they have an escort. It is common for deaf unmarried women to bring their fathers or brothers to the clubs. The men watch television while the deaf women chat with the other females. The deaf women may play sports only in special enclosed areas. Whereas recreation for deaf women in Iran today is largely restricted to entertaining close family and female friends at home, deaf men may leave without an escort, play games with their buddies out in the countryside, and spend their evenings with each other at a local cafe.

Sign Language

There are three sign languages in the Iranian deaf community. The first one is cued speech or Baghcheban's phonetic hand alphabet, which for more than thirty years has been used by schools and social clubs. In 1925 (1304), Jabar Baghcheban invented this phonetic hand alphabet to help deaf pupils become literate. The second sign language is Tea House Sign Language (Ghahveh Khaneh). This sign language is named after a popular place where deaf people, both literate and illiterate, get together to chat in the afternoons or evenings after work. The tea house, unfortunately, was not a safe place for females to attend. The third one is the natural sign language called Persian Sign Language, which splintered from cued speech. Persian Sign Language was heavily influenced by Tea House Sign Language as well.

The research on Persian Sign Language began in 1973 (1352), with the support of both literate and illiterate deaf people. In 1978 (1357), this research was interrupted by the death of Julia Ann Oliver Samii, the American wife of an Iranian businessman. She had immigrated to Iran and joined Samineh Baghcheban in expanding the Persian Sign Language dictionary in spite of a meager salary. Sadly, Julia was killed along with her sons and a friend in a small aircraft crash on a visit to northern Iran. After a short suspension, deaf people resumed research on Persian Sign Language. To honor Julia, the research center that Julia established with Samineh's assistance was renamed Julia Samii Research Center. Julia was the impetus for Iranian deaf individuals recognizing that there was a need for the publication of a Persian Sign Language dictionary to preserve deaf culture. For this reason, Julia is considered to be the mother of Persian Sign Language. She will always be remembered for her contributions to the Iranian Deaf Community, particularly the research done for the Persian Sign Language dictionary.

Deaf Associations and Organizations

Many deaf people who established deaf organizations came from the more than fifteen Baghcheban deaf schools in Tehran. It was common for deaf people to have a social life and to do activities together after graduation as part of deaf culture. They also established deaf organizations after graduation in other cities, such as Isfahan, Tabriz, Mashhad, Zahdan, Kermanshah, Ahvaz, Dezfool, and others. The deaf organizations became more popular when members could get involved in many different kinds of deaf sports. A few members who graduated from the universities in Iran became leaders of the Iranian deaf communities.

There are several deaf organizations and associations: Iranian National Center for the Deaf (Canon Karolalhay Iran), Association of Deaf Families (Anjoman Khanevadeh Nashenavayan), Iranian Deaf Sports Federation (Federation Varzeshi Nashenavayan Iran), Iranian Parents Association of the Deaf (Jammiat Oliay Nashenavayan Iran), Youth Palace (Kakh Javanan), Youth Cultural House of the Deaf (Anjoman Park Shafagh), and the House of the Deaf. There were also a few deaf organizations that later collapsed because of lack of support and political conflict. Those were the Iranian National Association for Welfare of the Deaf (Sazman Meli Refah Nashenavayan Iran), Sandbags of Literacy for the Deaf Organization (Sazman Sangar Roshanfeker Nashenavay Iran), and the Society for the Protection of Deaf Children.

The most important deaf organizations are the Iranian National Center for the Deaf and the House of the Deaf. These organizations provide assistance to deaf people regardless of their income during the joined political and religious regime. Examples are (1) Iranian females getting together for a cup of tea and networking with each other to gain communication access to hearing agencies, (2) pantomime, playacting, and storytelling by deaf actors and actresses, (3) workshops on crafts such as sewing and knitting, (4) computer literacy and training workshops, (5) education and exposure of hearing people and agencies about deaf culture and the abilities of deaf people to assimilate into hearing society, (6) arranged marriages, wedding parties, and funerals, including donations and financial assistance for deaf people who cannot afford them otherwise, and (7) deaf people traveling to the holy cities in Syria and Turkey to pay respect to the imams or Islamic leaders' graves, particularly those who were assassinated.

Conclusion

In conclusion, the education of deaf people in Iran has a long history and a strong influence over all of Iran. It was due to the pioneering efforts of Baghcheban, Samineh, Julia, and others like them. The results of their actions had a favorable effect on many deaf Iranian individuals and groups. Regardless of recent religious and political conflicts, deaf schools have been operational and have experienced constant expansion throughout Iran.

Acknowledgments

Thanks are due to Rebecca Orton and Mary Thornley, tutors at English Works!/Tutoring and Instructional Programs at Gallaudet University, for their editing contributions; to Deaf studies professors Arlene Kelly, Dirksen Bauman, and Benjamin Bahan for supervision and advice in my internship, to the Centre of Global Education director, Robert Mobley, for work supervision and financial support for travel, and to Lindsay Dunn, special assistant to the president, for his advice on my internship. For more information about Iranian deaf culture, visit the Web site http://www.geocities.com/abehmanesh/Abbas.htm.

References

Baghcheban-Pirnazar, Samineh. "Challenge in the Past and the Future." Presentation at Gallaudet University, Washington, DC, November 1993.
Baghcheban-Pirnazar, Samineh. Interview by author (e-mail), 2001 and 2002.
Baghcheban-Pirnazar, Samineh. Interview by author (written correspondence), 1997, 2000, 2001, and 2002. Washington DC.
Ghahrman, Rouzbeh. Interview by author, August, 2001.
Ghahrman, Rouzbeh. Interview by author (e-mail), 2001 and 2002.
Ghahrman, Rouzbeh. Interview by author (written notes), 2001 and 2002.
Ghazarbekian, Bonnie. "Iran's Gardener of Little Flowers." Paper presented at Deaf World Convention in Tehran, Iran, October 1977. Available from http://www.geocities.com/abehmanesh/BaghchebanDen/JabbarBio.htm.
Mahdavi, Habib. Interview by author (written notes), August, 2001.

Mahmoudi, Reza. Interview by author (written notes), August, 2001.
Mosavi, Muhsen. Interview by author (written notes), August, 2001.
Pirozi, Morteza. Interview by author (written notes), August, 2001.
Tehranizadeh, Habib. Interview by author (written notes), August, 2001.
Vazir Safavi, Ali. Interview by author (written notes), August, 2001.
Zahmati, Mohammad Reza. Interview by author (written notes), August, 2001.

Our Civil Rights Movements: A Guide for All

KELBY BRICK

To fully implement the deaf civil rights movement, it is important to look at the civil rights movements of other groups to understand their advocacy efforts and strategies so that we can copy successful advocacy strategies and learn from others' mistakes. The earliest group was the National Association for the Advancement of Colored People (NAACP), which was established in 1909. One of its main objectives is to advocate against discrimination imposed upon its group. How did the group do it? It filed lawsuits against the offenders and litigated court cases on various issues including employment, housing, and education, among others. Even so, the NAACP realized that filing lawsuits was not sufficient to accomplish its goals. It needed more power and unity and needed to get more people involved in its efforts. Members contacted other minority groups and established a coalition of organizations, called the Leadership Conference on Civil Rights (LCCR), in 1950. The LCCR coalition was composed of thirty organizations including different women's organizations, religious organizations, and ethnic minority organizations. With the LCCR coalition, the NAACP, as well as each minority group, attains the desired power by working together as a large group, advocating for the same issues against discrimination and for equality.

One of their biggest successes was the U.S. Supreme Court's favorable ruling in the 1954 case, *Brown v. Board of Education of Topeka*. For many years, there were two separate school systems, one for blacks and the other for whites. This usually meant that black schools did not get their fair share of educational funding for staff, books, and buildings. Segregated schools also promoted a sense of inferiority for those schools serving black students. The Supreme Court agreed that the segregated school systems were "separate but not equal" and ruled that there should be no segregated school systems.

The coalition also went to the U.S. Congress and advocated for the enactment of various laws including the Civil Rights Act of 1957. There were some weaknesses in the act, so they came back and advocated the inclusion of new language to strengthen the act, not once but twice over several years, leading to the enactment of the Civil Rights Acts of 1960 and 1964.

How did they get the attention and support from many people on these significant issues described? They were involved in a number of public demonstrations and marches that received a lot of attention. One of the two well-known marches occurred in Washington, D.C., in 1963, where the Rev. Martin Luther King gave his famous "I Have a Dream" speech, in which he described his dream that all the people would be treated equally, regardless of race, gender, and physical appearances. The other well-known march, the Selma-to-Montgomery March, occurred two years later in 1965. The protest march took several days from Selma to the state capitol building in Montgomery, Alabama, and marchers demanded the right to vote as citizens. The U.S. Congress was under pressure to respond and passed the Voting Rights Act of 1965 within a few months.

These marches were effective in raising public awareness of and support for issues in education, employment, and housing. Members of Congress were pressured to respond positively to resolve inequality. A number of laws were passed over the years, including the Fair Housing Act of 1968, which bans the discriminatory practice of excluding certain individuals from living in a house or apartment on the basis of race or gender.

Let us now look our movement. I refer to "deaf" people in an all-inclusive sense: people who are deaf, hard of hearing, late deafened, and deaf-blind.

The National Association of the Deaf (NAD) was established in 1880, or twenty-nine years before the establishment of the NAACP. It is the first and oldest organization representing people with disabilities in the United States and the largest organization representing individuals with hearing loss. Like the NAACP, the NAD was established to advocate for equal rights in education, employment, telecommunications, housing, health care, and social services.

The NAD has experienced many struggles in its advocacy efforts and acknowledged the need to work with a larger group of people to give it a more powerful stance and to heighten public awareness. A coalition of organizations, called the Consumer Action Network (CAN) and now known as the Deaf and Hard of Hearing Consumer Advocacy Network (DHHCAN), was built. The coalition includes a variety of deafness-related organizations representing deaf and hearing people in several areas such as sports, religion, deaf racial minority groups, parents, interpreters, and others.

Through the NAD's advocacy efforts over many years, a number of federal laws were enacted, including the Rehabilitation Act in 1973. The Rehabilitation Act essentially mandates that any organization or entity that receives federal funding must make its programs and services accessible to deaf and other disabled individuals. Key sections of the Rehabilitation Act are as follows:

§501: Affirmative Action: Federal Employees
§502: Architectural and Transportation Barriers Compliance Board (ATBCB)
§503: Affirmative Action: Federal Contractors
§504: Any Federal $ = Non-Discrimination

The Rehabilitation Act also provides funds and support for programs and training for disabled individuals for gainful employment.

In the area of education, there have been problems with access for children with disabilities at public schools. Deaf children not enrolled at schools for deaf students experienced serious barriers to communication at public schools that do not provide qualified interpreters, note takers, captioned videos, and other support services. In response, the U.S. Congress passed the Education for all Handicapped Children Act in 1975, now known as the Individuals with Disabilities Education Act (IDEA). The law requires that public school programs must make the necessary accommodations to ensure equal access to education for all children with disabilities. Otherwise, federal funding would be withheld from schools and programs.

After 1975, it was relatively quiet on the legislative front until after the week-long Deaf President Now (DPN) protest in 1988. As some of you probably remember, the DPN protest at Gallaudet University drew a lot of attention and support from many people not only in America but from around the world as well. During the protest, the students shut down Gallaudet University to protest the Gallaudet Board's decision not to select a qualified deaf president. There were marches in Washington, D.C., interviews with newspaper and television reporters, presentations made at the steps of the U.S. Capitol, and meetings with certain members of the U.S. Congress. Initially, the students started the protest, with support from the National Association of the Deaf, but by the end of the week, many organizations—including Gallaudet alumni, faculty, and staff; local and national deaf and hard of hearing organizations; disabled individuals organizations; and even labor unions—announced their support for the DPN protest, contributed money, and joined the students in the protest. This earth-shattering protest has no equal in heightening public awareness and sensitivity to discrimination and oppression experienced not only by deaf people but by all individuals with disabilities as well.

After the DPN protest, a number of significant laws were enacted. One of them was the well-known Americans with Disabilities Act of 1990 (ADA). There are several titles in the act. In employment in government agencies or private businesses, individuals with disabilities cannot be discriminated against, and they must be provided equal opportunities to gain employment. In access to government or public buildings, offices, sports arenas, and so forth, necessary accommodations must be made so that individuals with disabilities have equal access to these facilities. In telecommunications, telephone relay services (TRS) must be established so that deaf individuals can use the greater telecommunications network to make calls to their doctors, or to order pizzas, just like anyone else. Today, with the new video technology, we are able to use videophone to make calls through a video relay operator, using our natural language, sign language. The ADA also mandates equal access in other areas including transportation, health care, libraries, and other for-profit or not-for-profit organizations and facilities.

The Television Decoder Circuitry Act of 1991 (TDCA) mandates that all televisions with screen size 13 inches or larger that are manufactured in or imported into the United States must include a built-in captioning decoder chip. Previously we had to purchase an expensive external captioning decoder to watch closed captions at home or bring it with us when traveling, because most hotels and motels do not have the external captioning decoders. The built-in decoder chip is relatively cheap, and now most hotels and motels have them. As it turns out, many hearing people enjoy this closed captioning feature as well, including many senior citizens with progressive hearing loss. An increasing number of restaurants, bars, and sports arenas turn on the captions on their large video screens so that people can follow the conversations in a noisy place or from a distance.

The Telecommunications Act of 1996—a large telecommunications deregulation act that allows telephone or cable companies to provide a bundle of phone, data, and video services—includes a number of provisions mandating telecommunications access for individuals with disabilities in several areas. As described previously, the TDCA requires that built-in decoders be installed in televisions but does not require any minimum amount of programs to be captioned. The Telecommunications Act includes language requiring a schedule of increased captioning over several years that it would start at a minimum of 25 percent, before increasing to 50 percent, then to 75 percent, and then finally approximating 100 percent by the year 2006. Only a few local programs operating on shoestring budgets may be exempted from the required captioning.

Now, let us compare the similarities between efforts promoting racial equality for African Americans and efforts promoting equal access for deaf people. Initially, the NAACP advocated alone, before building a coalition, the LCCR, for greater power and unity. Similarly, the NAD, after years of advocacy work, found it advantageous to build a deafness-related coalition, the CAN, to do more on the legislative agenda. Both the NAACP and NAD are alike in that each organization advocates for affirmative action in employment. They both know that employment opportunities are important, because without jobs people would not have any money, which means no money for housing or food and ultimately no money for quality education.

Both groups and their respective communities relied on public events to heighten public awareness. African Americans' efforts, including their marches in Washington, D.C., and from Selma to Montgomery, eventually led to the enactment of several federal civil rights laws. Likewise, deaf people made at least two DPN protest marches in Washington, D.C., within a week, which eventually led to the enactment of several federal laws promoting disability access and equality. To be sure, both groups have had other marches not mentioned here. These events have proven to be very effective strategies for both groups.

Both groups have advocated for equality in education. One of the NAACP's early actions was to promote equality in education, as indicated in the favorable Supreme Court ruling in the landmark case, *Brown v. Board of Education*, against segregated schools. Although the law promotes educational equality, because of some economic factors full equality has not yet been achieved for African American children. Similarly, the IDEA promotes education equality for deaf children by requiring full access to communication at public schools. However, because of some shortages of support services, accessible materials, and qualified interpreters, full equality has not yet been realized for deaf students at the public schools.

There have been a number of federal laws passed promoting equality in housing, health services, and other areas that were advocated for by each group. Each deaf group looked at the language of various civil rights acts promoting racial equality and used essentially the same language for similar laws promoting rights and access for deaf people and individuals with disabilities, but with references to deaf individuals or individuals with disabilities instead of references to race or minority groups. For example, the ADA copied a lot of legislative language from the Civil Rights Act of

1964. The copying is done not because we are lazy. On the contrary, copying is an important strategy for use. Why reinvent the wheel, when there already is an effective language for an important law that we want to emulate? More important, when we approach members of the U.S. Congress for their support, we are better able to convince them that there is nothing new in the bill, because essentially the law has already been passed for another minority group. Why should our group be treated differently, merely because of our individual disability? Congress then is very likely to give the support we need.

Again, I cannot stress enough the importance of using other legislation to take down the barriers we need to overcome. If we do that by using practically the same language and were questioned or challenged by a member of Congress or by a government official, then we could ask why we are being treated differently. We could ask whether we are not deserving of an equal status. We could argue that all individuals should be treated equally, irrespective of individual disability. Most often that works well for us. The same strategy can work in other countries.

Have we achieved the long-term successes that we had sought?

Poverty rates have slightly decreased and median income has slightly increased for minority groups and individuals with disabilities. However, they are still far from being comparable with the entire population. Unemployment and underemployment are still major issues. There has been a large increase in the number of government employees who are members of a minority group or who are individuals with disabilities. One should not underestimate the importance of government employment, because it leads to many good things. Government employees are better able to gain experience and knowledge of how government works and then share what they have learned with their groups. Also, many of them eventually leave the government sector, enter the private sector, and establish businesses providing services and products beneficial to their groups. Many of these businesses have contracts to provide services or products to government agencies, too. We have seen that happen with deaf individuals here, who started with government employment before entering the private sector.

There are many deaf students being mainstreamed in isolation. In spite of the IDEA, most programs of "one" do not provide the necessary support services or communication access to a single deaf student. For deaf students to obtain total education inside and outside of classroom, there is a need for critical mass found at large programs serving deaf students within a public school system or at schools for deaf students. The meaning of "most appropriate education" evidently needs to be strengthened especially as it relates to deaf students. Better education for deaf students results in better employment opportunities for them, and this in turn results in better quality of life with comfortable housing and healthy eating.

We have seen a large increase in the number of elected government officials among African Americans, Hispanics, women, and other minority groups. They have been elected at local levels (city council, mayor, etc.), state levels (legislature, governor, directors, etc.), and federal levels (Congress, federal officials, etc.). Unfortunately, however, currently there are no elected deaf officials in America. As far as I know, historically, there were only two deaf elected officials in America. One was elected in a small town in Virginia many, many years ago. The other one, named Kevin Nolan, whom I personally know as a good friend, was elected to a three-year term in a city council in a small town in Massachusetts about fifteen years ago. Right now there are no deaf individuals in elected offices. Where are they?

It was heartening to watch the plenary presentation made this morning by a deaf member of the South African parliament, Wilma Newhoudt-Druchen. I believe there were few deaf government officials in other countries. We need many more of them. Why is it important to have government officials? When we meet with government officials, we often have to struggle to convince them of the importance of our issues. We have always been working from the outside. Deaf officials could gather up support from within for our cause.

It is extremely difficult to get deaf people elected. The deaf candidates need to represent both the deaf and hearing constituencies to have a fighting chance of getting elected. Each of us needs to give all-out support to a potential deaf candidate, by volunteering, contributing monies to the candidate's campaign, distributing flyers, and putting up signs. It would be great if we could get a good number of deaf elected officials so that we could have them working on our behalf from within the government system.

In spite of some of the shortcomings, we should appreciate all the efforts deaf organizations, deaf leaders, and deaf people—and our hearing friends—have done to bring us to where we are now. But as you can see, our work is far from finished. We must continue to work.

Houses out of Sand: Building a Deaf Community in Israel

MEIR ETEDGI

Israel was established as an independent state in 1948. A few years before, a Deaf club was established in 1944, named the Jewish Association for the Deaf and Dumb in Tel Aviv. In its early days, the association functioned as a community center, which housed a variety of social and cultural activities.

There are many different ways that I could talk about the history of the Deaf community in Israel. As an architect, I present a particular view of the relationship between the community and the buildings that have housed its institutions, mentioning also how those are related to the early buildings of the state. In tracing the history of this Deaf community and its headquarters, many fundamental questions arise: What is a community? What makes it a community? Could the Deaf community survive without a building in which to meet?

There are very few articles or written documents about the history of the Deaf community in Israel. It is the people themselves, the elder members of the community, who can unfold its history for us. I have interviewed many senior Deaf adults and share our history from an architectural perspective, because there is a relationship between the development of the buildings and the growth of the Deaf community.

In the 1930s in Tel Aviv, there was a big expansion in buildings because there were a lot of Jewish immigrants coming to Israel. It was called the "white city" because of all the cement that was used in the building of the city, and the buildings were painted in white.

The Jewish people arrived for two reasons. First, because of ideological reasons, they wanted to go back to their Jewish roots. The second, more important reason is because of the widespread anti-Semitism that forced them to look for a safe haven.

There was a large influx of immigrants, some of whom were Deaf. Deaf people came and expected to find other Deaf people and Deaf culture like they had in Europe. However, there were very few Deaf people in the country then and no place for them to gather and meet.

Israel Savir told me that the "the European immigrants thus would go to the movie theaters to meet and socialize with each other. They would also meet in restaurants. At that time, there was no common language and it was difficult to communicate with each other or with hearing people. There was no access to interpreters, either."

Deaf people needed to find a reliable way to transfer information between them. They found an original solution: In the center of Tel Aviv, there was large plaza, where many people would pass by daily. One of the people who came to the plaza regularly was a Deaf shoe shiner, who sat there and polished the shoes of the passers-by. Because he was located in such a central place, he became a one-person communication or information center. That is, Deaf people would leave messages with the shoe shiner, and he then would relay or share the messages to other Deaf people who came by.

I interviewed one of the central figures in the emerging Deaf community, Moshe Bamberger. Mr. Bamberger was born in Frankfurt and went to a school for Deaf students in Berlin. I asked him why he came to Israel at 1943. As a teenager, he was inspired by a book written by Theodor Herzl, titled *Altneuland* (*Old New Land*). He came to Israel and immediately tried to find out how to meet other Deaf people. He met a former teacher from his old school in Berlin, Richard B. Hexter, who immigrated to Israel and became the principal of the first school for Deaf students in the country, founded in 1932. Mr. Hexter gave Mr. Bamberger the addresses of some Deaf people. Moshe Bamaberger went to those addresses in Jerusalem and met a few Deaf people. From a core of eight people, the community began to grow. Then several members of the community moved to Tel Aviv, and Tel Aviv became a meeting place. Deaf people started to meet every Friday at a restaurant. They also had Hanukkah parties and played games.

Keep in mind that this was in 1944. At the time Israel was under British occupation. Any kind of private organization needed to have approval from the British protectorate. The hard core of the Deaf community numbered forty-four members, who worked very hard to get a lawyer to write a constitution for their organization. The British officials approved it, and the municipality gave the Deaf people permission to use a gymnasium as a meeting place. That was, at that time, the Deaf center or club.

Many Deaf people could not read or write, so they turned to some of the older members of the community for help. One of those people was Haim Apter, who had immigrated to Israel in 1933, right before Germany ended emigration for Jews.

Mr. Apter was a tailor, and he opened a tailoring business in Tel Aviv. Deaf people came to his house, and he spent so much time translating for them and helping them with the language that he gave up his profession as a tailor and began exclusively working with Deaf people.

During that time, in 1944, the association formulated its statute, which constituted a major milestone in the formation of the Deaf community in Israel. The document is of great importance to this day, because it reflects the early days of the community. The statute has five sections, and I give a short description of each one of them.

The first section dealt with who could become a member of the organization. Most people were new immigrants.

The second section focused on the social benefits and rights of working Deaf people. At that time, Deaf people were not aware of their rights. For example, they were often not paid for overtime. This section of the statute explicitly demanded the improvement of the working conditions of Deaf people.

The third section discussed cultural activities, such as learning Hebrew, learning the Bible, history, and taking field trips. For example, Deaf people could not read

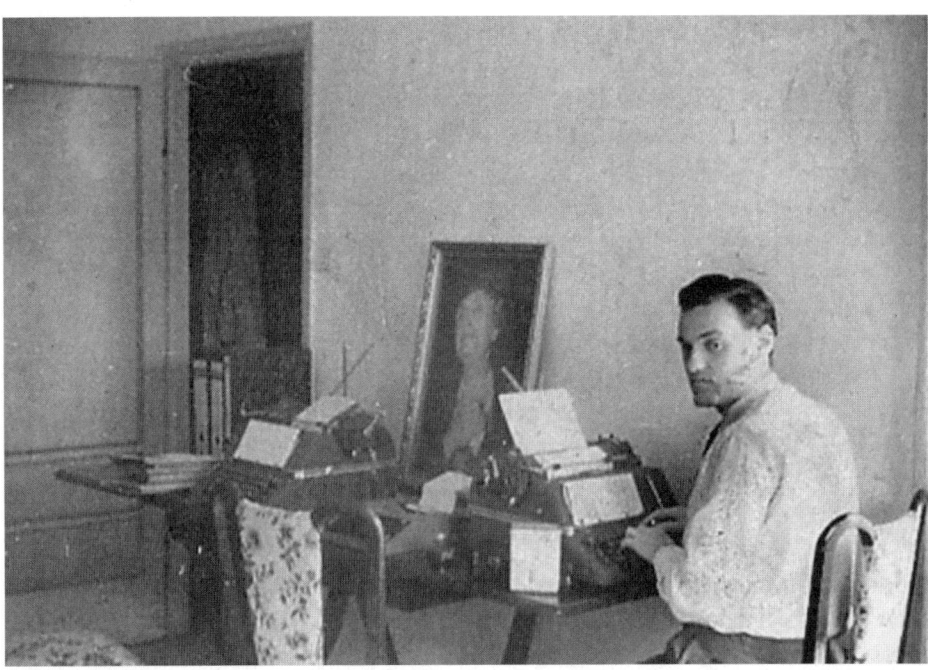

Haim Apter

Hebrew. They would come to the club and learn to read and write Hebrew. In addition, they had different theatrical events, played ping-pong, and went to the beach.

The fourth section had to do with Deaf awareness and explained to hearing people who Deaf people were and how they communicated using sign language. A central issue at that time was the inability of Deaf people to get driving licenses. Deaf people were very frustrated because they were not allowed to drive, which seemed to them to be a very ridiculous prohibition. Deaf people were seen as ignorant and therefore unable to drive. However, the association came across a study that showed that Deaf drivers are safer drivers, better drivers, and more careful drivers than hearing drivers. The association showed the report to the government, and the government finally allowed Deaf people to get driving licenses.

The fifth section discussed contact with different Jewish organizations outside of the state of Israel and the possibility of some cultural interchange. Interestingly, from 1944 until 1957, not much really happened in that arena except for tourists coming to visit Israel. That seemed to be the only contact at that time. For example, a delegation of Deaf people from South Africa visited Israel during that period. After 1957, the first Deaf Israeli basketball team went to the Deaf Olympics in Milan. This was the first event in which an official delegation represented the Israeli Deaf association.

In the first general meeting of the Deaf association, held in February 1944, the constitution was confirmed by the members, and an executive committee was appointed. Moshe Bamberger, standing on the stage with a poster of Theodor Herzel in the back, gave a speech in which he asked for "full support, both physically and spiritually, for the new association."

The new association needed a logo, so a competition was held to that end. Most of the suggestions were characterized by Jewish symbols—the Star of David, the Torah, and a branch of an olive tree. The logo that eventually won was shaped as an arch, with the name of the association, "The Association of Deaf and Mute," written in it. Below that, there is a phrase that says, "Be Strong and Be Brave," which was intended to give Deaf people hope. To this day, we use the sign of the arch to refer to the Deaf Association.

In 1948, the War of Independence broke out. The Deaf club had to stop its activities, and Deaf people once more had to meet at coffee shops, restaurants, or other informal places. They realized that they needed a permanent home where people could meet, but they also realized that they needed help and support from hearing people. They invited several members of the Kneset (the Israeli Parliament) to their meetings. The entire community took part in the efforts to raise money for building a home for the association.

Two events that took place in those years are considered significant in the process of building the Deaf club. The first was the screening of the movie *Johnny Belinda*, which tells of the hard life of a deaf young woman in the United States at the beginning of the twentieth century. The movie was quite popular, and many Deaf as well as hearing people saw it. One copy of the movie was donated to the Deaf association, which held a special screening open to the general public, with all the proceeds going to the building fund.

The second major event took place in 1952. It was Helen Keller's visit to Israel. During her one-week visit, she gave lectures in various places. She agreed to give a talk for the Deaf association, which gave Deaf people the chance to talk to her. Helen said "that the life of deaf people is very difficult, more difficult than the life of blind people." Her interpreter used tactile finger spelling to convey to Helen what the people in the audience said, but Helen Keller could also tactilely lipread her interpreter, which astonished and inspired the Deaf audience. She was a role model and a very inspiring person.

One of the issues that had to be resolved was the location of the future Deaf center. Some people suggested that it should be located in the center of Tel Aviv, whereas others suggested the outskirts. Most Deaf people preferred a central location, but the public committee voted for the outskirts, because they knew that Tel Aviv was a growing city and that soon peripheral locations would become integral parts of the city. The architect who designed the building was very old and wanted to retire, but the Deaf people begged him to take this project on himself. He agreed, and this was his last project.

In December 1953, the cornerstone-laying ceremony for the building took place, which was attended by many people. Although it was a very hot day, people kept coming, including people from the Deaf community and important people from the government and other authorities. Rachel Yanait Ben Zvi, wife of the president of Israel, congratulated the audience. Rabbi Toledano, the chief rabbi of Tel Aviv-Jaffa, gave a speech as well.

There were no sign language interpreters then to interpret the speeches for the Deaf audience. We tried to figure out how to convey the content of the speakers' presentations in signs. A Deaf person read the written script of the speeches and then signed them in Israeli Sign Language.

Houses out of Sand

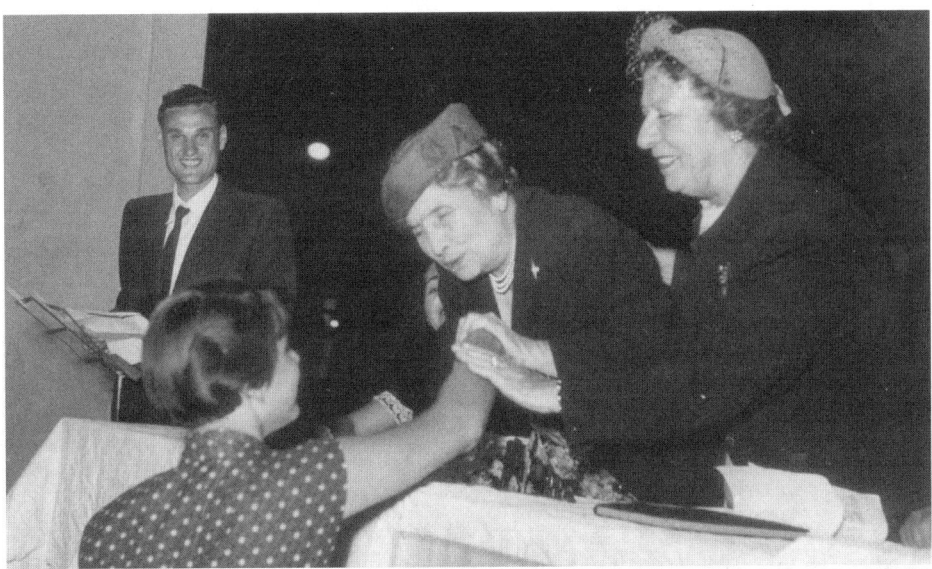

Helen Keller (center) and Haim Apter (far left)

In the period that followed the ceremony, the rest of the building was built. The finished building was in white concrete, very much like the rest of Tel Aviv. It was functional, clean, and simple. It contained offices, a lecture hall that holds hundreds of people, dorms, and the Deaf club. The opening celebration took place in 1958, after the completion of the building. Both the Israeli and the American flags decorated the building. Many American people donated money for the building, so we wanted to honor them by displaying their flag.

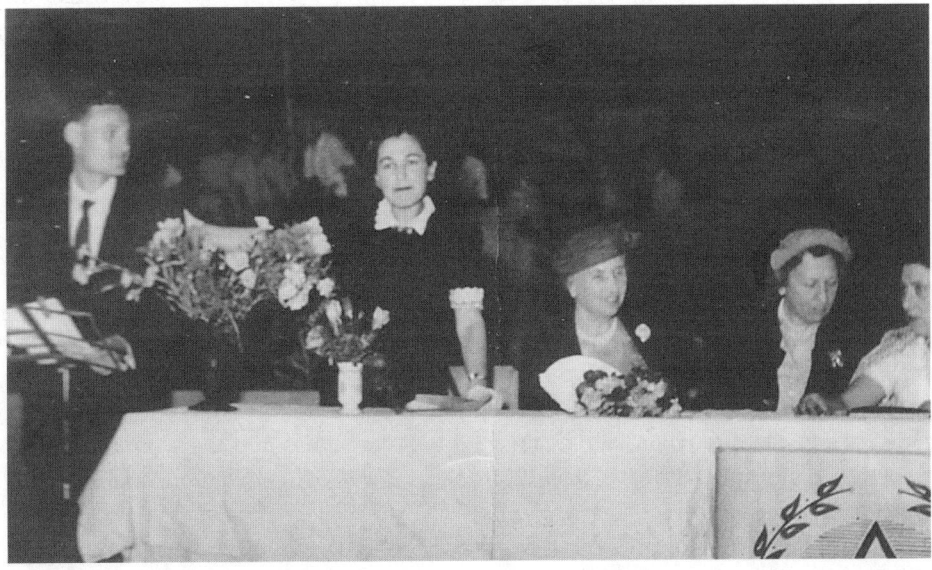

Helen Keller

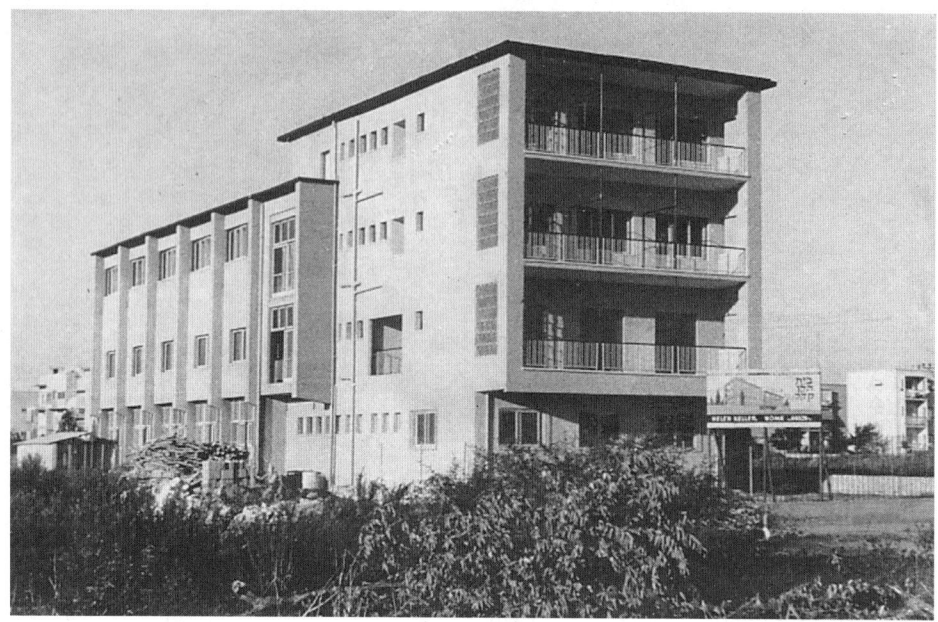

Helen Keller Home

My father told me that he lived in the dorms as a young man. The dorms and the Deaf club were situated in different parts of the building. When he wanted to talk with Deaf people at the club on the other side of the building, he would sneak around through the porch at night so that the security people could not see him. He would chat with the Deaf people and then sneak back into his dorm.

We named the building the Helen Keller Home. We used the term *home* rather than *house* or *institute* because a house is just a place to live, but a home has more intimacy and warmth. Many Deaf people were very inspired by this home, which has become a new symbol for Deaf people.

The next project was another building for the Deaf community in Beersheba. Other clubs were built in Haifa and Jerusalem. The one in Beersheba was municipally funded. It collapsed in an earthquake some years ago.

We see that the Deaf clubs and communities developed in the major cities—Tel Aviv, Haifa, Jerusalem, and Beer Sheva. I was curious to know whether there were any attempts to build a Deaf community in the periphery, such as a Deaf village or a Deaf kibbutz. In the 1960s, the Deaf association bought a small motel in Mitzpe Ramon, a tiny town in the middle of the Negev area in the southern part of the country. The place was run by a group of Deaf people. This went hand in hand with Ben Gurion's vision of populating and transforming the desert into a lively community. However, in the desert area the distance to the main cities and the separation from the Deaf community made it too hard for the people in Mitzpe Ramon, and the place was closed down after two years.

I found a document presenting some statistics of the young Deaf community. In 1944, there was a large influx of immigrants. In the 1960s, the association had fifteen hundred members. A census shows how the Deaf community developed through that period.

Today, the story of the establishment and building of the Deaf community teaches us of the vision that led to its creation and development, the events that have shaped us. Every person is nourished by his or her past, and if we do not heed our past, it will be difficult for us to make sense of our present existence. This essay is a first attempt to develop a discussion in order to understand our past and how all these things affect us today. More than anything else, this reveals the importance of documentation through historical research. The history of the community teaches us that part of our desires and ambitions have not yet been realized, and we must continue to try and realize them in new ways.

I thank Moshe Bamberger, the family of Haim and Mazal Apter in Israel, Hava and Israel Shavir, Ezra and Ester Levi, for their assistance in the research. Special thanks to the Institute for the Advancement of the Deaf in Israel.

AUDIENCE: As far as Palestine or the Arab Deaf are concerned, do the Arab Deaf come together with the Jewish Deaf, or are they separate?

MEIR: That is really a good question. You cannot ignore the Palestinians. And our community is a community of Deaf people. There are a few Palestinian Deaf people who are involved in our organization. In Palestinian culture, the Deaf people are not encouraged to go outside their home. That is really a very separate topic. I do not know their language, and I cannot speak about or for them. They would need to do that for themselves.

AUDIENCE: Actually I have two questions. The first question is regarding Israel as a state, and Israeli Sign Language. Is Israeli Sign Language a real language and has the government recognized it? My second question is about the Israeli Deaf community. What is their agenda for the coming years?

MEIR: You have to remember Israel is only fifty years old, compared to the United States, which is more than two hundred. Deaf people want to be accepted the same as others, as Deaf people in other countries. Your second question was about our future agenda. Before there was only one place Deaf people could go to socialize or get information. Now there is much more freedom and choices available. People need to pick their own identities just as the same people need to select their own shoes. Admittedly, because of many choices these days, Deaf associations' power seem to be eroding somewhat. That is why it is important for Deaf history to be preserved and to be a living part of our world.

AUDIENCE: I am Marla Berkowitz, and I have a question about the Deaf association. You are saying that, unfortunately, the society is eroding. Could you talk a little bit about the reasons for this? Also I am wondering if the Deaf communities in different cities collaborate with one another. How are they receiving information about what is happening in the war?

MEIR: Regarding your first question about the association, more and more people are spreading outside of the cities, more than five thousand people, and so the original constitution for the organization does not seem to fit the way life is currently. It does not seem to be as relevant. It will take time to change things and adjust. It will not happen abruptly. I do feel that there will be positive advances for the association in the future.

Now, to your second question: there is not much bombing in Tel Aviv. Currently people use videophones for communication. There is a twenty-four-hour relay service that is open using the videophones. Not that many people have this service, but some do, and some interpreters are used. If Deaf people know how to use the Internet, then they can have access to the latest information. There needs to be a lot more research as far as that is concerned. We have instant messaging similar to your pagers that you have here in the States, plus we have television such as CNN, but that program is not fully captioned.

AUDIENCE: I have a friend from Israel who is here. I have a couple of questions. Somebody just mentioned the bombing, and I want to know if any Deaf people have been hurt in any of the bombings, to your knowledge. Second, in talking about Deaf culture in Israel, you did not really say much about how Deaf culture got itself established in Israel. You were talking about people coming from Germany and coming from all these different countries to congregate in Israel, but how did the Deaf culture get itself established in Israel?

MEIR: You see people walking and they could be Deaf, they could be hearing, and if they sign, is that culture? If a hearing person or a Deaf person were walking on the street, to the uninitiated, they look the same. But once one lifts one's hands, significant differences are noticed. There is a divide between the two, and what is involved in culture is language behavior. What you see in the lecture was something where you see Deaf people trying to build their own identity in a new land. Her question was if you have Deaf people from Russia, Deaf people from different countries, coming all to one country, what does their Deaf culture look like? You need to understand the atmosphere during most of this period from 1948 onward after the war for independence. At this time in 1948, people, both Deaf and hearing, came and worked together to produced an "integrated" person and a culture together. They developed their own unique culture together.

The Status of Deaf People in Developing Countries

RAPHAEL DOMINGO

This essay introduces the history of the Filipino Deaf people as a valuable record and model for young Deaf people. Many Filipino Deaf people achieved remarkable goals, but because these achievements were not recorded, they are not recognized as historical facts. I hope to recognize and record the history of Filipino Deaf people by collecting and preserving data provided by organizations, individuals, and service providers and by so doing, hope that there will be positive changes in perception of both Deaf and hearing people.

Individuals and service providers have been interviewed on video (including five out of forty-eight Deaf achievers in leadership, career, human rights, and beauty pageants, five of whom I'll describe here) and their written documents have been examined. They tell us how they went through hardships and successes in from their childhoods throughout their lives

One of our valuable recognizable leaders is Pedro M. Santos, who founded the Philippine Association of the Deaf (PAD) in 1926. It is high time that we give credit and due recognition to him. Santos was born in Atlag, Malolos, Bulacan, on May 20, 1900. He became Deaf when he was seriously ill with a severe cold and high fever as a child. He graduated from the School for the Deaf and Blind; as a student he showed such exceptional talent, keen intellect, and bright promise for the future that the school decided to send him to the United States for further studies. He had the distinction of being the first and only Filipino deaf *pensionado* sent by the Philippine government to study at the Gallaudet College in Washington, D.C. On his return to the Philippines in 1921, he was offered a teaching job at the School for the Deaf and Blind (SDB) in Pasay, Rizal (now Pasay City) with twelve Deaf pupils under his supervision and instruction. Aware of the deplorable and miserable condition of the Deaf population in his country, not to mention the unsympathetic attitude of a few toward them, and further believing in the old adage that "in union there is strength," on October 17, 1926, he gathered some of the Deaf graduates from the SDB to form an association that would look after their interest and well-being. Thus, the PAD was born. He became the first president and held that post in the association until the outbreak of World War II. One of his noble ambitions in life was to see the day when he could point his finger and claim, "That is the building of the deaf, by the deaf, and for the deaf!" He had not yet realized his dream when he passed away on May 31, 1970. His indomitable courage will serve as a perennial source of inspiration for all the Deaf people in this part of the globe, and his memory will not fade in the hearts and minds of his associates. The former president of the World Federation of the Deaf (WFD), Dragoljub Vukotic, said, "the Philippine Association of the Deaf belongs among pioneer organizations of the Deaf in the world, which have been the first to start an organized and creative work on satisfying the needs of the Deaf in the sphere of their rehabilitation."

The Katipunan ng May Kapansanan sa Pilipinas, Inc. (KAMPI) once hired a Deaf bookkeeper (who is now a financial officer) after hearing about his two successful cases against the unfair labor practices. His fellow Deaf co-workers relied on his knowledge because of his triumphs in labor court. He is Jose Sales, born in Santiago City, Isabela, on May 4, 1961. His deafness started when he was ten years old, just after finishing third grade in school, and is attributed to high fever and medicine overdose. He graduated from hearing schools, namely Cabulay Elementary School and Santiago Vocational and Industrial School. He was insulted by his classmates from the time of his deafness until fifth grade. When he entered sixth grade, he made a vow to himself that never again would they insult him. They started to make friends with him when they realized that he was improving his studies. Even if he could not hear in the class without an interpreter and often relied on visuals and written instructions, he did very well. He was valedictorian from sixth grade through the fourth year of high school. What fascinated them was that he bested them all despite being the only Deaf student in a class of about two hundred hearing students. His parents decided to send him to the city of Manila for college. After two years in FEATI University, he majored in fine arts as an undergraduate and worked part time in a furniture firm, advancing from utility helper to quality controller. He completed computer studies at the STI College, where he majored in accounting. He was then promoted to work in a recruitment agency as a filing clerk under the same manager.

After eleven years of employment in that agency, he was terminated unfairly, leaving him with no recourse but to file a complaint in labor court for unfair labor practices against him. The hearing of his case took about four years, during which he nearly lost, but he fought for his rights until he won. His former employer paid for his termination pay and back wages. Before his labor court case was finally concluded, he found work in a bank as a money counter and sorter, together with about fifty-two Deaf people, some of whom had worked there three to five years. At that time, he started to learn sign language through his fellow Deaf co-workers. When they learned of his triumph in Labor Court, his Deaf co-workers started to inform him of maltreatment and abuse in the bank, including nonregularization of employment, lower pay, sexual harassment, and unfair deductions. They complained to the bank for almost one year to no avail, so the majority of the Deaf workers filed a class suit in the labor court. This action led to their termination, one after the other. It took them about six years in labor court litigation. They lost in the lower courts, and so they brought their case to the Supreme Court, which reversed the ruling of the lower courts by applying the passage from the Magna Carta for Persons with Disabilities in the Philippines. They finally won (S. Jose, personal communication, 2001).

Her students, friends, and even hearing co-workers went to her for counseling help when she taught at the Catholic Ministry to Deaf People, Inc. It took her a long time to enter her final career as a mental health counselor. She is Maria Tanya Lindain de Guzman, who was born in Pasig, Rizal, on July 16, 1972, to her beloved Deaf parents Gil P. de Guzman Jr. and Arsenia Lindain and her Deaf eldest sister Maria Theresa de G. Yulo. She became deaf after a falling accident as a child. She was a born leader because her Deaf parents were also very active members of the Filipino Deaf community. She graduated from the Southeast Asian Institute for the Deaf, Technological University of the Philippines, with a bachelor of fine arts in advertising. Imagine how she overcame her painful experiences. Her relatives still looked down on her because of her deafness and poverty, but she overcame this. She served the needs of the Filipino Deaf community by teaching religion, leadership, and gender awareness in Baliwag, Antipolo, and the provinces. She was finally accepted to Gallaudet University, where she is now currently working on a masters of arts in mental health counseling. She is the first Deaf Filipina mental health counselor (G. Maria Tanya, personal communication, 2001).

She reigned as Miss Masskara Queen 1981. Ma. Cecilia C. Villacin was born in Manapla on August 10, 1965, to a hearing family. She graduated from Andres Bonifacio Elementary School; Bacolod City National High School, Bacolod City; and La Salle De University, Bacolod City, where she majored in computer studies. During her high school days, she once played lawn tennis with her fellow hearing schoolmates and she acted exactly like a tomboy. Before the pageant, the board members of Volunteers for the Rehabilitation of the Handicapped and Disabled organization went to her school and visited her class. They asked her to enter the Miss Masskara Queen Pageant 1981 but she declined, so they asked the permission of her mother. Her mother encouraged her to join. Later, she was startled when she met fellow hearing contestants, and she expected to lose because of her deafness. Eventually, she received many awards such as Best in Talent, Miss Congeniality, Miss Photogenic, and Best in Casual Wear, and she finally won the crown as Miss Masskara Queen. She cannot believe that she won the competition against fourteen hearing candidates (V. Cecilia, personal communication, 2001).

Her height, fair complexion, and charm can be seen among the Deaf Filipinas. She is one of several empowered Deaf feminists who pressed a sexual harassment case against a prestigious bank. She is Maritess Raquel A. Estiller and was born in San Luis Nabua, Camarines Sur, on July 24, 1966. She graduated with primary and secondary diplomas from the University of Northeastern Philippines. She is now an emergency laborer (recorder) with eight years of service at the Philippine Postal Corporation. She was very lonely, unloved by children who bullied and abused her when she was child. Her father and grandmother comforted her and encouraged her self-esteem. When she was the only Deaf student in school, she faced many obstacles and wanted to quit her studies because her classmates hurt her pride, but her father told her to be brave and ignore them. She did not give up until she finished high school, in spite of the hostile atmosphere. She found a job in a factory with many Deaf workers and started to learn sign language from them. She was promoted to trainer of new applicants. After three years, she quit working because the chemicals affected her health. She got another job in a prestigious bank as a money sorter, along with many Deaf co-workers. They filed a complaint of sexual harassment against the security guards even though the anti–sexual harassment law was not yet legalized. However, the evidence was very poor, and they lost their the case. Despite this, they eventually won in the labor court because of the bank's unfair labor practices. Recently, Congress approved the proposed anti–sexual harassment law and her case was one they examined before finalizing the legislation (E. Marites Raquel, personal communication, 2001).

Many of these people achieved remarkable goals. They should be recognized as historical figures for future generations. After my presentation in United States and the Philippines, I hope these facts become part of the history of the Filipino Deaf community.

PART SEVEN

Language and Culture

The Domino Effect: Changing Values = Changing Language = New Styles of Training

CLARK DENMARK AND FRANCES ELTON

In the early 1970s there were 330 residential schools for Deaf students scattered throughout the United Kingdom. There are now only 34 such schools left, and often they enroll Deaf children who have disabilities. Nondisabled Deaf children, who would previously have been placed in Deaf schools, are now sent to mainstream facilities or attached units for Deaf children. The latest figures show that the majority are currently in mainstream education (British Association of Teachers of the Deaf, 2003).

Deaf schools were the bedrock for transmission of British Sign Language (BSL) and Deaf culture. Ladd (2003) claims that the Deaf community emerged and developed in these schools and was further strengthened in the Deaf clubs. Changing trends have affected the demographic of Deaf populations. Residential schools usually sprang up in the United Kingdom's principal cities and towns, and this greatly influenced Deaf people's choice of residence after leaving school. Consequently, there were greater numbers of Deaf people and Deaf clubs in the urban areas than in the countryside. People had more frequent contact with each other, and regional variations in BSL saw their heyday during this period. Now, with the emphasis on mainstream placements, Deaf children are more widely scattered throughout the country and separated from their peers; hence the steady decline in regional variation that BSL once enjoyed. This paucity of input and influence from regional residential Deaf schools could bring about a definite move toward a standardized BSL, which will be discussed further later.

Social Life

Changes in education since the Education Act 1981 (Warnock, 1978) meant that more Deaf children stay within their local area and that the umbilical cord that residential Deaf schools and Deaf clubs provided has been lost. Increasingly, Deaf children stay inside the home because they have no peers in the local community and many of them are unaware of the existence of Deaf clubs or the Deaf community. They may know a few other Deaf children at school but have no more contact than that. Deaf clubs are consequently dwindling at an alarming rate, especially in the main cities (Denmark, 2001).

As the younger generation grows up and leaves school, local Deaf clubs are no longer popular. Although most Deaf clubs do have their own bar facilities, young people prefer to meet in mainstream pubs.

Members of the Deaf community have observed that an additional reason for the disappearance of young people in Deaf clubs is that the young people do not wish to take on the responsibilities of running the clubs. They wish to be among their own age group, without older generations telling them what to do or how to behave. Sometimes there are drugs or other illegal substances involved, and they wish to indulge in these without the prying eyes of older Deaf people.

Broader cultural influences are also having an effect, such as wanting to go "clubbing" like other people of their age. Also, as more hearing people learn to sign, younger Deaf people are more comfortable outside the safe haven of Deaf clubs. A painful generation gap is developing within the Deaf community whereby the young tend to respect older people less than before.

Signing styles are also changing. Possible reasons for such changes include that fact that young Deaf people are taught in mainstream schools (or attached units) by teachers who only have beginner-level signing skills (British Deaf Association, 1996). Consequently, signs often have to be invented because the young do not have access to native signers. As a result, some of these new signs have now spread into the Deaf community and have affected the use of BSL.

Language Change

All "living" languages, both spoken and signed, change over time. Significant changes in BSL have been observed in lexical items and the use of mouth patterns and finger spelling (Sutton-Spence & Woll, 1999). In BSL, it is worth noting the effect of the massively increasing numbers of people who now learn the language.

Thousands of hearing (and nonsigning deaf) people learn BSL each year (Council for the Advancement of Communication with Deaf People, 2004). The majority of these attend BSL classes, which are available throughout the country. A large number of the tutors are untrained, and many of the signs used by untrained tutors were created by "language planners" or borrowed from other regions. The result of this is that many "hearing" signs are now being used and have had an influence on signing within the Deaf community through the effects of using communication support.

An additional influence comes in the form of signs adopted from other countries and through the impact of the media and increased access to travel. Recent changes noticed in finger spelling include borrowing from ASL (American Sign Language), whereby certain ASL letters are mixed in with the usual BSL production. An example of this is commonly seen when fingerspelling B. S. L., where the "B. S." is produced using British fingerspelling but the "L" is American. Along with the letter L, frequently borrowed ASL letters include O, C, B, and E. Since the closure of residential schools, there are fewer role models to pass on traditional regional signs and finger spellings.

Media Influences

The media is also a major source of language change. Since 1981, there has been a weekly Deaf magazine program on British television. Consequently, the Deaf community has now had more than twenty years of exposure to some sign language variations that were traditionally more localized. One classic example is the sign NEWS; a Scottish dialect for NEWS is almost standardized now because of its frequent use on television. Similarly, the London sign MOTHER has become widespread.

Styles of BSL production have also changed. One example is the heavy use of finger spelling seen in the early days of television programs compared to the minimal use preferred in more recent times. Three distinct phases of influence have been observable over the past twenty years. The first phase concerned a northern flavor, because presenters were mainly from the north of England or Scotland. In the second phase, more presenters were from the south and from the younger generation. An explosion of overuse of signs, such as one that can be glossed as FANTASTIC or BRILLIANT but came to be used for almost everything positive, is an example of the type of impact seen in this second phase. There was also a move to a wider signing space by younger presenters. During this phase, further influences came from exposure to "in-vision" signers who, until recently, were mainly hearing sign language interpreters. Hence, some English-like grammatical structures became commonplace on television. However, there has recently been a reversal of this trend as a result of increasing numbers of Deaf "in-vision" signers working in this field.

The third phase sees even greater challenges looming. Virtual signers will increasingly replace human "in-vision" signers (Sign Language Channel Working Party, 2003). Who will be the source of all the signs in the database? What type of language structure will develop in this way? What will happen with the advent of the videophone, the use of signs being transmitted electronically, that is, over the phone or the Internet? All of these are bound to affect the use of language—hence, more changes.

Aside from the media, there are also signs borrowed from the European continent or the States, which have become part of our language through increased opportunities for travel. Some examples of these borrowed signs are ATTITUDE (Danish), GOVERNMENT (Scandinavian), and CHARACTER (United States), to name but a few. These signs have now become standardized even though resistance still exists and a renaissance of local signs is being promoted.

All of this can have profound effects on changing styles and attitudes in some professionals, for example, sign language interpreters, BSL tutors, teachers of Deaf students, and sign language users. This, in turn, can cause division and confusion.

Interpreter Training

The examination or assessment format for interpreters has now changed from a more traditional examination to National Vocational Qualifications (NVQs). NVQs are primarily for assessing the application of skills in the workplace. They rely on the assumption that the person already has acquired the necessary skills to an appropriate level and can then produce a work-based portfolio to demonstrate the application of those skills in the relevant domain. The use of NVQs for interpreters has brought about a difficult development in the teaching of BSL. Once students gain a conversational competency, their only choice for language progression is to move into the vocational assessment system. This means that there is very little actual language training at the higher levels, and interpreters are qualifying with much less sign language competency than before. Similarly, the majority of interpreters have difficulties adapting to the use of regional variations and consequently try to standardize some signs.

The new examination format has implications at lower levels of training, too. There is a serious shortage of qualified interpreters in the United Kingdom. Consequently, those who are still developing their skills are also used as interpreters, typically in educational settings but also, to some extent, in health services and other community-related work. Previously, under the old exam system, students would have to achieve stage 2 BSL and be training toward stage 3 to take this kind of work. When these stages were converted to NVQ levels 2 and 3, they were not kept as close equivalents. The NVQ level 3 is only equivalent to the previous stage 2, but the requirement remains that those working in education be training toward level 3, and therefore people go on to become communicators or CSWs (communicator support workers) at a lower level of training than before.

BSL Tutor Training

In 1985 the first BSL tutor training course in the country was established at Durham University in the Deaf Studies Research Unit. This was foundation level training, and it was hoped that further levels (intermediate and advanced) would follow, up to and including the training of interpreters. Unfortunately, this never happened, but a master of arts and an advanced diploma in BSL/English interpreting were established instead. The Deaf Studies Research Unit closed in July 2001, and the tutor training course therefore came to an end. Consequently, there was no intermediate or advanced training for BSL tutors, who were in desperate need of education beyond the foundation level. This situation has not been resolved to date. Since this closure, the provision of tutor training courses has become a serious problem.

The introduction of the new NVQ structure has had serious effects on BSL tutors, who are now being forced into mainstream training to obtain certain qualifications necessary for training/assessing students and to prepare portfolio work, which is rather complicated. There is little interpreting support in these establishments.

According to the CACDP's 2001 annual report, approximately twenty-six thousand hearing and nonsigning deaf people have taken examinations in sign language at various levels in the year 2001. Not every class is registered with the CACDP, so the actual figures of people who have been taught BSL could be as high as fifty thousand or more. Some centers have their own examination structures.

BSL Stage 1

In 1998, 20,400 candidates took the stage 1 examination; it was a record number of entries. In 1999, the numbers dropped to 18,300, and then in 2000 increased slightly to 18,550. In 2001, it dropped again to 16,692.

The pass rate dropped from 79 percent in 1996 to 74 percent in 2000, and then decreased again to 67 percent in 2001. Chart 1 in the appendix shows the pass rates since 1996.

BSL Stage 2

Numbers of candidates entering the BSL stage 2 examination have been increasing since 1996, when 2,100 people applied, to just more than 4,000 for 2000, but the overall pass rate has dropped. This is the figure for the period between 1996 and 2000, but the 2001 figures show an increase to 4,814. The pass rate for 2001 has also increased slightly (see chart 2 in the appendix).

There are four possible reasons for this drop:

1. Colleges are not following the recommended guidelines, and therefore
    a. students are using one tutor instead of the recommended two,
    b. students are using unqualified tutors, or
    c. learners are trying to complete courses in fewer hours than is stipulated in the CACDP's guidelines.
2. Candidates are not ready for the exam.
3. Examiners are becoming more experienced in using and understanding the linguistic structures of BSL, but tutors do not have access to an equivalent level of training and knowledge.
4. More candidates achieve low scores in section 2 of the examination because they are not sufficiently skilled to deal with the question structures required of them.

Tutor Policy

The CACDP is an examining body and is not responsible for tutors. However, because there is no established institute for tutors, CACDP has drawn up tutor guidelines. Tutors are expected to have at least one subject qualification and at least one teaching qualification, as listed in the policy. Any other qualifications would be an advantage.

British Deaf Association's Sign Language Policy

British Deaf Association members have been expressing strong concerns about an increasing number of hearing people teaching BSL. Most of them are non-native BSL users or have low-level signing skills, and they are taking potential employment away from Deaf people. The Sign Language Policy Task Group has drawn up some recommendations to meet the members' concerns.

The Institute of British Sign Language is currently being set up to monitor the standard and status of BSL and, as part of this role, is currently preparing a new tutors policy.

Future of Tutor Training

The BDA is seeking funding to establish a Tutor of BSL training course with a new outlook to meet the needs of modern times. The group of tutors who were trained at Durham University are now more experienced and have gained in confidence in teaching and developing appropriate curriculum structures. We now need to look at the overall teaching situation and our requirements for the future. It may be necessary to make more use of remote teaching, online learning, and tutorials. The materials, of course, will have to be updated.

The BDA's new Institute of British Sign Language aims to monitor and protect the status of BSL by giving advice and support about the language, Deaf culture, the Deaf community, and other related information the public would like to know. The panel consists of BSL experts from throughout the United Kingdom, both Deaf and hearing.

The generally poor examination results for BSL raise grave concerns about the quality of language being used. This will probably prompt new tutor training courses to be set up in the future. A new examination format will also be explored.

Even though the BDA's and CACDP's tutor policies recommend and encourage Deaf tutors to teach BSL, increasing numbers of hearing people are teaching BSL. It has been quoted that at least 60 percent of the tutors in Scotland are hearing (ABSLT, 1998).

Standardization of BSL?

BSL is increasingly moving toward standardization because of borrowing, media impact, lexicons created by language planners, and signing used by hearing people. BSL tutors are also partly responsible for these changes because of lack of knowledge and training in sign linguistics.

Do people want standardization of BSL? If so, who is going to benefit greatly from this? Can we compare this to the effects of spoken languages? How will it work in sign language? Who will decide which regional signs to use and which to discard?

Conclusion

Immense pressures for change are currently experienced by many of the world's languages and cultures. Most of these have seen dramatic alterations in relatively short periods of time. BSL is affected similarly. There is currently a research proposal under way to preserve the London Sign Variation of BSL, which is in danger of extinction. However, something much more wide-reaching is needed.

We desperately need funding to set up new BSL tutor training courses, perhaps something futuristic, such as a virtual training institute to cater to Deaf sign language tutors in Europe and internationally. At present there is an urgent need for funding to establish interpreter training courses, and it is widely publicized that educational institutes are trying to obtain funding for this provision. The need for tutor training courses and research into BSL teaching and learning are often ignored or overlooked.

Tutors involved in teaching interpreters ideally need previous training and a very strong background in sign language teaching and sign linguistics.

Improved tutor training would mean more hearing people would be taught a better standard of BSL and assessment procedures could be looked at in more depth. Consequently, teachers of Deaf children, interpreters, and other professionals would communicate in a more richly informed level of the language and, given that mainstream education seems likely to be with us for a long while yet, children would benefit from this immensely. In this way we would hope to see a reversal of the current domino effect.

References

Association of British Sign Language. (1999). *Annual report.* Surrey, U.K.: Author.
British Deaf Association. (1996). *Education policy.* London: Author.
British Association of Teachers for the Deaf. (2003). *Survey 2003.* Retrieved from http://www.BATOD.org.uk/publications.
The Council for the Advancement of Communication with Deaf People. (2001). *Annual report.* Durham, U.K.: Author.
The Council for the Advancement of Communication with Deaf People. (2004). *Annual review 2004.* Durham, U.K.: Author.
Denmark, A. C. (2001). *Membership of Deaf clubs.* Paper presented at the Deafhood Conference, Royal Association for the Deaf, London, July 12–14.
Ladd, P. (2003). *Understanding Deaf culture: In search of deafhood* (chap. 7). Clevedon, U.K.: Multilingual Matters.
Sign Language Channel Working Party. (2003). *Do we want our own channel?* British Deaf Association. London: Author.
Sutton-Spence, R., & Woll, B. (1999). *The linguistics of British Sign Language: An introduction.* Cambridge: Cambridge University Press.
Warnock, H. M. (1978). Special *educational needs: Report of the Committee of Enquiry into the Education of Handicapped Children and Young People.* London: Her Majesty's Stationary Office.

Appendix 1

BSL stage 1 pass rates:

1996: 79 percent
1997: 77 percent
1998: 78 percent
1999: 75 percent
2000: 74 percent
2001: 67 percent

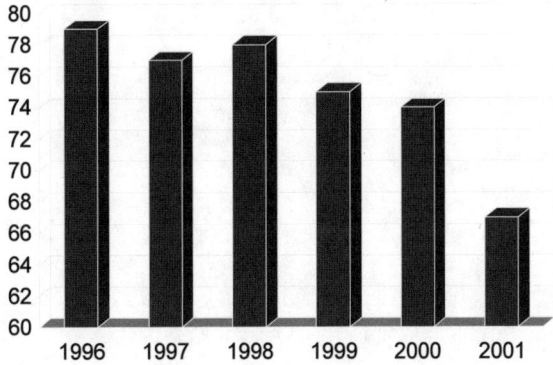

CHART 1: Stage 1 pass rates

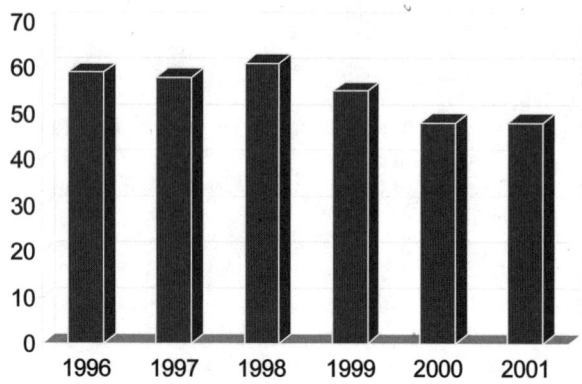

CHART 2: Stage 2 pass rates

BSL stage 2 pass rates:

1996: 59 percent
1997: 58 percent
1998: 61 percent
1999: 55 percent
2000: 48 percent
2001: 52 percent

How Is Asian Deaf Culture Different from American Deaf Culture?

STEVEN CHOUGH AND KRISTINA DOBYNS

Although we have a relative wealth of documents in American Deaf culture that we have developed in the past three decades, we are acutely aware of how little knowledge we have of Asian Deaf culture at the moment. Before beginning the discussion in depth, we advise against using the term "the deaf" (Chough, 1978). Our Deaf and hard of hearing citizens are a cultural group of human beings with emotional sensitivity like anyone else. They want to express themselves as human beings, not as an abstract entity. They sincerely ask to be called "Deaf people" or "Deaf individuals" rather than "the deaf." In addition, we ought to identify a difference, first advocated by James Woodward: the term "deaf" refers to the audiological condition of the inability to hear, whereas the term "Deaf" refers to a cultural group whose members do not hear but share a common language, for example, American Sign Language (ASL), common culture, and common values (Woodward, 1972). We are therefore using "Deaf" to refer to both Deaf and hard of hearing individuals.

In the mid-1880s, an international conference on education of Deaf children was held in Milan, Italy, where participants voted to forbid the use of sign language at special education programs serving these children. Those who attended the conference favored the pure oral method, opposed only by the American and British contingent (Gannon, 1981). This ruling in Milan was responsible for the "dark age" for Deaf children and adults all over the world! This was the first official mandate to suppress sign language, though oralists have long suppressed its use, thereby depriving Deaf persons of their natural, native language. For a long, long time—more than seven decades—sign language was stigmatized. As a result, Deaf people were not proud of being Deaf, felt oppressed and ashamed, and suffered from collective low self-image until the late 1960s and early 1970s. Nevertheless, they stubbornly persisted to believe in the benefits of utilizing their sign language and continued to use it outside the classroom.

In the late 1950s, Dr. William C. Stokoe launched a research project studying sign language at Gallaudet College (now known as Gallaudet University). His colleagues—even Deaf faculty members—mocked his belief that sign language was "indeed a language in its own right" (Gannon, 1981). With the assistance of research associates, in 1965 he published the famed *A Dictionary of American Sign Language on Linguistic*

Principle and was the first scholar to give our sign language a formal name: American Sign Language!

When it was proven that ASL was a true language, it became visible in public schools, adult education, colleges, and universities almost overnight. Deaf people began to feel proud to be Deaf and wanted to learn more about their own culture. Deaf studies grew rapidly. More specifically, the first Deaf studies department was established in this nation at Boston University in 1980. Another program followed at California State University, Northridge (CSUN), shortly thereafter. A new Deaf studies department was set up much later (1995) at Gallaudet University (Ben Bahan, personal communication, June 25, 2002). In other words, we Deaf Americans wanted to separate truth from stereotype, fact from misconception, and reality from myth about us.

Now we have developed literature and research on American Deaf culture; nevertheless, with Asian Deaf culture we have only very little, probably because so few Deaf culture scholars, particularly Asian Deaf people themselves, have explored the new field of such a microculture within the Deaf community in the country. We hope to expand our limited information about Asian Deaf culture in terms of both Deaf people in Asia and Asian Deaf people in America (Chough, 1998).

The early history of Asian Americans begins as follows: "the first Asians to set foot on American land were Filipinos in the mid-1700s" (Cao & Novas, 1996). Many Chinese people immigrated to the United States in the mid-1850s during the gold rush for new adventures, but several laws were later passed by the Congress to prevent or restrict an influx of immigrants from the Asian regions. However, thanks to the Hart-Celler Act in 1965, which abolished the quota system that had been enormously discriminating against Asian people, more and more Deaf fortune-seekers were able to come over to this nation from Asia, and some Asian Deaf individuals were born here in the United States. At this point, we have observed that those who were born here or who moved at an early age and have lived in this country for quite a long time have demonstrated behavior and thinking more or less similar to other Deaf Americans, unless being raised and affected by their traditionally or culturally strict parents influenced their thinking.

Recently, we have become more aware of the features that distinguish Asian Deaf and non-Asian Deaf culture, thanks to slowly increasing articles and lectures in the Asian Deaf field. A new course here at Gallaudet University's Deaf Studies Department, Asian Deaf Studies, was first offered in spring 2000. Each year the students who took the course were asked to prepare a list comparing Asian Deaf culture with American Deaf culture. When preparing this essay, we reviewed those comparisons and agreed with some, disagreed with others, and created our own analysis.

Here we discuss in what ways both cultures differ. We hope this pioneering discussion will help initiate additional research comparing the individual cultures and result in new insight for the entire Deaf studies field. Now, let us focus on the comparisons between American Deaf culture and Asian Deaf culture. We describe general differences although we understand that there will always be exceptions. We have organized the contrasts into three categories: political-economical, social, and communication. Please note that some characteristics overlap and apply to other categories as well.

Before further discussion about these fascinating contrasts, we cannot overemphasize the concept of *karma*. Karma is the "moral law of causation by which all the acts of a person have good or bad effects in some future period, generally in another existence" (Welty, 1984). Asian people in Hinduism, Buddhism, and other faiths believe that an individual's karma still carries on and remains after death. Thus, many people in the Asian regions accept the concept that deafness or disability is a fate caused by the parents' and/or their paternal parents' bad behavior or wrongdoing.

Tables 1–3 list the main differences between Asian Deaf culture and American Deaf culture. We encourage you to continue the discussion in comparing the two

TABLE 1. Political-Economical Differences between American Deaf Culture and Asian Deaf Culture

American Deaf Culture	Asian Deaf Culture
Deaf Acceptance by Society	
Deaf people are more accepted by society, thanks to the democratic ideology and the egalitarian spirit.	It is more difficult for Deaf people to be accepted by society as first-class citizens because of Asian culture and religions, particularly the extensive influence of the concept of karma.
Deaf Teachers	
Many Deaf teachers in schools and colleges are hired as a result of the educational advancement for Deaf students in this nation.	Relatively few Deaf teachers are employed; the majority of hearing people in many Asian countries still do not believe in the intellectual ability of Deaf people.
Financial Support	
A number of Deaf students and adults depend on government support, e.g., disability or Social Security Insurance, which has been long developed in the Western hemisphere.	Many Deaf adults still depend upon their parents or siblings for financial assistance while being unemployed, because the Asian family is responsible for the welfare of its members.
Automotive Driving	
Deaf people can drive anywhere in the country, special thanks to the Deaf leaders in Michigan who fought for the deserved privilege to drive.	Deaf people are still not permitted to drive in developing countries on account of the "cannot syndrome" among hearing government officials.
Opportunity and Oppression	
There is greater opportunity and less oppression for Deaf people, and better economic conditions and education in this exceedingly wealthy nation, along with high humanitarian spirit.	There are worse feelings of oppression, lower self-esteem, more difficult economic conditions, more limited educational opportunities, more emphasis on oralism and forbidding sign language in many Asian regions than in America.
Religion	
Somewhat less religious, but more churches/temples for the Deaf population, with more Deaf clergymen.	More religious, but having fewer religious institutions; however, the longer the immigrants stay in America, the less likely that they are to remain very religious. (This issue is debatable and needs further research.)
Education	
Deaf students have access to mainstream programs, residential schools, can go to any college with interpreter services, can go to colleges with Deaf programs, or colleges for Deaf students, such as Gallaudet University and National Technical Institute for the Deaf.	Education in many Asian regions is generally poorly funded and "behind," especially in Nepal, Tibet, and Vietnam. This has considerable impact on jobs and the economy. It may also weaken Deaf culture because Deaf students lack the educational awareness, advancements, and opportunities to be exposed to material in Deaf culture classes that foster Deaf pride.

TABLE 2. Social Differences between American Deaf Culture and Asian Deaf Culture

American Deaf Culture	Asian Deaf Culture
Assertive/Passive Behavior	
Americans are more assertive than Asians, who tend to be more passive or silent (this applies to hearing people as well).	Society has had a long history of male superiority. This is due to the Confucian philosophy, which delineates strict social orders where the man is superior and the woman is taught to be submissive and avoid eye contact. In short, Asians are more passive.
Deaf Pride	
Americans have more Deaf pride, due to Dr. Stokoe for proving ASL to be a true language, which has helped the Deaf community feel proud.	Asians have much less Deaf pride and more feelings of shame because of the influence of bad karma.
Marriage with Deaf/Hearing	
Americans marry fewer hearing partners than Asians.	Asians marry more hearing spouses because either hearing persons are thought to be superior to Deaf persons or because their parents put pressure upon them to marry hearing partners to avoid the birth of possible Deaf grandchildren.
Social Class Consciousness	
Americans are less conscious about social class/status in the egalitarian society, with an illustration of the diversity in metropolitan areas, e.g., Washington, D.C., where many different individuals of different social statuses interact easily without self-consciousness.	Asians value higher social status because of the caste system in India and the Confucian ideology, which emphasizes social stratification.
Graciousness	
Americans often take small gifts or hospitality for granted; for example, they may not frequently send a thank-you response to the giver.	Asians use many good manners because of the long tradition of etiquette.
Deaf Family as Source of Pride/Shame	
Deaf parents with Deaf children consider themselves as fortunate, happy and "royal."	Deaf parents feel stigmatized for having Deaf children, occasionally hiding these children in rooms isolated from the general public.
Old/Young Interaction	
Old and young Deaf people interact socially in a small-sized Deaf community.	Old and young are more separated from each other because of the long history of traditional respect for the elderly.
Perspective on Friendship	
Americans tend to have fewer very close or special friends, probably influenced by the ideology of individualism.	Asians consider friendship to be an obligation they will not take lightly. In several Asian regions, the special friend is as equally important as the spouse, but it should not be surprising that the longer the immigrants live here, the fewer close friends they tend to have.
Visit Friends	
Americans often frown upon the last-minute visitors at home; an appointment of visiting ahead of time is necessary. Everyone in this country is very busy.	Asians are not quite surprised and are hospitable to visitors at the last minute, but in the American metropolitan areas, they tend to frown on such last-minute visitors, just like other Americans.

TABLE 2. *Continued*

American Deaf Culture	Asian Deaf Culture
Deafness as Scientific/Spiritual	
Americans regard deafness as scientific; for example, when a child is born deaf or becomes deaf at an early age, the cause is inspected from a medical perspective—either the deafness is hereditary or occurred through a rational exogenous source.	Asians consider deafness as spiritual or a result of bad karma.

TABLE 3. Differences in Communication between American Deaf Culture and Asian Deaf Culture

American Deaf Culture	Asian Deaf Culture
Useful Technology for Deaf Citizens	
Deaf people have a great deal of technology such as pagers, TTY, e-mail, closed/open captioning, flashing clocks, and doorbells that are manufactured for Deaf needs.	All the technology that is available to Deaf Americans is not widely available in several parts of Asia. In some places, there are e-mails and faxes, but for the most part the technology for Deaf consumers is insufficient.
Communication Style	
Deaf people have a direct or blunt communication style; this is more blunt than hearing Americans as well as Deaf people in Asia.	Asians are more subtle, ambiguous, polite, more reluctant to say "no." Yet, those who live in the United States a long time, tend to become more blunt or direct like other Deaf Americans.
Touching and Hugging	
Deaf Americans use much more touching and hugging than Asians and even hearing Americans.	Touching, hugs, and kissing can be inappropriate or rude.
Visual and Physical Noise	
Deaf Americans are more visually and physically noisy in the presence of hearing people than their Asian counterparts. They bang, stomp, yell, or wave.	In hearing Asian culture, this is considered rude, and this is reflected in Asian Deaf culture.
Nonmanual Expression	
Deaf Americans use more nonmanual expressions than Deaf Asians at first, and then when intimacy and comfort level increase, their facial expressions correspondingly may decrease.	At first to assimilate like the hearing, they do not use facial expressions that much, but as they become more comfortable in their environment, they increasingly use nonmanual behavior. (This is our theory, which welcomes debate and needs further research.)
Manual Alphabet	
Deaf Americans heavily use the manual alphabet to mention human names, technical vocabulary, and any unfamiliar words for more accurate information, at the same time as moving their lips. From time to time, we may see their exaggerated lip movement while signing.	Deaf Asians use much less finger spelling and much more signed vocabulary than Americans.

cultures, and perhaps come up with good points of your own to enhance Asian Deaf studies and to help the literature and research on Asian Deaf culture grow. The 1989 Deaf Way conference proceedings had only a very small section for Asian Deaf culture. We hope the 2002 Deaf Way II conference will increase the size of Asian Deaf studies literature and build the awareness of the two cultures. One is from the East and the other from the West, and both are included under the label of Deaf culture, but each has its own unique characteristics that deserve further examination and analysis.

References

Cao, L., & Novas, H. (1996). *Everything you need to know about Asian American history*. New York: Plume.

Chough, S. (1978). New era of Deaf first-class citizenship. *The Deaf American, 28.*

Chough, S. (1998). The fascinating Asian/Deaf cultures in America. *Deaf Studies V: Toward 2000—Unity and Diversity.* Washington, DC: Gallaudet University Press.

Gannon, J. (1981). American Sign Language: Our natural language. *Deaf heritage: A narrative history of Deaf America* (pp. 359–376). Silver Spring, MD: National Association of the Deaf.

Welty, P. (1984). *The Asians: Their evolving heritage*. New York: Harper & Row.

Woodward, J. (1972). Implications for socioliguistics research among the deaf. *Sign Language Studies* 1:1–7.

Sign Language Use among Indigenous Populations

JEFFREY E. DAVIS

Deaf people's strong inclination to develop and acquire sign language can be traced through history and is evident worldwide. In addition to being some of the primary languages in Deaf communities, signed languages have been used by hearing indigenous communities around the world as alternatives to spoken languages. This chapter presents some instances where sign language has been used and handed down from one generation to the next among indigenous populations—particularly North American Indians.[1] Contemporary and historical cases are considered in light of new evidence and current linguistic theory. Some of the historical connections between sign language use among American Indian and Deaf communities are presented.

In a 1913 lecture presented in sign language, George Veditz stated, "As long as we have deaf people on earth, we will have signs." Based on numerous accounts (as early as Socrates in Greece), signed languages, like spoken languages, have existed throughout human history. The existence and acquisition of sign language, however, is not necessarily based on the single condition of hearing loss. Historically, hearing aboriginal peoples also have signed—even when Deaf people were not present. For example, it has been well documented that the signed systems used among the Aboriginal peoples of Central Australia, and some indigenous groups of North and South America, were highly elaborated alternatives to spoken language. The role of Deaf individuals who were born into communities where everyone signed warrants further consideration (see Davis, 2006; Davis & Supalla, 1995; Groce, 1985; Kendon, 1988, 2002; McKay-Cody, 1997; Umiker-Sebeok & Sebeok, 1978; West, 1960).

In industrialized societies, signed languages are acquired and transmitted primarily by members of the Deaf cultural group. In contrast, in some indigenous communities around the world, signing has been acquired by both Deaf and hearing members of the community. One of the best-known historical cases occurred on the island of

---

1. Various terms are used to refer to members of the First Nations cultural groups. "Native American" may be considered politically correct; however, members of these groups generally refer to themselves as "Indian" or "American Indian." The specific tribal affiliation or cultural-linguistic group is acknowledged whenever possible—for example, Assiniboine, Blackfoot, Eastern Cherokee, Inuit, Lakota, Northern Cheyenne, and so forth. "Aboriginal" and "indigenous" are synonyms used to refer to the original native inhabitants who inhabited the continent prior to foreign immigration and colonization.

Martha's Vineyard, Massachusetts. From the seventeenth through twentieth centuries, for more than 250 years, both deaf and hearing inhabitants of the island reportedly used sign language for everyday communication purposes (Groce, 1985). Martha's Vineyard was an example of a preindustrialized indigenous community where sign language was handed down from one generation to the next.

It is also of historical relevance that prior to the arrival of the first European immigrants in the early 1600s, the inhabitants of Martha's Vineyard were the Wampanoag. It is not known if these Native American Indians were a source for the sign language that was eventually widely used by both deaf and hearing people of the island. However, the Wampanoag were members of the Algonquin cultural and linguistic group, who were, and remain today, among the most fluent signers. Because there was contact and exchange between the European immigrants and the native inhabitants, it is plausible that they were exposed to the Indians signing (Pritchard, 2002).

Further research is needed to determine these connections; however, it appears that no illustrations, linguistic descriptions, or films were made of Martha's Vineyard Sign Language. Consequently, little is known about the lexicon or grammatical structure of the historical Martha's Vineyard sign language variety, which some scholars hypothesize formed the basis for modern American Sign Language (ASL). In other words, Martha's Vineyard Sign Language became extinct. Such endangered languages must be stabilized, documented, and maintained—lest they be lost forever (Crystal, 2000).

The language and cultural genocide among indigenous communities brought on by colonization eventually culminated with nineteenth-century industrialization. The social and educational forces of this historical period also threatened the signed languages of Deaf communities. George Veditz and his colleagues with the National Association of the Deaf (NAD) were concerned that sign language was endangered. To preserve sign language, the NAD produced a series of films in the early 1900s (Supalla, 2001). Although these films were made of formal signed presentations, they provide a view of how ASL was signed at the nexus of the nineteenth and twentieth centuries. Another invaluable source for comparative historical linguistic data comes from the written descriptions, copious illustrations, and extensive films made of North American Indian Sign Language. Preservation of these language documents are critical to prevent further language loss and contribute to our understanding of language origin and change.

Sign Language Use among American Indians

Much has been written about the clash of cultures that occurred following massive European immigration and colonization (or invasion, as it came to be considered by the Indians). Some scholars have hypothesized that signed communication was already used among indigenous peoples across the North American continent prior to European contact (Campbell & Mithun, 1979; Goddard, 1979; Wurtzburg & Campbell, 1995). The earliest accounts of Indians signing come from the 1527 expedition for the conquest of Florida, led by the Spanish conquistador Cabeza de Vaca, who reported numerous occasions of native groups signing with each other along the Gulf Coast region.

The origins of American Indian Sign Language remain uncertain.[2] Sign language, or "hand talk" as some Indians called it, was documented for dozens of distinct linguistic groups inhabiting the Great Plains cultural areas. Based on these accounts, it was called Plains Indian Sign Language. However, the historical linguistic documentation shows that varieties of sign language were used beyond the Great Plains geographic area, spanning most of the major American Indian cultural areas of North America, including Mesoamerica and the subartic regions (Davis, 2006).

The vast expanse of the North American continent was once an area of extreme linguistic and cultural diversity. There was frequent contact between numerous indigenous communities speaking hundreds of distinct and mutually unintelligible spoken languages. Sign language appears to have evolved as a way to make communication possible between individuals speaking many different mother tongues. Signing was so prevalent and widespread that early scholars considered it a lingua franca—that is, a language variety used for communication among groups of people who did not otherwise share a common language. This was well documented by some of the earliest nineteenth-century anthropologists and linguists (previously known as *ethnologists* and *philologists*) who studied the sign language used among the American Indians (e.g., Boas, 1890/1978; Clark, 1885/1982; Mallery, 1881/2001). These early scholars laid the groundwork for sign language among the North American Indians to be considered a preexistent, full-fledged language. Based on extensive fieldwork, they have provided a rich legacy of historical linguistic documentation to support this claim.

National Treasure

The richest source for these historical linguistic data comes from archival sources—particularly the 1930s motion pictures produced by General Hugh Scott with support from an act of the U.S. Congress. These films documented chieftains and elders from thirteen distinct spoken language groups who were communicating with each other through sign language. Produced during the historical three-day Indian Sign Language Council (September 4–6, 1930), these films documented the Indian participants engaged in lively, natural, and unrehearsed signed language discourse. Davis (2006) has studied these films extensively and found evidence of several types of discourse, for example, making formal introductions, showing the sign names for the participants and the tribes represented, signing traditional cultural and medicine stories, and making whimsical and metaphorical comparisons.

Therefore, sign language was not limited to communication with "foreigners" or for use between individuals from tribes speaking distinct languages, nor was it restricted to ceremonial purposes. Sign language was used for everyday communication purposes *between and within* tribes. In the 1930s films, the participants were predominately signing without the accompaniment of spoken language. There may have been some variation from tribe to tribe, and likely not all individuals were

---

2. The ways that native users name their languages should be considered. The varieties of sign language used among American Indian groups have been named in different ways—for example, Plains Indian Sign Language, Indian Sign Language, North American Indian Sign Language, and so forth. In this essay, "Sign language among the American Indians" or "American Indian Sign Language" is generally used.

equally proficient in sign language. The preliminary research conducted by Davis (2006) finds striking similarities between the linguistic structures of Indian Sign Language and ASL (e.g., marked and unmarked handshapes, symmetry and dominance conditions, and classifier forms). Further research is needed to determine the historical connections, similarities, and differences between these varieties of sign language. Sample clips of the historical films of Indian Sign Language can be viewed at this website: http://web.utk.edu/~jdavis49/.

It is noteworthy that among the most proficient signers of the First Nations were the tribal chiefs, elders, and medicine men. Sign language served a variety of discourse purposes—storytelling, jokes, gender-specific activities, ritual and ceremonial practices, and times when speech was difficult or taboo (e.g., during hunting, in the presence of one's elders, and in times of mourning the death of someone). There is substantial evidence that sign language was a rich part of the storytelling and cultural traditions of the American Indians. Sadly, contemporary sign language use among the Indians has virtually vanished. Spoken English has replaced the role once served by a signed lingua franca. However, there is evidence that varieties of American Indian Sign Language are still used today by some Deaf and hearing Indians. Although endangered, the language remains preserved through the rich sources of historical linguistic documentation (Davis, 2006). Hopefully, Indian Sign Language will not be lost but will be reintroduced and maintained for this and future generations.

The Earliest Accounts

The earliest known descriptions of the lexicon formed the basis of a paper titled "Sign Language of the Indian Nations to the West of the Mississippi River," presented by Thomas Jefferson, president of the American Philosophical Society (Dunbar, 1800). Descriptions were included for more than fifty signs used among the Indian nations. Reportedly, Jefferson presented this paper in 1801, the same year he became U.S. president. The title and content of the paper reflects that Jefferson recognized the significance of the sign language used among the "Indian Nations." In 1803, the year of the Louisiana Purchase, President Thomas Jefferson ordered the expedition from St. Louis, Missouri, to the Pacific Ocean, led by Captains Meriwether Lewis and William Clark. The historical linguistic evidence supports that sign language was used among the tribes encountered on the expedition. See Goff-Paris and Wood (2002) for further accounts along these lines, including the role of Sacagawea as an interpreter for the expedition.

Major Stephen H. Long led the next official U.S. expedition from Pittsburgh, Pennsylvania, to the Rocky Mountains in 1819. In 1823, an account of the expedition was published that included one hundred descriptions of Indian signs. It is noteworthy that Thomas H. Gallaudet, cofounder of the first school for Deaf students in the United States in 1817, studied and published papers about these descriptions of Indian Sign Language.

The Natural Approach

In 1848, the first known article published by Thomas H. Gallaudet was titled "On the Natural Language of Signs: And Its Value and Uses in the Instruction of the Deaf and

Dumb."[3] In this paper, Gallaudet used Indian Sign Language as evidence of the value of "the natural language of signs" for teaching and communicating with deaf people. He did not write, however, that Indian Sign Language itself was used as the language of instruction. His line of reasoning was that, similar to the Indians, the originators of sign language were Deaf people themselves. Gallaudet pointed out that sign language "naturally" occurs "when necessity exists" and that this "prompts the invention and use of this language of signs" (p. 59). This seminal 1848 publication included the detailed descriptions of some signs used by the "aboriginal Indians" taken from the account of the "Expedition from Pittsburgh to the Rocky Mountains" in which 104 "Indian signs" were described (Long, 1823, pp. 378–394).

Gallaudet's study of Indian Sign Language makes its introduction to Deaf students a possibility. However, this is not certain from reading his 1848 essay. He wrote:

> Major Long's work contains an accurate description of many of these signs, and it is surprising to notice how not a few of them are almost identically the same with those which the deaf and dumb employ to describe the same things, while others have such general features of resemblance as to show that they originate from elements of this sign-language which nature furnishes to man wherever he is found, whether barbarous or civilized. (p. 59)

Clearly, Gallaudet considered that Indian Sign Language was a natural occurrence and that signing was the most effective way to communicate with Deaf people. More research is necessary before conclusions can be reached about the outcomes of language contact between the varieties of sign language used among the American Indians and the Deaf populace of that historical period.

Thus, many questions remain. Did Gallaudet or other teachers incorporate the published descriptions of Indian signs to enhance the sign language used to teach deaf students? What contact did Deaf people have with Indians who signed? What contact was there between the earliest European immigrants who were Deaf and the Native Americans? What were the linguistic outcomes of a deaf child being born and raised in a community in which most or all of the hearing members used sign language? Were there connections between Indian Sign Language and the emergence of Martha's Vineyard Sign Language? These are some of the questions that have led scholars to hypothesize about the historical linguistic bases for modern ASL.

An Endangered Language

Tragically, by the end of the nineteenth century, most of the treaties made between the U.S. government and the First Nations had been broken. Continued western expansionism, the California gold rush, the Civil War and the reconstruction that followed, and completion of the first transcontinental railroad served to further the genocide of the languages and cultural ways of the First Nations. Education policy of that period was full "cultural and linguistic assimilation," which translated into loss

---

3. This paper appeared in the inaugural publication of *American Annals of the Deaf and Dumb* (vol. 1, nos. 1 and 2, 1848). Composed nearly 160 years ago, following early nineteenth-century conventions, it includes some terms considered archaic and patronizing by today's conventions.

of native language and cultural traditions for many American Indians—sign language included.

For example, Indian children and adolescents were systematically removed from their families and placed into residential Indian schools. The children were taught in English only and in most cases were forbidden to use their native languages or practice cultural traditions. Along with the decline of native language and culture came the loss of the sign language that was once a widely used alternative to spoken language and a way of storytelling. Although greatly diminished today, varying degrees of sign language use among some North American Indian groups continue, leading some researchers to suggest that it is an endangered language (Davis, 2006; Farnell, 1995; Kelly & McGregor, 2003; McKay-Cody, 1997).

Current Language Preservation Efforts

This major part of North American Indian history and culture must be preserved and maintained through language education. It is encouraging that current sign language education programs have been reported for the Assiniboine, Stoney, Blackfeet, Piegan, Blood, Crow, and Northern Cheyenne tribes (Davis, 2006; Farnell, 1995). Most notably, the Intertribal Deaf Council; the Department of Blackfoot Studies at Blackfoot Community College at Browning, Montana; and the National Multicultural Interpreting Project at El Paso Community College have been educating others about the experiences of American Indians who are Deaf, Indian Sign Language, and the historical connections of sign language in Deaf communities.

Conclusion

Signed language communities that were predominately hearing have existed around the world throughout history. This essay focused on North American indigenous communities. Signed communication also has been observed among the indigenous peoples of South America and Australia. Furthermore, this linguistic phenomenon has been evident within some occupational settings and monastic traditions. Signed language has evolved as a universal linguistic observable fact, prevalent among both Deaf and hearing communities. For further descriptions of sign language use in these communities, see Davis, 2006; Davis and Supalla, 1995; Farnell, 1995; Johnson, 1994; Kelly and McGregor, 2003; Kendon, 1988, 2002; Umiker-Sebeok & Sebeok, 1978; Washabaugh, 1986; Washabaugh, Woodward, and DeSantis, 1978; and West, 1960.

Clearly, signed language is a universal linguistic phenomenon. "Universal" does not mean that these various signed languages were mutually intelligible. It is a popular misconception that "one" sign language is used and comprehended universally. Both signed and spoken languages universally occur. In fact, more than 6,700 distinct living languages have been documented—that is, thirty times more languages than countries (Gordon, 2005). Language encompasses all communication modalities. It is not limited to oral-auditory channels but is equally and richly expressed through kinesthetic-visual means. Signed languages have evolved as full-fledged languages and as alternatives to spoken language. This demonstrates the innate human drive for language.

References

Boas, F. (1890/1978). Sign language. In D. J. Umiker-Sebeok & T. A. Sebeok (Eds.), *Aboriginal sign language of the Americas and Australia* (Vol. 2, pp. 19–20). New York: Plenum Press.

Campbell, L. (2000). *American Indian languages.* Oxford: Oxford University Press.

Campbell, L., & M. Mitchum. (1979). *The languages of Native Americans: Historical and comparative assessment.* Austin: University of Texas Press.

Clark, W. P. (1885/1982). *The Indian Sign Language.* Lincoln: University of Nebraska Press.

Crystal, D. (2000). *Language death.* Cambridge: Cambridge University Press.

Davis, J. E. (2006). A historical linguistic account of North American Indian Sign Language. In C. Lucas (Ed.), *Multilingualism and Sign Language: From the Great Plains to Australia* (Vol. 12). Washington, DC: Gallaudet University Press.

Davis, J. E., & Supalla, S. (1995). A sociolinguistic description of sign language use in a Navajo Family. In C. Lucas (Ed.) *Sociolinguistics in Deaf communities.* Washington, DC: Gallaudet University Press.

Dunbar, W. (1800). On the language of signs among certain North American Indians. *Transactions of the American Philosophical Society, 6*(1–8). Presented by Thomas Jefferson, president of the Society (January 11, 1801).

Farnell, B. M. (1995). *Do you see what I mean?: Plains Indian sign talk and the embodiment of action.* Austin: University of Texas Press.

Gallaudet, T. H. (1848). On the natural language of signs; and its value and uses in the instruction of the deaf and dumb. *American Annals of the Deaf and Dumb, 1*(1), 55–60.

Gallaudet, T. H. (1852). Indian language of signs. *American Annals of the Deaf and Dumb, 4*(1).

Goddard, I. (1979). The languages of South Texas and the lower Rio Grande. In L. Campbell & M. Mithun (Eds.), *The languages of Native America: Historical and comparative assessment* (pp. 355–389). Austin: University of Texas Press.

Goff-Paris, D., & Wood, S. (2002). *Step into the circle: The heartbeat of American Indian, Alaska Native and First Nations Deaf communities.* Monmouth, OR: AGO Publications.

Gordon, R. G. (Ed.). (2005). *Ethnologue: Languages of the world* (15th ed.). Dallas, TX: SIL International. Retrieved from http://www.ethnologue.com/.

Groce, N. E. (1985). *Everyone here spoke sign language: Hereditary deafness on Martha's Vineyard.* Cambridge, MA: Harvard University Press.

Johnson, R. E. (1994). Sign language and the concept of deafness in a traditional Yucatec Mayan village. In C. Erting, R. Johnson, D. Smith, & B. Snider (Eds.), *The Deaf way: Perspectives from the international conference on Deaf culture* (pp. 102–109). Washington, DC: Gallaudet University Press.

Kendon, A. (2002). Historical observations on the relationship between research on sign languages and language origins theory. In D. Armstrong, M. A. Karchmer, & J. Van Cleve (Eds.), *Essays in honor of William C. Stokoe: The study of signed languages.* Washington, DC: Gallaudet University Press.

Kendon, A. (1988). *Sign languages of aboriginal Australia: Cultural, semiotic, and communication perspectives.* Cambridge: Cambridge University Press.

Kelly, W. P., & McGregor, T. L. (2003). Keresan Pueblo Indian Sign Language. In J. Reyhner, O. Trujillo, R. L. Carrasco, & L. Lockard (Eds.). *Nurturing native languages* (pp. 141–148). Flagstaff: Northern Arizona University.

Long, S. H. (1823). *Account of an expedition from Pittsburgh to the Rocky Mountains.* Philadelphia: Edwin James.

Mallery, G. (1881/2001). *Sign language among North American Indians.* Mineola, NY: Dover Publications.

McKay-Cody, M. (1997). *Plains Indian Sign Language: A comparative study of alternate and primary signers.* Unpublished master's thesis, University of Arizona.

Mithun, M. (1999). *The languages of native North America.* Cambridge: Cambridge University Press.

Pritchard, E. (2002). *Native New Yorkers: The legacy of the Algonquin people of New York.* San Francisco: Council Oak Books.

Scott, H. L. (1931). *Film dictionary of the North American Indian Sign Language.* Washington, DC: National Archives.

Umiker-Sebok, J., & Sebeok, T. A. (Eds.). (1978). *Aboriginal sign languages of the Americas and Australia* (Vols. 1 and 2). New York: Plenum Press.

Supalla, T. (2001). Making historical sign language materials accessible: A prototype data base of early ASL. *Sign Language and Linguistics,* 4(1/2): 285–97.

Washabaugh, W. (1986). The acquisition of communicative skills by the deaf of Providence Island. *Semiotica,* 6(2), 179–190.

Washabaugh, W. J., Woodward, J., & De Santis, S. (1978, March). Providence Island Sign Language: A context-dependent language. *Anthropological Linguistics,* 95–109.

West, L. (1960). *The sign language: An analysis* (Vols. 1 & 2). Unpublished doctoral dissertation, Indiana University, Bloomington, Indiana.

Wurtzburg, S., and Campbell, L. (1995). North American Indian sign language: Evidence of its existence before European contact. *International Journal of American Linguistics,* 61(2), 153–167.

Onomatopoeia in British Sign Language? or, The Visuality/Sensation of Sound

DAVID FOWLER AND MARK HEATON

In texts written about British and other sign languages, there seems to be little or no reference to the way Deaf people represent sound in their languages. This is not surprising—Deaf people do not, of course, hear sound. Some may hear a little, but it is not in the way that hearing people understand the concept of sound. Padden and Humphries (1988) report on the Deaf fascination with sound and on the general hearing misconception that a Deaf life is one without sound. Despite this stereotypical belief in a "silent world," Deaf people *do* use sound, and, in British Sign Language (BSL), many signs actually incorporate an element of sound—in some cases, could this be the sign language version of onomatopoeia?

Is sign language onomatopoeia simply the iconicity of sound? Some have suggested that iconicity in signed languages serves a similar purpose to onomatopoeia in spoken languages, and that onomatopoeia and iconicity run on parallel but different tracks. In the oral/aural world of spoken language, onomatopoeia represents a perceived sound; in the visual world of sign language, therefore, a similar function is served by the visual iconicity of many signs, which actually *look* like the thing they represent. We suggest that it is not quite as simple as this. From a hearing perspective, yes, it would appear that iconicity equals sign language onomatopoeia, and that if onomatopoeia exists in sign language, it is of necessity iconic. To a certain extent, this is true; however, one difficulty is that it is just that: a *hearing* perspective.

Spoken languages make considerable use of onomatopoeia, where the word represents or imitates the sound made. The word *onomatopoeia* itself comes through Latin from Greek, from the old Greek *onomat*, "name" and *poios*, "making." In spoken language, onomatopoeia refers to words created because they resemble the sound of the actual thing they represent. Examples include *pop, whoosh, pow, gulp, gurgle, crash, bubble* (as in boiling), and so on. The noises animals make are prime examples (or at least how hearing humans perceive those noises): *cluck, quack, woof, meow*; and it is interesting how these vary from country to country, dependent upon both individual language phonology and cultural variation. This is discussed (see Valli & Lucas, 1992, p. 210 ff, and Sutton-Spence & Woll, 1999, p. 165) in the context of the arbitrariness of spoken language, especially English, where there usually seems to be no real reason for why words are what they are, with the exception of onomatopoeia, where the origin of the word can be heard in the sound it makes. It is possible that in spoken languages, onomatopoeia is a cultural representation of sound as perceived by hearing people; if this is so, and if sign language onomatopoeia exists, is sign language onomatopoeia also a cultural representation?

Taub (1997, 2001) would say that the reason for the lack of iconicity in spoken languages is that their modality is expressed through sound, which means that there is, of course, limited possibility for iconic representation. Therefore, the speaker's voice must represent what in sign language would be iconic—and in the case of spoken language, it is onomatopoeia that serves to represent the linguistic and cultural understanding of, for example, a dog *woof*ing or a duck *quack*ing, water *splash*ing, or a bomb going *boom*.

Could there be a similar origin for some of the signs used in BSL—that they are based on the sound that is linked to the meaning of the word—or, at least, to the sound *as perceived by Deaf people*? Many signs contain an element of sound, but whereas spoken onomatopoeia is an indirect copy of the sound, with sign language it incorporates more: an extra element of sound as perceived through visual and physical senses rather than through hearing. It is seen and felt, not heard: it replicates and conveys the Deaf sensation of sound.

In the case of spoken onomatopoeia, the speaker gives the listener a direct experience of the sound represented; in sign language, the "listener" clearly does not *hear* the sound the signer makes to represent the sensation but experiences it nonetheless. To a hearing person, this may seem to be on a different level, once removed from the direct experience offered by spoken onomatopoeia, but the directness of communication is, to a Deaf person, immediately recognizable. The signers make the sound themselves; obviously the "listener" cannot perceive the sound itself but instantly recognizes it for what it is, a representation of the sensation that Deaf people experience.

An example that comes to mind is BOILING, where the progression from a SIMMER, through a ROLLING BOIL, to BOILING FURIOUSLY are shown visually by increased speed and intensity of hand movement, changing facial expression (phonology), and an oral component of sound. SIMMER uses a slow popping noise made with the lips; BOILING RAPIDLY incorporates hissing and bubbling sounds to represent the sound made. Sutton-Spence and Woll refer to oral components in their discussion of signs and "enacting mouth movements," in which the role of the mouth in sign production is an important part, but they do not mention the use of sound. Yet it is certain that sound *is* used in sign language, and although the Deaf "listener" may not hear the sound as such, it is also certain that they perceive and comprehend it just as directly as a hearing listener understands spoken onomatopoeia.

From a hearing perspective, it would seem to be a mystery—why, when they do not hear, do Deaf people use sounds in their signing? One might suppose that the sounds are used as a courteous cultural nod toward the hearing person or as an aid to understanding; however, this is clearly not the case. It is not only when signing to hearing people that sounds are used; sound is also used between Deaf users, perhaps even *more* than when they sign with hearing people. Natural use of BSL—that is, between fluent users without critical hearing onlookers—certainly involves the use of sounds, often used more openly and loudly than when Deaf people are signing to hearing BSL users. Perhaps, it could be because Deaf-Deaf communication has none of the restrictive politeness of Deaf-hearing communication and less inhibition.

Nevertheless, one might still ask *why*, when both do not hear the sounds, do Deaf people use them when signing with other Deaf persons? What do the sounds represent, and what is their function? ROAD-DRILL and WALL-DRILL are both iconic signs accompanied by sound: puffed cheeks for intensity and a pursed-lip mix of a hiss and *FFFFFF*, which does not actually sound like a drill but is a perception of the sound the drill makes *as felt through vibration* by the user. However, the sign TIRE-GOING-FLAT, which uses a long *SSSSS*, is probably not based upon the sensation of vibration, because few people are actually holding a tire when it deflates; rather, perhaps it comes from the Deaf observer's perception of the rush of air from the deflating tire.

GASOLINE-FILL-UP is another example of a sign that uses a sound naturally as an integral part of itself, not to increase intensity or emphasis, but just as a normal part of the sign. The iconic handshape indicating the gasoline nozzle is accompanied by pursed lips, clenched teeth, and a *SSSSWOOOOOSSSSH* sound of the gasoline gushing; the moment when the tank is full and the pump stops is represented by hand movement and a *PRRUP-CLUNK!* sound, which accurately imitates both the sound and the physical sensation. Yet most sign language users do not have enough hearing to *hear* the actual sound of the gasoline flowing or the nozzle jamming—it appears to be based upon the *feel*, the sensation of the sound rather than the "real" sound itself. Deaf people *feel* the gasoline *SSWOOSSH*ing through the pipe; ask a hearing person to imitate the sound and they usually come up with gurgling or *glug-glug*. Hearing learners of BSL tend to apply an English structure to GASOLINE-FILL-UP: they will sign FULL-UP MY CAR, without the accompanying sound, with the result that this is not true BSL. Deaf people use the iconic gasoline-nozzle handshape and the onomatopoeic *SSSSWOOOOOSSSSH*, with the inherent or innate cultural knowledge that this is an essential part of the language.

Sign language onomatopoeia may be based upon perception and expectation. Look at the sign GOAL-SCORE, as applied to British football (soccer). Here the signer represents the footballer kicking the ball; it soars through the air, then *PRRRP!* hits the back of the net. (This sign varies: some Deaf people do sign this silently, while others use the sound.) Yet in reality, the ball hitting the net *makes no real sound*: the net is soft and flexible, and the ball is silent on impact. Ask a hearing person to describe the same scene and the sound will most probably be a cartoon-like *pow!* as the boot hits the ball, and any sound as the ball enters the net will be cheering, not the sound of the ball itself. A Deaf person puts his or her perception of the central moment into this sign, and the sound comes with the all-important net-contact.

Strangely enough, the converse applies to basketball POINT-SCORE; whereas a hearing person may add a sound—*plop*—to a description of this, in BSL the sign is a silent one. This is because the net or basket is open, has no bottom, and therefore Deaf people see this as having no impact *and therefore no sound*. Consequently, it is rather a restrained sign. This could reflect British culture—basketball is a relatively new sport with a small following compared to soccer—and it could be very interesting to look at the American Sign Language sign to see if that incorporates an element that could be described as sign onomatopoeia.

What exactly these sounds signify, or their function, is open to question; it could be that the sounds in themselves have a morphemic function. In the sign GASOLINE-FILL-UP, the handshape itself is not sufficient to give the full meaning; alone, the handshape is flat and empty, and suggests the gasoline pump is not working. It is only when the sound element *SWWOOSH* is made that the sign has the desired meaning. Similarly, it is only when the *CLUNK* is added that the sign sequence is complete, and the nonmanual jerk feature does not make sense without the morphemic sound.

This is an area that invites research to see how cultural and linguistic differences between, for example, users of BSL and other sign languages around the world affect the use of sounds in sign and thereby sign-onomatopoeia, that is, if it exists. The literature mentions onomatopoeia, but only in relation to spoken language, and only in comparison. Nowhere, to our knowledge, is the use of sound in BSL discussed in any depth, yet it is a part of BSL, as any hearing visitor to a Deaf club will attest. Deaf people in their own environment, confident and uninhibited, do use sounds in their signing. Could it be that researchers have not yet gained the trust and openness from Deaf people that allow them to feel comfortable making sounds? Observe some older Deaf people signing: they are more "tight-lipped" about it, having been brought up to feel ashamed of their signing. Younger people are less self-conscious, more sure of their identity, more Deaf-and-proud . . . and *noisier*. This could be the effect of openness in society or of equal opportunity—or even the result of years of looking at comic books and watching television cartoons, with their added speech and exclamation balloons.

Whether sign onomatopoeia exists is a question we could consider. It is clear that iconicity is, in its way, a sign language equivalent of spoken onomatopoeia, but this does not account for the use of sound in many signs. Sutton-Spence and Woll (1999) discuss how different languages and cultures affect onomatopoeia in different spoken languages, with the result that a United Nations pig says *oink* to the British delegates but *bu* to the Japanese. When Americans see Superman striking the bad guy, they perceive the sound as *ZAP!*, whereas French viewers hear *PAF!* Similarly, Deaf and hearing people have different perceptions of sound, affected by how they perceive it and by the culture and language they bring to that perception. Perhaps now could be the time to research this area and to add new linguistic categories of signs: multichannel signs, oral components, and *sign onomatopoeia*.

References

Padden, C., & Humphries, T. (1988). *Deaf in America: Voices from a culture*. Cambridge, MA: Harvard University Press.

Sutton-Spence, R., & Woll, B. (1999). *The linguistics of British Sign Language*. Cambridge: Cambridge University Press.

Taub, S. (1997). *Language in the body: Iconicity and metaphor in American Sign Language*. Unpublished doctoral dissertation. Berkeley: University of California, Berkeley.

Taub, S. (2001). *Language from the body*. University of California Press.

Valli, C., & Lucas, C. (1992). *The linguistics of American Sign Language: An introduction*. Washington, DC: Gallaudet University Press.

What Is Deafhood and Why Is It Important?

PADDY LADD

I developed *Deafhood* as an English term to counter other negative English terms describing Deaf people. We already have our own signs that capture much of what might be seen as Deafhood, which we use in our own discourses. However, to take on and change the discourses of those who have colonized us, we need a term that interrupts the patterns they have established. Colonial discourses are framed within terms such as "hearing-impaired" and "deafness." As Alker (2000) has said, when one uses the word *blindness*, the idea that the term might include all those who wear glasses is absurd. Yet Deaf people are still trapped inside *deafness*, which includes everyone with a hearing loss. This has had many consequences for us, as Ladd (2003) shows.

Deafhood in History

A powerful effect of developing the Deafhood term is that it sets off a whole new set of thought processes. We start to ask, "What is *Deaf*? What does this word actually mean?" We realize that we have to take into account whatever damage has been done to our idea of "Deaf" by the 120 years of oralist colonization. After a century of having all things Deaf denied or denigrated, how can we be sure we are thinking and behaving to our full Deaf potential? One way we can answer this is to find historical evidence of how Deaf people thought before oralism. Because sign languages could not be recorded, much evidence has been lost, but there are examples showing how in those days, Deaf people did discuss ontological questions such as "What is *Deaf*? Who am I and why am I here on earth? What might my role here on earth be?" They developed positive, powerful answers and conclusions.

Although I have found examples in the United Kingdom, my focus is on preoralist France and the decades of thoughts and perceptions by French Deaf people, from Desloges around the time of the French Revolution in 1789 (Lane & Philip, 1984), through Massieu and Clerc (de Ladebat, 1815), to the Paris banquets started by Berthier and colleagues in the 1830s, whose beliefs have been made available to us by the pioneering work of Mottez (1993). Because of space limits, I focus only on the latter.

This essay is dedicated to the lifeworks of Sharon Wood and Joseph Castronovo.

In the 1830s, Berthier's group believed in bilingual education, with intense struggles in the Deaf school where the group taught, which even then was moving toward oralism. One strategy was to enlist support from outside the school by holding annual banquets to which the press was invited. These became so famous that Deaf people traveled from as far as the United States to attend. A key part of the banquets was the sign presentations, which were printed in book form and thus have remained accessible ever since. The tone of these speeches is truly impressive (cf. Ladd, 2003, pp. 108–112). I argue that they reveal seven preoralist Deafhood principles, which are as follows:

1. Deaf people possess a gift of languages so special that sign languages can be used to say things that speech cannot.
2. The languages are even more special because they can be adapted to cross international boundaries, where spoken languages fail. (There is also strong evidence that Berthier and others believed that there was one global sign language and that each national sign language was a single branch on this tree.)
3. Consequently, Deaf people manifest the potential ability to become the world's first truly global citizens and thus serve as models for the rest of society.
4. Deaf people were intentionally created on earth (whether by God or Nature) to manifest these qualities; thus the reason for their existence should not be questioned.
5. Sign languages are a gift offered to hearing people, so that if they joined with Deaf people and learned them, the quality of their lives would be improved. The strongest proponents of this belief would go as far as to state principle number 6.
6. "Sign languages are an art of the body. Deaf people, the 'Peoples of the Eye,' may have developed them, but these skills form part of what constitutes full human beings—people who can use all their senses to communicate. If all the available senses are not used, humans are incomplete beings."
7. All Deaf people are fundamentally equal, and those more fortunate are obliged to fight for the others to have the same opportunities.

After oralism, Deaf people lost sight of most of these or no longer used them in public discourses. You could consider which ones are still covert beliefs or values.

The belief in "Nature-ism" implicit in the seven principles became our downfall in the eras of science, industrialization, and colonialism. We were seen only as natural as all the other "savage" races of the earth (that is, not fully human) and fit only to serve the white man, who has ruled the world ever since—with disastrous consequences wherever we look. Now there is a swing toward the "natural" again, toward respect for the riches of the Earth and its earth-valuing peoples, who are its true custodians. Thus the time is ripe to begin to open dialogue with them to regain respect for ourselves as men and women "of Nature."

Deafhood after Colonization, and the Deaf Culture Concept

As my research into Deaf culture progressed, I realized it was possible to reexamine our community through the lens of the term Deafhood, and I identified ways in which some Deaf children and adults fought to maintain their ideas about their strongest Deaf selves, to keep their Deafhood alive, whereas others remained mentally colonized (cf. Ladd, 2003, chaps. 7–9).

It seems that many Deaf associations around the world are still mentally colonized. This is partly because they *embody* traditional Deaf cultures, which is of course valuable. However, they cannot change as swiftly as colonialist organizations can, through simply importing new hearing professionals, because culture is a living, breathing, organic force and can only change slowly. It can speed up if a culture examines itself, learns to understand itself, and makes changes based on what it has found: to study ourselves formally, engage in (Deaf) consciousness-raising workshops, and the like.

This is where the idea of Deafhood is helpful to us. We can posit that during colonialism, examples of what we might term "hearing culture which has become part of Deaf culture" multiplied. If we want to change our present Deaf culture and find the biggest Deafhood self that we can, here are four examples from many:

1. Many members of Deaf cultures see it as the Deaf way to criticize rather than praise. Those norms were learned from oralism, where Deaf children were criticized every day for innumerable small transgressions, such as signing.
2. The "crab theory" is also seen as the Deaf way. (The "crab theory" refers to the tendency of some Deaf people to criticize or put down the success of other Deaf people. The analogy is to a bucket of live crabs: Whenever one crab attempts to escape by climbing out of the bucket, the others reach up and pull it back down.) However, it can be argued that this was learned from the process of resistance, of pulling down those "successful" oral Deaf students whom the teachers used as sticks with which to beat the others.
3. Deaf cultural suspicion or dislike of hearing people can also be attributed to oralism. Deaf children and adults did not know that oralists were not typical of hearing people and that there were thousands out there who wanted to be their friends.
4. A very different example is Deaf theater. We can ask whether it uses "real BSL," for example, whether it has "real BSL" Deaf characters and real types from Deaf life, whether it shows real internal Deaf community lives and issues, and so on. The answer until very recently was no. The focus was outward, toward translation of hearing plays and styles, rather than inward in a search for our own styles. Ironically, in the nonprestigious domain of sign storytelling, we can find these features and can witness on informal levels some wonderful skills, which are not overtly valued. Because the idea of Deaf community and history was denigrated by oralists, the ability to cherish ourselves, to comment on ourselves in a public way to ourselves, as happens in hearing drama, has disappeared over the years.

One can continue like this through many different Deaf cultural patterns. How does one break the patterns? One step is to realize that they *are* patterns. The next step is to draw a line under Deaf culture as it is presently understood and say, "Yes, these are the Deaf traditions we have inherited following colonization. We respect them, but we must also continue to aim to realize a larger Deaf self." That larger self can be seen as our search for Deafhood. If we take such a double-headed approach, we can open up new worlds to ourselves, while still being aware of our traditions and know that they still operate on us. In the process, we decide which of those traditions are still valuable to us and should be retained and which should be cast aside. One can try an exercise to get a sense of the difference in scale by imagining what the Deaf world would be like if oralism had never happened:

We would have one hundred years of literate, strong, proud Deaf people. Many Deaf heads and Deaf teachers. Many more interpreters. Many more hearing people would have been signing and part of the Deaf community. Our relationships with our own parents and other hearing parents of Deaf children would be radically different. There would have been much more BSL and many more Deaf people in film and television, much more Deaf art, Deaf theater, Deaf poetry, and so forth. This amounts to a totally different world: not just a few Deaf people with better jobs, but whole communities on a different level of existence.

That is what Deafhood could have been. And that is what it still can become!

International Aspects of Deafhood

Let us now return to what Deafhood might mean from an international perspective, that key theme of the Paris banquets. One place we can find a deeper Deafhood is on the international level. There, signed communication must be kept as visually clear and pure as possible. If we slip into anything linguistically unique to our national cultures, communication breaks down. In this respect we have a global metalanguage, one of pure genius, and the accompanying wonderful feelings of global citizenship is something millions of people admire in us and aspire to. In such an environment, one can feel one's Deafhood growing into a larger size, another dimension. What we have yet to do is to appreciate that dimension fully and bring back to our own countries the Deafhood lessons that it opens up to us.

U.K., European, and U.S. Deafhoods

My research also covered comparisons between U.S. and U.K. Deaf cultures. I briefly describe some features, as seen through the lens of Deafhood.

When we examine American Deafhood, we notice greater Deaf pride, greater confidence and belief. As any one Deaf foreigner who has lived in the United States knows, one can feel oneself growing inside with a realization that Deaf people can do everything except hear.

One manifestation is a much greater appreciation of good/beautiful signing. This can extend so far that Deaf leaders can be chosen *because* they are powerful signers. That idea simply does not exist in British Deafhood. One effect of this is that many Deaf Americans work hard to improve their signing skills. Another is that Deaf signing art has many more skilled practitioners, in poetry, storytelling, cabaret, theatre, and so on. It was this rich soil that enabled Dot Miles to flourish, and she had a hard time when she came back to the United Kingdom and was underappreciated. Clearly for Deaf Americans, deeper ASL skills mean deeper Deafhood.

To put it another way, American Deafhood accords a higher priority to these skills than to some others.

Many of us have seen or heard many stories about how Deaf Americans do not mix well with other Deaf people at international gatherings. We can interpret that another way: that for most Deaf people, their idea of their own Deafhood is based on acting out their identity as global Deaf people. This does not seem to be the case for Deaf Americans. Incidentally, it has also been said that the British are not that much more sociable. There is a sense in which both are seen as putting their national identities first and their Deaf identity second.

It also appears that Deaf Americans are not very involved in overt political activity. The Gallaudet campaign seems to have been an isolated incident. In the United Kingdom, Deafhood seems to be much more linked to political action.

In the United States, there is more of an emphasis on individuals and on status than on equality and community. If one comes from an American Deaf family, one effectively inherits a "crown." In the United Kingdom, this respect still has to be earned by service to the community. Again we can see these as different types or priorities of each country's Deafhood—one is focused on individual achievement and the other on community.

Another example is the European focus on campaigning for Deaf programs in sign language on television, that is, a means of communication that the whole community can access. In the United States, the fight is almost entirely for captions. Because it is unlikely that all American Deaf people read perfectly, this suggests that the focus is on access for individuals, a percentage of the community but not the entire community.

This kind of analysis can help us understand our own Deaf selves better through understanding how and why other Deaf people frame their Deafhood differently.

Deafhoods and Implications for the Future

It is important to realize that Deafhood is not a finite, fixed state, but one that can change, grow, or shrink. It is natural for different groups of Deaf people to interpret Deafhood in different ways, and that debate is healthy. Our overall task is to make sure we understand as many of these as possible so that we can try to and draw on the best of each to improve, develop, or redevelop our national and international communities.

We need to be aware that many of these processes happen, as with all cultures, unconsciously. Likewise, there are still many Deaf people around the world whose Deafhood is operating on more limited levels, including many young mainstreamed Deaf who have barely begun to set foot on the Deafhood path.

Other important implications are the need to make Deaf services more Deaf centered, social and mental health services assessing and treating Deaf people by Deafhood-devised criteria, Deaf television run according to Deaf visual perceptions and Deafhood values, and Deaf organizations aspiring to the highest goals of Deafhood.

Perhaps even more important, let us imagine Deaf education run according to these values. This is a fascinating challenge because when we come to educate Deaf children, we can use intuitive cultural knowledge to shape their development, but we also have to realize that, unlike ourselves, these children can go on to become something we could not be ourselves. We have to *imagine* what they can become and try to nurture that. In the process, we ourselves grow too.

All these decolonization stages mean that we are in for another transition period of greater Deaf-hearing tension in such workplaces. We know that we do not yet have enough qualified Deaf managerial professionals to take charge of all necessary positions, compared with the increased level of desire for this control. One way that Deafhood ideas can help to speed up this transition period is for both Deaf and hearing people to workshop ideas about what "Deaf" could mean, for example, by asking what types of Deaf people are working in each establishment, by being open to whether what a strong Deaf person is saying or doing is right, or by seeing if they are acting from negative cultural patterns.

Likewise, we might ask whether hearing people are more comfortable working with Deaf people who do not challenge them and thus either do not employ strong Deaf people, limit their roles, or denigrate them as angry extremists. There will be as many different situations as there are people, but such cultural workshops may help to defuse this tension and turn it into a positive, life-enhancing process.

Finally, there is the vital importance of Deafhood concepts to the coming threat of genetic engineering, which in effect challenges us by asking "Why should we allow you Deaf people to live? What do you offer to humanity?"

Our ancestors from preoralist Deafhood have shown us how we might answer such questions. Because the Deafhood concept enables us to seek and develop those largest dimensions of Deaf existence, it is in the expansion of those dimensions that many of us, both Deaf and hearing, will learn lessons for creating positive change rather than continuing to obsess about the usual aspects of oppression. It is coming close to the time when Berthier's unique combination of political and spiritual (ontological) dimensions of Deafhood must be developed once more. Until we provide geneticists—or rather, influence the public—with the largest, most celebratory Deafhood answers we can find, the very existence of all of our people will hang in the balance.

References

Alker, D. (2000). *Really not interested in the Deaf?* Darwen, U.K.: Darwen Press.
De Ladebat, L. (1815). *A collection of the most remarkable definitions and answers of Massieu and Clerc.* London: Cox and Bayliss.
Ladd, P. (2003). *Understanding Deaf culture: In search of Deafhood.* Cleveden, U.K.: Multilingual Matters.
Lane, H., & Philip, F. (Eds.). (1984). *The Deaf experience.* Cambridge, MA: Harvard University Press.
Mottez, B. (1993). The deaf mute banquets and the birth of the Deaf movement. In R. Fisher & H. Lane (Eds.), *Looking back: A reader on the history of Deaf communities and their sign languages* (pp. 143–156). Hamburg, Germany: Signum Verlag.

Deaf View Image Art: A Manifesto Revisited

BETTY MILLER, DEBORAH SONNENSTRAHL, ALEX WILHITE, AND PAUL JOHNSTON

BETTY: It is time to revisit Deaf View Image Art because it has been almost thirteen years since the first Deaf Way. Initially I discuss a brief history of how we even came to establish Deaf View Image Art.

It was spring of 1972 when I had arranged for an exhibit of my work, and it was the first time an exhibit was specifically arranged to express the Deaf experience. After the exhibit, it was evident that people were totally unprepared with what they saw at the exhibit. They were actually quite shocked and angry and felt insulted by the imagery they saw. I did not expect to receive such a strong reaction, and it became apparent that my work was ahead of its time in expressing Deaf feelings and experiences.

It also gave a real-life window to our experience as Deaf people. We had a piece of work called "The Hearing Test," in which a child was literally being put through a hearing test. The artwork was showing our discomfort, our dislike in these oral and audio-based situations at schools. Many of the pieces showed different perspectives of our experience growing up in a world that is not Deaf. I did not anticipate and was not prepared for the strong reaction. After that exhibit, there was not much follow-through action on my part—I did not do any drawings, paintings, or exhibits until the early 1980s. I do not wish to go into details, but the strong reactions and criticisms did adversely affect me back then.

Nevertheless, from 1972 to 1989, I wanted to see the day when we would establish a "manifesto" to let people know that we have Deaf artists expressing their experiences through artwork. During that period, I met with many Deaf artists from all over the United States. I traveled a great deal and had in-depth conversations, and some not-so-in-depth conversations, with other Deaf artists.

There was nothing formal until 1989, when I submitted a proposal to the first Deaf Way. I wanted a four-day workshop specifically to discuss the issues facing Deaf artists. I had several artists in mind who I wanted to include, one of whom was Paul Johnston. He and I actually created the initial agenda and the plan for the four-day weekend. We personally invited various artists from across the country to attend. Not all of them could come, but we ended up with nine attendees, including Johnston and myself.

Let me tell you who those artists were: Johnston, Nancy Creighton, Sandi Inches Vasnick, Guy Wonder, Alex Wilhite, Chuck Baird, Deborah Sonnenstrahl, and Lai-Yok Ho. By the way, Sonnenstrahl is now selling her recently published book titled *Deaf Artists in America: Colonial to Contemporary*, which is a wonderful coffee-table book worth buying.

For four days, we shared our personal experiences as artists, the frustrations we had experienced and the struggles we encountered. We showed each other our work through slides, and some brought the actual pieces in for us to view. We talked about what we liked to do in our artwork and why we liked to do our artwork.

We discussed our purpose of coming together. We talked a lot about our personal experiences, our experiences as artists, our frustrations, our struggles, and so forth. Many of us felt we could do artwork related to our Deaf experience. We discussed the elements, the creative piece, to put our art into the category of Deaf art. We wanted to develop a visual and written manifesto. I am very disappointed that I cannot show you these slides because we have pictures that represent the visual manifesto. Unfortunately, the piece was stolen from an exhibit at the Washburn Art Building. It was unbelievable because it was a tremendously large piece. I have not seen it again since then.

We talked about what we meant by "manifesto." We brainstormed about different elements we wanted to encompass. We wanted a name for the movement that would look good in American Sign Language (ASL) and would translate well in English. Thus, we ended up with "Deaf View Image Art." Some of the artists like to use De'VIA as the acronym. I personally do not use that acronym very much unless I am writing a piece on the movement and use the term repeatedly throughout the writing. If I am in conversation or presenting on the movement, I prefer to use ASL sign for "Deaf View Image Art" in its entirety.

The manifesto focused on basic elements that are universal among Deaf artists, in the use of colors, shapes, lines, composition, and the different characteristics that show up in the images that are chosen. There may be more elements we add to that list as time goes on.

There are common elements when you view a collection of Deaf artists' work. One of them is the use of strong contrasting colors. Another is contrasting textures, for example, rough versus smooth. Often, the pieces have a centralized focus, such as focusing on the center figure as the most important piece of the composition and downplaying the background. Sometimes there is an exaggeration or emphasis on ears, eyes, or mouth; physical gesture or hands; an exaggeration of those features or other means of emphasizing those features.

Another thing we noticed about Deaf artists in the past—not so much now but definitely in the past—was a tendency to focus on figures or people as the central point of the work. There was little attention paid to the background because it was not what the artists wanted to emphasize. It was often rather unclear, purposely ambiguous, to emphasize the central figure.

That weekend, we sat and talked a great deal about not only Deaf View Image Art but also the overall perspective of Deaf art. We started early in the morning, taking a simple meal break and going for the rest of the day into the evening hours. It was more than just a nine-to-five workshop. I think the only day we broke before what normally would be time for bed was that last day, when we finally decided to close up late in the afternoon.

I found the four-day workshop to be an outstanding experience. We got the opportunity to finally share how we felt as artists and as Deaf people and to find how much commonality there was in our shared experiences and frustrations. It really added to our inspiration and enthusiasm to establish the De'VIA Manifesto as a recognized category. Most of the artists in this category are painters who paint about the Deaf experience as a subject matter. There are also other artists who paint on very different subject matter such as landscapes and abstract painting. We certainly respect their work as artists but those are not pieces that would be representative of De'VIA artwork. Let me make it clear that De'VIA artists do not reject the professionalism of other Deaf artists and their artwork on different subject matter; it is just that De'VIA artists want to recognize their artwork as part of Deaf culture, in the same way African Americans, Hispanics, and other minority groups have recognized artworks that represent their ethnic cultures or heritages. Now the De'VIA category of artwork has become a wonderful part of Deaf culture, and Deaf studies programs have recognized such artwork as something that Deaf artists have done successfully.

We announced the official manifesto during the first Deaf Way in 1989. The artists were very touched and inspired to have such an official manifesto in place. However, there were also many criticisms. People asked: Why was it necessary to have such a manifesto? Were there even enough artists to produce enough work to legitimize the manifesto? Why not simply call the work Deaf Art as before?

We needed to clarify that Deaf Art is a very broad genre, which includes Deaf artists producing any artwork, and many of those do not necessarily address their experiences as Deaf people as a cultural linguistic minority. Again, we offer no criticism of those artists and their product, but they are different and need to be delineated from the people we are defining and the work we are defining in the De'VIA Manifesto. If they choose to produce a particular work that represents their Deaf experience that may be an exception to the body of their work, that piece would be included as an exhibit piece for De'VIA.

We are not forming a movement or an organization of particular Deaf artists. On the contrary, De'VIA is a new concept that was derived from the four-day workshop involving nine Deaf artists, who unanimously agreed on the manifesto. We are not here to cause a controversy but merely to delineate a concept or category. We have respect for all artists, and it is not our intention to reject anyone's work.

We have gone through thirteen years of some pretty intense criticism, but that criticism has faded over time, and Deaf View Image Art has remained strong and become known throughout the country.

Now it is starting to spread internationally. Deaf artists from other countries are openly expressing their artwork representing their Deaf experiences and have shown interest in the manifesto, the concept behind it, as it represents Deaf people. It has proliferated throughout the world and thus is not unique to the United States. The De'VIA Manifesto was originally conceived for American Deaf artists, but we are certainly open to having the manifesto used by any country and modified to become their own, because the basic concepts of the manifesto are the same in different countries.

Several years ago, Gallaudet University began offering a course specifically on Deaf View Image Art. In Rochester, New York, the National Technical Institute for the Deaf also has Deaf View Image Art studies as an option for students. That means that two accredited universities are offering this as a means of coursework as an outgrowth from our initial conversation back in 1989. They are collecting artwork from many different artists to use in the materials to teach those courses, and so people can clearly compare the original work to the current work that artists are producing under De'VIA.

Paul Johnston, Deborah Sonnenstrahl, and Alex Wilhite are in the audience, and I would like to bring them up on the stage with me to entertain questions from the floor and to have an open discussion with audience members about the future for Deaf artists. We would like to take some time to share ideas and talk with you about those future visions for our work under the De'VIA category. These were three of the original artists who attended the four-day workshop back in 1989. Unfortunately, the other members are not able to be here at this moment.

DEBORAH: That was a wonderful summary bringing us up to date. It puts things in the appropriate perspective as we look back to the first Deaf Way workshop, and everything Betty said is absolutely on target.

BETTY: I would like to add that when we worked on the manifesto back then, we did discuss the appropriateness of including hearing artists whose artwork reflects Deaf experience. It was a new experience for me to work with a hearing artist who has successfully exhibited his work, "Hearing Aids Are Not Like Glasses," at the Millennium Arts Center in Washington, D.C. Admittedly, this wonderful experience makes me think twice about whether the manifesto should include such hearing artists.

DEBORAH: I have seen more widespread interest in and acceptance of the concept of De'VIA than ever before. I personally find myself finger spelling DEVIA instead of signing Deaf View Image Art.

PAUL: More people are accepting the concept of Deaf View Image Art than ever before, but I find myself finger spelling the acronym DEVIA as opposed to using the ASL sign for Deaf View Image Art. People would ask me, "Are you involved with De'VIA artwork?" instead of signing the entire phrase, so I am wondering whether we should sign it or use the acronym? It is hard because we do not really want to criticize the way people sign and it appears much easier to finger spell the acronym than to sign all four words. I think the acronym is behaving almost like a word we recognize, like most people would say UCLA instead of the University of California at Los Angeles. You may not know what each of those letters necessarily stands for, but you know the meaning of the acronym. I personally think it is okay and convenient to use or finger spell the acronym these days.

The reason we came up with that four-word phrase in the first place is because those nine artists had involved ASL as their primary language, and we were trying to formulate ASL signs to reflect the concept of artwork expressing Deaf people's experiences or views. From the formulated ASL signs, we came up with the corresponding English translation, Deaf View Image Art, or for short, D-e-V-I-A, or simply De'VIA, and thus finger spelled DEVIA.

ALEX: Before this, we did not really have a concept of the Deaf art history. After we established this Deaf View Image Art, we began to be recognized more, and we borrowed the concept from the hearing community, from different styles and lines and colors. We then got our artwork spread out to the Deaf community and started showing our culture. It was a way to bridge artworks done by Deaf artists and hearing artists as well.

AUDIENCE: My name is Angelina. I am from the state of Washington. I know there was a gallery exhibit that you mentioned back in the 1970s. How did your artwork at that time impact the Deaf community? I have heard that when Deaf people came into the exhibit, they were very confronted, had very strong reactions to the pieces they saw and the messages conveyed. I wonder if you could share a little bit more about that.

BETTY: It was in 1972, specifically, and I had been asked to arrange for an exhibit of my pieces. I was teaching at the time at Gallaudet University. None of us, including the faculty and staff, expected my exhibit would cause such uproar. We had the opening and had good attendance. Deaf and hearing people came up to me and did not hesitate to tell me how angry I was, as exhibited through my artwork. Hearing people were more likely to tell me that it was wrong for me to do such artwork, and they found them to be insulting, not nice, and not pleasant. They were indeed shocked and found my work upsetting, and their comments affected me greatly. At the same time, the Deaf experience message carried a lot of weight and got many unwary people thinking defensively afterward.

There is a pen-and-ink drawing I did that seemed to become the famous "signature" piece at that exhibit, which has become widely known worldwide these days. This work, titled "Ameslan Prohibited," exhibited the hands in handcuffs with lower parts of fingers chopped off, representing the time when sign language was forbidden in the educational systems in residential schools. Initially, I thought that my work was unique but I found out that was not true when the various artists I mentioned of the original manifesto group brought their work. Alex Wilhite and Chuck Baird did this, and so did several others including Ann Silver and Harry Williams. There was an article in 1972 in the *Washington Post*, which I have a copy of. It was actually a very well-written review. I was very pleased with the coverage on the exhibit I gave. I started painting again in the 1980s.

AUDIENCE: This is Barbara Kannapell. People call me Kanny, and I have known Betty for forty years. I remember exactly what was going on at that 1972 exhibit. There was quite a stunning reaction to her work, and I remember there was the one painting of hands in shackles you mentioned earlier. Actually, it was a very large picture. It was a pen-and-ink piece that was at Gallaudet University. There was another one of a person who had a head with no eyes, and yet another one about a child with a mouth that would open and close like a wooden puppet. Betty indicated to me that the puppet child picture is still here, hanging on the first floor near an elevator in Gallaudet University Kellogg Conference Center. There is the fourth one I will never forget, which was about a hearing aid box that was nailed to the body of a child as if the child was crucified by the hearing aid. It was a very powerful message with a strong knockout punch that shook and affected many of us within the Deaf community.

My questions to you and the panelists are these: How do you see yourselves since 1989? Do you think things have changed? Is the movement growing slowly? I know that there are courses now in Deaf View Image Art. Could we have an explanation from you about this? I know Sonnenstrahl had a book published. What is its impact on De'VIA over the past thirteen years since the first Deaf Way?

PAUL: We as Deaf artists are so grateful to the Deaf studies departments at Gallaudet University and elsewhere, which have given a strong impetus to our work and our movement by including some Deaf artists in their studies. Through word of mouth, the inclusion of Deaf artists becomes important in any Deaf studies program anywhere. Indeed, many schools for Deaf students around the country have included this concept as part of Deaf studies curriculum. Students are able to see that Deaf identity, experiences, and pride can be exhibited through our artwork.

Let me talk about the De'VIA courses at Gallaudet University. I should explain that for many, many years in art history courses, we looked at many artists and studied their masterpieces. We found it embarrassing to not know much about Deaf artists and their works throughout history, probably because there were no earlier research attempts to collect data on Deaf artists. We thought it was time to offer a course so that students can gain appreciation of Deaf artists—as well as hearing artists—who were there before us. Not all of De'VIA artwork is political either. Actually, its themes vary from something humorous all the way to something political.

Many people write poems, stories, or plays about Deaf people and their experiences. Why cannot the Deaf artists do the same through their drawings or paintings? So, in the course, we try to cover all of the art forms.

In the past, we did a number of interviews with several Deaf artists who had produced artwork about their experiences and learned that because they were not confident or comfortable about their Deaf identity, they hid their artwork rather than show them at certain exhibits. After seeing that many Deaf people are proud about their identity and have pride and confidence in themselves, more and more Deaf artists have done De'VIA types of artwork for exhibits all over the country.

BETTY: Susan Duper is another artist who is Deaf and teaches art as well at the Wisconsin School for the Deaf. She uses the children's Deaf experiences, their unique experiences, to foster their own expression artistically and fosters that growth through the years.

ALEX: I was an artist in residence at that school at one point and I think that work is still ongoing.

DEBORAH: I would like to add a response to Kanny's question. She asked us about the Deaf View Image Art. I have known Betty for many years. We were college classmates, and I know that she has also grown a great deal. I personally admit I was one of the people who were incredibly shocked and did not like her art at first viewing, but I am also here to admit that I am a human being. My first reaction was that she was making fun of deafness and that she insulted the fact that we are Deaf. It was a horrible experience for me. Naturally, I have grown, thanks to Betty.

Now it is wonderful to see this art gain widespread acceptance. It started very small and then has grown. But it has also given me trouble because I was writing a book on the history of Deaf artists in America, and I had to start my book from scratch because there was no such book prior to the one I was doing. Now I had to know how to put these artists in their proper framework and structure within the history of Deaf artists.

Like she said, there are many fine Deaf artists who deserve equal recognition, so it became important to distinguish these two groups of Deaf artists in some way. I finally found a solution. I put in both groups into the late-twentieth-century and twenty-first-century artists, but I did it in separate sections because I wanted to clearly separate those artists who are using their Deaf experience in their artwork from those Deaf artists who do not. It was a happy conclusion.

I think some of you may be a little confused. You know, some people ask if you are a member of De'VIA, and they ask, "Can I paint pictures that have nothing to do with Deafness?" Some people appear to see a gray area between the two, and sometimes it is not quite clear to them. Like Betty said, De'VIA is not a club or an organization. You do not have to pay dues. You do not have to join it in any way. It is sort of like the French impressionists in Europe. They did not have a club that they joined. It was more like a concept. They would talk about how they would paint in a certain way, how they would approach art as a concept. That is what the Deaf View Image Art is: a concept.

Most of you know of a famous hearing artist named Picasso. His style changed throughout the years: there was the blue period, there was the red period, and there was his cubism. Similarly, any Deaf artist certainly can change style within or without the concept of De'VIA.

ALEX: In 1989, I was a very young graduate student, and I did not really know any other Deaf artists. I was very, very isolated. At that time, I did not know enough about the history of Deaf artists. I was focused on the New York school groups and the abstract art group, and that was a hearing group. I was looking for other Deaf artists, and it seemed that Betty came to me as an angel. She asked me to be involved in this Deaf Way discussion group, and so I took the train down from New York, stayed for a few days, and got involved. I had never felt such support from the artists of the Deaf community, for which I have been grateful. There was no written history of Deaf artists or of Deaf culture in art at the time. It was a bridge that allowed me to grow. It seemed like Deaf culture in art was sleeping, waiting to be woken up.

After we developed the concept of Deaf View Image Art, we have been teaching the Deaf community about their own art as well as offering a bridge by expressing our art and our view of art to the hearing world.

AUDIENCE: Hello. I am from England. It is interesting, I agree, that although there are differences over the world in Deaf experiences, there are also commonalities as well. It is interesting to try and have an art category specifically for the Deaf experience. There are some people who may not identify with that because they have a different experience. If you are going to have a gallery and hearing people are going into an exhibition, they might not really understand the concepts that you are trying to convey in your artwork. I feel privileged when I am in that position to be able to teach hearing people a new perspective on the world. My question is slightly different from that, however. You said that hearing people were shocked and outraged, and there was quite an extreme reaction to your artwork. Now there seems to be greater Deaf awareness and greater information out in the community. I was wondering if people's responses now are the same as they were in 1989. Is there still such outrage and shock, or do you find that people are more accepting?

BETTY: It is difficult to say, but there are more and more hearing people involved in the Deaf community overall. I notice that the more I show, the more people are involved who are also hearing. Remember, my work comes from my heart and from my inner self. It is the way that we express who we are. I think that today, the interaction between Deaf and hearing people and their perspectives on our work would be more positive, unless you encountered the person who had no understanding of the Deaf community at all. I do not know if you would agree with that. I personally do not have any experience with reactions from a hearing person who did not have any contact with the Deaf community. Perhaps one of you can share such an experience.

DEBORAH: I am not an artist myself, but my observation is that hearing people are much more fascinated than critical. I believe they are more open to our work now.

ALEX: Hearing people love to buy artwork for investment purposes or as a means of preserving history. I do not see why they would not continue to invest in work that represents different communities and cultures, including ours.

PAUL: Our artwork is also a historical document of our experiences, which will last for many years. When hearing people see it, it does have an impact on them. As Deborah said, when she first saw your work many years ago, she had a reaction to it and then it became more acceptable. I think nowadays many hearing people look at Deaf people not as a cultural group, that is, they still see us as people with disabilities. In fact, I have two hearing friends who are affected by my work. They find it very powerful. It does engender some pity from them, rather than having them express joy with our messages. They have not really grasped the pride we have being Deaf.

A lot of hearing people are now involved in the Deaf community one way or another. They take sign language classes, and I think they are becoming more accepting and understanding of our work as well. Also, I know that one person does not represent the entire hearing world, so we should not make any generalizations but rather look at each individual's reaction.

ALEX: I have a question, actually. When you talk about Spanish artist Goya, do you feel he represents Deaf artists as a De'VIA artist or as an artist who is Deaf? He painted in the early 1800s and he was Deaf, but does his work actually fall into a representation of what could be considered a Deaf View Image Art product?

DEBORAH: Well, briefly, the eighteenth-century Spanish artist named Goya became Deaf at the age of forty-two. All art historians agree that his art changed after he became Deaf. It is very clear. Before his Deafness, he basically painted the outside world. He painted what he saw and he painted the carefree happy life of Spaniards. After he became Deaf, which occurred at about the time when Napoleon led his army toward the invasion of Spain, his worldview completely turned upside down, and he began to paint what he called his inside world. In other words, he was talking about his own internal experience, which was a Deaf experience. He was already Deaf at that time.

Earlier, Betty explained several elements commonly found in De'VIA artwork. The elements of De'VIA art were seen in Goya's work. If you look at his etchings, you can see that the hands are exaggeratedly large. There is one etching that shows a prison. It was a Spanish government prison. The figure in the drawing was shackled with his hands behind him, with locks over his ears. If that is not a Deaf experience, I do not know what you would call it.

So I would say, yes, we do have Deaf artists expressing Deaf experiences who came before us, but I am not sure you can call their work as part of the Deaf View Image Art because that concept was not talked about at that time. As a historian, I

Deaf View Image Art: A Manifesto Revisited

would limit that term to twentieth-century and later art. For artists before that time, I would use the term, pre-De'VIA, like I did in my book.

AUDIENCE: I enjoyed your presentation, particularly your comparison of Deaf View Image Art as a concept being parallel to the French impressionists. I am wondering if there is going to be further discussion of the rules or criteria that define art as a piece falling into a specific category or subcategory. For example, specific imagery such as hearing aids, sign language, or handshapes that would further define and delineate that piece as belonging to that specific category.

DEBORAH: I do not like the term "rules." I am hesitant and fearful to impose rules on artists. Generally artists create artwork using free expression. I do not see how we would want to have hard and fast rules. There is no question in my mind that the acceptance of De'VIA art will continue to grow and spread. As long as you have a Deaf experience—and each individual has a different Deaf experience—and then if that is what the art is expressing, we could identify it as falling within the concept of De'VIA art.

BETTY: Susan Dupor also established classes in De'VIA, in which she taught children specific ways of approaching their experience and placing it in their artwork. More and more universities accept coursework on Deaf View Image Art, and I think there are going to be more discussions of the parameters around the product, but not so much exactly what that product is supposed to include, because that would inhibit the artist's freedom of expression.

AUDIENCE: Do you think of yourselves as painting a visual language? When you look at your paintings, do you sometimes wonder if you are a painter or a poet? How much did your relationship with text change during the ten years between Deaf Way I and Deaf Way II, because I am very conscious that in contemporary poetry there has been a total turn toward visual and kinetic art and I wonder if you take part in that? Poetry is expressing itself differently than it used to. I am talking about the border between text and picture because sign language is obviously a visual language. How much do text and picture come together in your paintings? Would you say your paintings are textual, and are they becoming more textual or less textual?

BETTY: Well, first of all, we have to remember that American Sign Language is not a visual language. Although ASL is a language that is visual, it is not called a visual language per se. ASL is a language in its own right used by Deaf people, and it has its own grammar and syntax. It is no more visual in that sense than Spanish, so I just wanted to clarify that use of the word "visual language."

Our painting is very different than poetry. Poetry is language based and might use English text or other language text to express inner feelings. When we express our feelings through paintings, it is based on our Deaf experience, without even thinking about using any form of text. Our inner experiences are shown directly as art images, rather than through textual forms commonly found among products by poets or playwrights.

AUDIENCE: When we talk about this topic, there are things that have bothered me years and years before the De'VIA concept actually started. I know I want to express my experience as a Deaf person. I do not paint; I build. I construct. Now, there were several artists I met years ago. There was one artist named Kowalski from Poland who has passed away, and his work was produced back in the 1950s. He got me interested in art. I have lost the record of where his work has been, so I think we are having trouble finding some of these pieces of the earlier Deaf artists. I actually went to this artist's house and saw the artwork on mechanical hands he had created. Unfortunately, he did not have a good relationship with his wife when he passed away. She burned his artwork, and so there were no remaining archives of his work. Whatever was left was taken or stolen. So, how do we keep track of these collections and create backups of their work?

BETTY: Deaf View Image Art, again, is a concept. I know it is difficult to remember that we are not an organization. We do not have any means of creating archives or maintaining collections. To have such an organization responsible for collecting and preserving the artwork in galleries or other appropriate places to keep them from vandalism or theft is something to consider.

ALEX: Art is often stolen, and private collections are where an artist's work usually is kept. It is impossible for any gallery to keep all the work of all the Deaf artists. What we are trying to do is find the right person to buy our work, and then we can get the work out there among the public. I suggest that you all teach other communities about Deaf artists and ask that their work be included in permanent collections, perhaps at galleries, museums, private homes, and other places.

PAUL: Everyone is welcome to buy and put art into one's own artwork collection. There is no barrier to you producing a piece that could be considered part of the De'VIA. It can include anything from children's work all the way up to professional artists. There are many options, and we certainly could not imagine collecting all of the pieces in one place that represent what we are defining as Deaf View Image Art.

BETTY: One thing we do need to work on is a means of critiquing work to determine whether it falls under the De'VIA concept. Those criteria and means of having that conversation have not yet been addressed. It is sort of like the recognition of American Sign Language as an official language. When Stokoe finally printed his research work and publicly recognized ASL as an official language in the 1960s, the dark ages for our community were finally coming to an end. The same is somewhat true for our artwork. It basically remained an unrecognized product until De'VIA Manifesto was developed. Just as there is more to be done in American Sign Language research and recognition, the same is true of De'VIA art.

AUDIENCE: I think that there is something lacking in what you are discussing. I think you are lacking discussion about art theory. You are not considering theoretical perspectives of art in any of your discussions, and I was wondering if you had any comment on that. If you go to any library, you will find many, many books on art history and art theory, and so I am wondering whether we should think about establishing some more research into Deaf art theory. When I see a lot of Deaf art and I compare it to what art theorists have to say, I do not think it is real art. Art is rich. It should include history, yes. It should include culture. But if we think about art theory from a more purist perspective, this kind of Deaf art is not what we would see as true art. It is an important impoverished form of art.

BETTY: Are you talking about theory typical in terms of critique or criticism?

AUDIENCE: Potentially, it could be a form of criticism, a way to critique the art based on theory, yes.

PAUL: That is exactly what we would like to discuss further, and we do discuss it in my course here at Gallaudet on Deaf View Image Art: teaching the students to analyze a piece, to be able to express a criticism, to discuss composition, line, use of color. We have many tools that we offer the students to take apart and assess a given art piece. One semester or even two semesters is not enough. It would take several years to give them a full handle on how to critique Deaf artwork.

I am hoping, in the future, to involve graduate students in research, to really do some analysis of current work versus previous periods, and eventually publish a book on exactly what you are mentioning, theory and critique, of De'VIA.

AUDIENCE: I am from Europe. I am very pleased to see what you have been doing here in America. I am fascinated that your art actually incorporates cultural reference. I have also seen that with Jewish artists expressing their experience from the Holocaust. I do not know if there is something unique to a Deaf Jewish artist's product from that period.

BETTY: Are you talking prior to or after the Second World War?

AUDIENCE: This was artwork produced after World War II. These were Deaf people who had survived the Holocaust. There was an exhibit by David Bloch. I think the actual pieces were produced in the 1960s and 1970s. Perhaps this is just part of this theory conversation; do these artists and their work fall under Deaf View Image Art or are they simply Deaf artists?

DEBORAH: There is a group of Holocaust survivors whose work parallels the issue of Deaf View Image Art. Now, if there are in addition elements of De'VIA, then there are Deaf Jewish artists whose work can be explained in terms of Deaf View Image Art as well because they use their Deaf experience.

AUDIENCE: I want to teach a class on history regarding the Holocaust, which is going to be a new course, and I want to make sure to incorporate things that talk about the Holocaust in general, but also from a Deaf perspective, and potential artwork that was produced as a result.

BETTY: As long as the pieces are following the basic elements outlined in the manifesto, you could legitimately categorize a person's pieces as part of the De'VIA concept. But I understand your question. If a Deaf person's experience from the Holocaust is what informs their figures and their composition, it becomes a question of which culture is dominant in that particular piece, their experience as a Deaf person or that of a Jewish person. It would be important to look at a given piece and a given artist and assess the specific elements to determine what category that piece could be classified under.

AUDIENCE: And I would like to respond to what this previous speaker said. There is an artist whose name was David Bloch. He was a Deaf artist, and he did sculpture or wood carvings about the Holocaust. There was an exhibit in a temple in Los Angeles a number of years ago. Perhaps you could look into that.

Theory leads to ideas and new discussions, and it is a wonderful thing, this exchange of ideas. Now, I myself am not a theoretician. I am a writer, and I have written some reviews of Deaf art. One person talked about art as a visual language, and I am not sure I totally agree with your comment, Betty. It is true that American Sign Language is a language, which is represented visually, obviously. It is not a visual language. When we look at art or sometimes we see, these images of the finger-spelled alphabet in art pieces, for example by Chuck Baird. Some of his work has that in it; it is not really text, but if I were to see images that were the finger-spelling symbols that went on in a piece for an extensive time and gave an actual text, that might be different. However, if you just see the alphabet as a symbol of something that the artist is trying to portray, that is probably one thing.

My question is this: somebody mentioned talking about pre-De'VIA and prior to the manifesto, but what about other artists in the past? They did what might be called De'VIA but that was before 1987, so I am not sure it is appropriate to dismiss them from this particular category or from this specific genre. What is your opinion about that? I think there were many artists prior to your 1972 exhibit. What do you think?

DEBORAH: I think you are right that there were many artists who used their Deaf experience to produce artwork long before we developed De'VIA Manifesto. I completely am in agreement with you on that. My only concern is if we call them the De'VIA artists, then it will create some confusion among people in trying to identify which time period these artists lived in.

Let me give you an example. There were Greek artists from the fourth century B.C. Later, there is an art period called the Renaissance period that technically started in the thirteenth or fourteenth century A.D. Those Renaissance artists in Italy used almost all the elements that originally were constructed in the fourth century B.C. by the Greek artists, but we cannot call the works of the thirteenth- and fourteenth-century Greek art because of the time differential. Otherwise, there would be confusion in terminology used or historical references made. Care has to be taken in the way we label these artists of different eras.

AUDIENCE: Is it only for American artists to be involved in that discussion, or is there the possibility and in what forums would it be possible for European artists to become involved in that discussion?

BETTY: We initially established it for American artists only, but if you want to establish a satellite movement similar to ours, and even with the same name, that certainly would be fine. We would be more than willing to share our manifesto, and I would suggest that you would probably then want to take it on and establish your own criteria, your own list of elements that represent the European Deaf experience as De'VIA because each of us as Deaf people also have our country of origin's culture. Our Deaf culture may be different than yours in some way, and that would impact your and our work differently as well. Our manifesto would not, at a hundred-percent level, translate to another country but certainly could be used the basis for establishing your own manifesto in England, for example.

PAUL: Please feel free to establish De'VIA in other countries. We want to encourage that. Certainly, again, we are not an organization. We are just a theme to be interpreted and used. In Russia, there are artists who obviously experience Deafness in their own country of origin and express it in their work. In America, we would often interpret a dog in artwork as a symbol of Deaf person, because the dog cannot speak and appeared obedient. We learned that a Russian Deaf artist would use a fish as a symbol of a Deaf person because a fish has no ears and can barely move its mouth. Every country is going to interpret Deaf art a little bit differently under the influence of different cultures.

AUDIENCE: Is Deaf art lower than other art? Of course I disagree. I have often wondered where a central warehouse for Deaf art might be, and I wonder what we can do henceforth to take care of that.

There is the World Wide Web; we can see Deaf artists work through the Web and we can share our experience in that way. But as we all know, there is not enough research on Deaf art and the Deaf artist's experience yet, but there is one way we can probably post our work on the Web. My husband and I are the webmasters of www.deafart.org. I helped set it up, so I am a little bit behind in my work. Web sites would be an opportunity for us to share our work and our experiences, and you can have links to any given Web site as well.

Another thing is that we could have exhibits of our work. You could contact your local galleries. Call any one of the panelists to come or provide assistance in setting up an exhibit in your own area and how to get the word out about Deaf art. There are a whole lot of things that we all can do.

There is not enough published about our work, even though our work is proliferating, and I think that also there is not enough research and resources. I think we need to really work together to do that.

AUDIENCE: I have a close family member who is Deaf and had a strong reaction to some of this art. I am wondering if you have seen your art used in therapy sessions? What I mean is using the art as a way to help someone express their feelings or to show that they are not isolated, that there is somebody who may have had a similar experience to the person in counseling or in therapy, as a catharsis for the affected person. Basically, what I mean is allowing the viewing of the work—not that the client would produce artwork as in a typical art therapy setting—but that the work itself would somehow trigger a means for the person to process their therapeutic concerns.

BETTY: The Model Secondary School for the Deaf (MSSD) in Washington, D.C., has bought and created a significant collection of Deaf art to show to young Deaf children different Deaf experiences expressed by Deaf artists. Deaf students would be able to identify with many of the artwork. I think this is a wonderful idea, and I hope that many other schools and programs for deaf students would create similar collections.

PAUL: I was a high school teacher at MSSD for one class, and I actually set up activities where the children were asked to express their Deaf experience through art. It certainly had value. We first discussed what we meant by Deaf experience. For the students, it really fostered a great deal of intense conversation—talking about family experiences, experiences of isolation, and so on. After they became clear on what we meant by Deaf experiences, they were ready to try and express them in art form. Hopefully that would foster future appreciation of art, as well as their own sense of self-esteem and identity. Many therapies include the arts, whether it is writing, performing, or producing fine art. Teachers can be creative in trying different forms of therapy to alleviate some form of distress or to enhance art appreciation.

BETTY: One example is when this gentleman, Alex, went to the Wisconsin School for the Deaf as artist-in-residence for one week. We have seen something similar being done in other schools and programs. We have also seen Chuck Baird do his work, and he travels around the country sharing his art and working with young children at schools or summer camps. There are many, many ways that the artists can be involved with that.

PART EIGHT
Literature

Crossing the Divide: Helen Keller and Yvonne Pitrois Dialogue about Vaudeville

RACHEL M. HARTIG

How do people living with a difference most effectively cross the cultural divide and explain themselves to mainstream society? This is a central question raised by Yvonne Pitrois in her biography of Helen Keller titled *Une nuit rayonnante: Helen Keller* (*A Shining Night: Helen Keller*) and responded to by Helen Keller in a fascinating letter that I discovered at the library of the American Foundation for the Blind. Although I focus, in particular, on these two texts in my analysis, my presentation attempts to go beyond these initial works and the conflict they reveal to indicate, albeit somewhat briefly, the respective views of Keller and Pitrois on living with disability and the personality and cultural differences that influenced their divergent views.

At the time that Pitrois' biography of Keller was published, in 1922, Helen Keller (1880–1968) was known worldwide as an extraordinary deaf-blind American writer, activist, and socialist. She had already written and published *The Story of My Life* (1902–1903), an autobiographical portrait of her early years. Yvonne Pitrois (1880–1937), although relatively unknown today, was almost equally renowned in her country, France, and in fact throughout Europe during her lifetime for her social service and her biographical studies. By 1912, Pitrois had already published her most famous work, her life of the first committed educator of deaf people in France, *La Vie de l'Abbé de l'Épée* (1912) (*The Life of the Abbé de l'Épée*).

Pitrois was, then, a singularly good choice to chronicle Helen Keller's life as a fellow literary artist. Further, as she, herself, had been stricken with both deafness and blindness at the age of seven, probably as the result of sunstroke, Pitrois can be considered Helen Keller's French counterpart. Although Pitrois regained her sight, she remained deaf throughout her life. She never forgot the years without vision and without hearing, however, and reflected throughout her career a passionate desire both to chronicle and to serve her deaf and deaf-blind contemporaries. Her biography of Helen Keller, in particular, reflects this empathy for, and understanding of, the issues that the disabled need to address in their lives. She focuses in particular on the tension between self-definition and isolation and the need for the disabled person to reconnect in an appropriate way with the larger society.

It is only in the last four pages of the largely positive sixty-one-page manuscript that Pitrois has any ethical disagreements with her subject. One single choice on the part of Helen Keller tarnishes her reputation for Pitrois and numerous other Europeans: her decision to allow herself to be drawn to the vaudeville stage and to perform with Anne Sullivan. For Pitrois, these theatrical performances were painful, offensive, and exhibitionistic.[1]

Pitrois herself sent the completed copy of Helen Keller's biography to her subject and friend across the seas. In the undated letter that I found at the library of the American Foundation for the Blind, Helen Keller responds to the analysis in the biography, particularly the previously discussed criticism. Although it represented only a small part of the otherwise glowing portrait of her in Pitrois' work, she was distressed by the harsh words. She valued Pitrois "sweet approval,"[2] for this friend in France had also led a silent life and knew the difficulties that deafness brought. She acknowledges the many similarities between their paths that Pitrois had indicated, particularly the roles of their respective mentors. Pitrois' mother, Marguerite Pitrois, an author in her own right known for her books for children, had served that function for her daughter. Because Pitrois had experienced "the wise ministrations of a gifted mother,"[3] she was able to understand how Anne Sullivan, Helen's teacher, had similarly freed Helen Keller from the spiritual bondage and the isolation that often encircle the disabled. Keller, consequently, recognizes the appropriateness of having Pitrois be her biographer.

Keller only takes issue with Pitrois' condemnation of her work in vaudeville. Her explanation and defense are intriguing. Far from seeing herself as being drawn against her will into vaudeville and being exhibited on the stage like a wild animal, as Pitrois had implied, Keller explained that it was she who chose the lectures and work in vaudeville and persuaded Anne Sullivan to participate with her.

She refuted Pitrois' negative characterization of vaudeville as only demonstrating extreme American publicity and theatricality, with no saving grace. Vaudeville, Keller believed, offered a means by which an actor, speaker, or artist could serve the society while at the same time earning his or her living. Keller spoke often of the educational facet of her vaudeville work. She was able to teach the public about the deaf and the deaf-blind. This was theatricality whose publicity, in her opinion, served a noble end. She herself, she said, continually learned about human nature as she traversed the country.

Not only had she been enriched, Helen Keller continued, but others had benefited, as well. Her expressed goal was to cheer, through the message of her performance, people who were deaf, blind, or poor and soldiers who had been wounded in World War I, among others. Moved throughout her life by these humanitarian goals and feeling that vaudeville offered her the opportunity to pursue them, Helen Keller strongly believed in the validity of her vaudeville experiences.

1. Yvonne Pitrois, *Une nuit rayonnante: Helen Keller* Neuchâtel: A. Delapraz, 1922. p. 58.
2. Helen Keller, letter to Yvonne Pitrois, n.d., Collections of the American Foundation for the Blind, New York City, 1.
3. Keller, 1.

What was the nature of these performances that had elicited such polarized responses from two exceptional women who otherwise appeared to have so much in common? The quest for answers led me back to the American Foundation for the Blind Archives in New York City to consult their extensive vaudeville file. Among the materials was the copy of an actual script that Helen Keller and Anne Sullivan had used in their performance, written in dialogue form. The script told Helen's story, depicting her evolution from an isolated child who had only a few gestures with which to show what she wanted, to a world celebrity, the master not only of English but of French, German, and Italian.

Ann Sullivan-Macy performed a larger part of the dialogue. She spoke of her pupil's indomitable spirit in overcoming formidable obstacles and told the story of Helen's struggles to learn her first word: "water." Following her teacher's introduction and discussion, Helen Keller appeared on the stage and, speaking for herself, concluded the twenty-minute act by offering a brief message of hope to humanity.

An analysis of the act itself would seem to give validity to Helen's assertion in a letter to her friend Daisy Sharpe that, "We had a dignified little act."[4] Enjoying this act, Helen Keller chose to remain in vaudeville between 1920 and 1924. Helen Keller fully accepted the American view and saw vaudeville as an acceptable, even a desirable, form of theater. Many actors who continued their careers on the legitimate stage had their beginnings in this unique theatrical form. Helen personally had a particular fascination with actors and the theater, and so when the opportunity to perform in vaudeville occurred, Helen did not hesitate. Always an extrovert, Helen loved the adventure of vaudeville and the people that it brought into her life.

Why did Yvonne Pitrois' feelings about vaudeville differ so dramatically from those of her friend and colleague? Of a more retiring nature than Helen Keller, Pitrois found this medium very alien to her. Her timidity is discussed in an article by E. Drouot, a critic who was her contemporary.[5] Was this shyness the result of the childhood trauma, the sudden loss of hearing and temporary loss of sight that she experienced at seven? Certainly, it is reasonable to assume that it was a significant contributing factor.

Yvonne's mother, to help her overcome this timidity, sent her out to various merchants to do the errands of the household. The strategy was successful in helping Yvonne not to become paralyzed by her shyness. In time, she developed the ambition to pursue a professional career as a writer and published her first work at the age of eighteen. Her personality, however, remained less expansive than that of Helen Keller. She was a private person, whose many acts of kindness were done with little fanfare. Thus, it is easy to understand why the concept and practice of vaudeville were very foreign to her psychologically.

What results might she have feared from a vaudeville performance? Based on her knowledge of eighteenth-century France's insensitivity toward the disabled, Pitrois sketches her nightmare scenario in one of her later works. Valentin Haüy, one of the three heroes featured in *Trois lumières dans la nuit* (*Three Lights in the Darkness*), was a sighted man who devoted himself to the cause of the blind. In this sketch, Pitrois portrays the moment of his decision to do so.

4. Helen Keller, letter to Daisy Sharpe, 19 December 1923, Vaudeville file, Collections of the American Foundation for the Blind, New York City.
5. H. Drouot, "Un auteur sourd," *Revue Générale de l'Enseignement des Sourds-Muets* 14, no. 5 (1912): 97–99.

In 1771, at the age of twenty-six, while walking through the streets of Paris, Haüy saw ten blind men grotesquely dressed in long robes, with pointed hats and fake eyeglasses, seated on a makeshift stage. They were being exhibited at a street fair, and the crowd was laughing at them. The organizers of the fair, in a final insulting touch, had the blind men playing violins, although they had no musical training. Haüy was horrified by the spectacle. He determined to make it possible for the blind to learn to read and, eventually, to earn a living in a dignified way. True to his vow, he developed a system of raised letters, a precursor of Braille, and spent most of his life teaching blind children.

Pitrois is clearly distressed in the retelling of this story. I believe that she saw theatrical spectacle, in general, as having the potential of going awry for the disabled people in France and, by extension, elsewhere. No wonder, then, that she disagreed quite vehemently with the notion that vaudeville could be a means of positive expression and activity for a deaf-blind person. Pitrois wanted respect and dignity for the deaf and the deaf-blind, as did Helen Keller. Unlike Helen Keller, she did not trust exhibitionism and spectacle to be the path that led to this respect.

Although the two women differed as to the manner in which to cross the social divide, they were equally impressive in their brilliance, in their passion for language and writing, and in their desire to serve others limited by disability. Ably educated and supported to overcome their limitations by their respective mentors, they became impressive human beings and impressive citizens of their respective countries. Because the achievements of both were considerable and their stances, although diametrically opposed, understandable, they illustrate the importance of not depicting one single means of self-realization as the correct one for any deaf or deaf-blind person.

Bibliography

Brooks, Van Wyck. *Helen Keller: Sketch for a Portrait*. New York: E. P. Dutton and Co., 1956.

Drouot, E. "Un auteur sourd." *Revue Générale de l'Enseignement des Sourds-Muets* 14, no. 5 (1912): 97–99.

Freeberg, Ernest. *The Education of Laura Bridgman: First Deaf and Blind Person to Learn Language*. Cambridge, MA: Harvard University Press, 2000.

Gibson, William. *The Miracle Worker*. New York: Bantam Books, 1975.

Gitter, Elisabeth. *The Imprisoned Guest: Samuel Howe and Laura Bridgman, the Original Deaf-Blind Girl*. New York: Farrar, Straus and Giroux, 2001.

Herrmann, Dorothy. *Helen Keller: A Life*. New York: Alfred A. Knopf, 1998.

Keith's Theatre News [Washington], May 24, 1920.

Keller, Helen. Letter to Daisy Sharpe. December 19, 1923. Collections of the American Foundation for the Blind, New York City.

———. Letter to Yvonne Pitrois. n.d. Collections of the American Foundation for the Blind, New York City.

———. *The Story of My Life*. New York: Bantam, 1990.

Lash, Joseph P. *Helen and Teacher: The Story of Helen Keller and Anne Sullivan Macy*. New York: Delacorte Press, 1980.

Pitrois, Yvonne. *Une nuit rayonnante: Helen Keller*. Neuchâtel: A. Delapraz, 1922.

———. *Ombres de Femmes*. Lausanne, France: Librairie Payot et Compagnie, 1925.

———. *Trois lumières dans la nuit, Valentin Haüy, Louis Braille, Maurice de la Sizeranne*. Strasbourg, France: Imprimerie de la Petite-France, 1936.

———. *La Vie de l'Abbé de l'Épée racontée aux Sourds-Muets*. Saint-Étienne, France: Imprimerie de l'Institution des Sourds-Muets, 1912.

Questions asked Helen Keller by Her Vaudeville Audience. n.d. Vaudeville File. Collections of the American Foundation for the Blind, New York City.

Script. Mrs. Macy and Helen Keller in Vaudeville. n.d. Vaudeville File. Collections of the American Foundation for the Blind, New York City.

The Poetics and Politics of Deaf American Literature

CYNTHIA PETERS

Colloquially termed "deaf lit," Deaf American literature is an evolving, polyglossic body of works comprising a wide range of vernacular (signed), written, and hybrid forms (those exhibiting both vernacular and written features). Deaf American literature therefore encompasses the following forms and genres: American Sign Language (ASL) stories and poetry, plays in ASL and printed English, stories in English (original or translated from ASL), and novels and poetry in English. The ABC story/poem, number story/poem, face story, drum song/story, literary night (as framework or vehicle), improvisation, slow-motion story/poem, and skits are some more nativist or indigenous forms that can be identified.

On a broader level, Deaf American literature, like African American, Hispanic, Chinese American, and Native American literatures, can be termed a minority literature. As is the case with other minorities, Deaf Americans exist within and without the mainstream American culture. What results is a body of works in which, in general, the majority language (English) and rhetoric seeks to dominate and extend its control, and the minority language (ASL) and rhetoric attempt to undermine and evade this control. In other words, Deaf American literature, in the vein of other minority literatures, rebels against mainstream American literature, in the process using it (in all senses and connotations of the word) to suit its own purposes and needs.

A time-honored method of rebelling is utilizing humor in various forms of expression, ranging from outright burlesque and parody to subtle satire and disingenuous comedy. MJ Bienvenu, a noted Deaf studies scholar, has said that Deaf Americans have five senses, as we know people generally do. Yet, how can Deaf Americans possibly have five senses? This is the answer: they do not have the sense of hearing—or have it fully—but they do have a great sense of humor (Peters, 2000). Thus, Deaf Americans resemble other minorities in that they tell and write humorous stories to a large extent. They laugh a lot—at the majority, at themselves, at both themselves and the majority. This can contribute to a sense of equality or even a feeling of superiority at times. Those members of the majority who can comprehend such culturally based stories will undoubtedly find much that is humorous in the various portrayals of majority or minority behavior, learn from it, and even act upon it in a way that can be beneficial for both.

An example of this is *Deafology 101: A Crash Course in Deaf Culture*, an entertaining mock lecture by Ken Glickman (a.k.a. Prof. Glick) on Deaf American culture. Prof. Glick pokes fun not only at mainstream society and its expectations of Deaf Americans but also at Deaf American culture itself. The action all begins when Prof. Glick, sporting baggy shorts, rumpled lab coat, big bow tie, disheveled hair, and thick, black-rimmed glasses, comes striding on stage smoking a pipe, his appearance obviously satirizing absent-minded professors and the educational system that nourishes them. The professor describes Deaf American culture and the mainstream culture of which it is and is not a part. He asks, "What is Deaf culture?" He answers with, "It is defined as a wonderful way of life that is unheard of. That will be on your test." Pacing back and forth between blackboard and podium, Glick goes on to state that deaf people interact with "those people who can't help but hear," noting that "the world is full of hearing people. Let's shorten that to hearies." He then abbreviates "deaf people" as "deafies." He further stipulates that in between are the "heafies"—deafies who look and act like hearies—and the hearies who act like deafies, or "dearies." "Oh, I love them," he announces. "Want an example? Here are two dearies." (He gestures at two interpreters sitting in the first row.) Glick continues, "After this lecture I'll get a piece of paper called an in*voice*. It's for their hearnings" (Glickman, 2000).

In poking fun at the majority (and themselves at times), Deaf Americans utilize another time-honored practice: rhetorically turning upside down the established order. Such a strategy entails stories of invasion and conquest, discourse featuring one or more people taking over or simply getting the upper hand, and ASL works showing up the majority language and rhetoric. In effect, the status quo is turned topsy-turvy; what was on top lands on the bottom, and what was on the bottom ends up on top. One well-known example of this is *Islay*, the Douglas Bullard novel about a small group of Deaf Americans, led by a federal worker with a dream—the mythic dream of a homeland—venturing into the economically depressed state of Islay and buying up property and businesses. Other Deaf Americans soon converge on Islay, and before long it is the Deaf Americans who are running things. Deaf mothers insist on their Deaf American sons and daughters attending the nearby local, public school rather than the Oral Institute. The Man with a Dream runs for governor and wins. Another example of inversion is Stephen Ryan's "Planet Way over Yonder," an ASL narrative about a young Deaf American boy who rockets off to a planet where the majority of inhabitants are deaf and a small minority is hearing. A third instance is the "Side Show" segment of the 1971–72 National Theatre of the Deaf (NTD) theatrical production, *My Third Eye*. In this production, a red-and-white-striped tent can be seen in the background and a large enclosure—akin to an old-fashioned birdcage—with two voice readers inside can be seen in the foreground. The ringmaster strides out on stage and promises to tell about "strange things . . . a strange people." At her behest, the acrobats go through their acts while the voice readers stand, virtually motionless. As the acrobats perform, the ringmaster extols the interaction, expressiveness, and freedom of ASL, which utilizes the face and the whole body. Implicitly and explicitly, she dismisses the poker faces, small mouth movements, and limp appendages of the voice readers (representing mainstream society). In effect, Deaf American culture is depicted as fluid and free—a little three-ring circus within an aural majority culture shown to be sadly limited, inflexible, and authoritarian (Bullard, 2000).

Western civilization often has the scientific and scholarly urge—in the Cartesian vein—to categorize, classify, and differentiate. This is reflected in literary studies by the analysis and dissection of Western literature in the attempt to label and define what a particular form of expression is and what it consists of. In effect, questions are asked and re-asked: What genres are there? What is a novel? What is a poem? How is a particular work a novel? How did the novel evolve? For instance, *Cane*, the early twentieth-century work by Jean Toomer, an African American writer, has a few narratives, a number of poems, and a play all built around a particular theme. Literary scholars have argued—and continue to argue—over its classification as a novel. Another example is *Borderlands*, a Hispanic novel by Gloria Anzaluda, which mixes fiction and nonfiction and plays English off of Spanish and vice versa. Modern-day scholars are similarly intrigued by the Native American novel *Ceremony* with its cyclical rather than conventional linear progression. Toomer, Anzaluda, and other minority writers choose not to heed genre distinctions; in other words, they break the rules when it comes to what is expected of a particular genre, turning upside down Western expectations of narrative, poetry, and drama.

Conventionally, a story is narrative that progresses forward from beginning, to middle, to end. Events that occur generally have a cause-and-effect logic. Bill Ennis' "Nitty" ASL narrative, however, defies these general expectations:

> My favorite . . . cat. I had a cat, this big. Bigger? This big. It was a tomcat and its name was "Nitty." It was born in the country: Staunton, Virginia. Gallaudet people brought it and gave it to us. Why call it "Nitty?" Why not "K?" Right. Can't pronounce "K." How did I find out? I wish you told me. The person who told me was the little one, John Mark. John Mark has seven children. True! Six girls and one boy, the last one. Six darlings! The boy is six months old now and called Mark, Jr. From the baby we go all the way up to the oldest girl who is seventeen and in high school. The second oldest girl is L. A. or Leigh Ann. Loves her aunt. She goes to her aunt and stays one week. Remember the cat Nitty? Her aunt decides to call it, "Here, kitty, kitty, kitty." I'm not using my voice. The cat may run here from Staunton, thirty miles away. The girl is fifteen, eleven? Twelve? No, fourteen. She tells her aunt that if she calls the cat this way, it won't come. Uncle Bill always pronounces it "Nitty." She caught it somehow. (Ennis, 2000)

Before there was writing, before stories became textualized, there was storytelling. Much storytelling exists in Deaf American culture because sign language has no generally accepted written form. In the "Nitty" narrative, Ennis goes off the point, adds personal information, and talks to the viewers without heeding the conventions of written narrative. Instead, Ennis adheres to the rules for "telling a good story," not those for "writing a good story." Generally, a written story progresses from beginning to end without unnecessary diversions or personal information, but Ennis is *telling* a story, employing tactics different from those for *writing* a story. Indeed, considering the different medium (live storytelling in front of a group), he has to do so in an effort to keep his viewers' attention and interest. Because, as Ben Bahan has remarked, "The storyteller *is* the story," who Ennis is, what he has to say, and how he says it are equally important (Peters, 2000). Hence, Ennis can include personal information from time to time and dispense with straightforward narrative progression as well as the transitional markers obligatory in written narrative.

Many Deaf American nativist or seminativist works defy standard genre classification and distinctions. Mary Beth Miller's "The Cowboy Story," in her taped *Live at SMI* performance, is based upon a slow one-two-three-four drum beat, and it frequently repeats signs and phrases.

> Boom boom
> Ride ride
> Ride ride
> Handkerchief handkerchief (handkerchief around the neck lifting in the breeze)
> Strings strings (hat strings sway in cowboy's face)
> Hat hat
> Pistol pistol
> Gallop gallop
> Dust dust (dust stirred up by horse hoofs)
> Gallop gallop
> Rise rise (rider rises off saddle)
>
> (Peters 2000)

The cowboy arrives in town and stops at a saloon where he espies a pretty saloon girl. They flirt, he wins her over, and the two depart, riding off into the sunset. Often, a scene uses the same handshape in many signs; for example, the V handshape is incorporated into the handkerchief waving, the hat strings lifting, and the riding and the rising off the saddle. The repetition of signs or the repetition of any aspect of a sign—its orientation, handshape, or movement—visually conveys rhyme. "The Cowboy Story" has elements of poetry and song, yet it is termed a "story" and progresses narratively from beginning, to middle, to end.

My Third Eye, staged by the NTD, is ostensibly a play. However, conventionally a play has acts: Act One, Act Two, Act Three, and so on. Also, it conventionally involves a plot of some kind. Yet, *My Third Eye* opens with a birthing sequence, which is followed by a couple of autobiographical anecdotes. "Side Show" succeeds, after which there is another autobiographical anecdote followed by an ASL tableau. A number of chorus presentations are next in which the NTD members first demonstrate various signs and then dance through "Three Blind Mice" and "The Quick Brown Fox." All in all, this production comes across as more of a musical or variety show than a conventional two- or three-act play. The reason for this may be that it is—more appropriately—a fairly indigenous Deaf American dramatic production. A characteristically indigenous dramatic production avoids the verbalism and the plodding narrative progression of a conventional play, instead taking into account, consciously or unconsciously, the visual needs of the Deaf American viewers. To clarify, Deaf American viewers use their eyes, and the *eye* likes visual stimuli—variable visual stimuli. It likes moving objects, and it likes variety. The *eye* also needs a break from time to time. Indeed, the traditional Literary Night, which *Eye* is undoubtedly derived from, is a feast for the eye. A kind of vaudeville production, it is a vehicle for diverse forms, genres, and rhetoric. It first came about when literary societies at schools and clubs for deaf students appropriated English stories and poems and adapted them to ASL and Deaf American viewers' visual needs. Not too soon thereafter, ASL stories and skits as well as other nativist or seminativist forms were developed.

When a printed English story or poem is adapted to ASL, a dynamic, hybridized form results. As was mentioned, before there was written literature, there was storytelling and drama. It was all people talking, acting, and moving around. The story or dramatic action could not be separated from the teller or performer. The teller or performer was present in person, meaning the *body* was an integral part of expression. Much of current discourse is in print or via the radio or Internet: the *body* has disappeared. Written discourse can thus be characterized as more abstract, literary, and objective rather than personalized. In other words, literature has evolved from performance into a written body of works. This evolution was facilitated by the rise of Christianity and the middle class because the former de-emphasizes earthly needs and the latter seeks a more decorous, clinical approach. Whereas in the past the storyteller was the story, the story is now just the story; the *body* has disappeared. However, when Deaf Americans adapt a printed English work to ASL, they put the *body* back into it, so to say, and this revitalizes the printed version.

In the past, deaf people were apprehensive about signing in public because sign language was not as well accepted as it is now. Now that it has been recognized as a legitimate language, Deaf Americans as a group, as a minority, want to display ASL, and in showing and publicizing ASL, they are not shy about showing the *body*. Deaf people tie sign language—their em*bod*ied means of communication—to "identity." They sign in public, request interpreters, and produce numerous ASL stories and poems for mass distribution. For instance, Ben Bahan and Sam Supalla, two noted storytellers, have produced two ASL narratives on videotape as part of the ASL Literature Series in an effort to show the world that a literature is possible in ASL. This parallels the African American identity-text connection. For a long time African Americans were denied reading and writing instruction. Because of this restriction, they wrote prodigiously upon emancipation to show that they could write and do it as well as whites—to show that they were human beings. Writing or text was a way to gain recognition, civil rights, and respect. "Identity" was tied to "text."

A final but not insignificant stratagem of Deaf Americans is corollary to "body as text." As a part of identity politics, many Deaf American artists do not shy away from more graphic discourse or portrayals. For instance, the Deaf American play, *A Deaf Family Diary*, includes a scene in which the future in-laws gather for an after-dinner talk. The soon-to-be groom asks how his future father-in-law is doing after his gall bladder operation, not expecting more than a brief report. The bride's father describes this operation in such detail that the groom's parents (who can hear) are appalled at his graphicness, yet the Deaf American characters and the viewers find much to appreciate in such ASL dexterity. In effect, because of the inherent graphicness of ASL, the literature can be deliciously indelicate at times. Deaf American artists often take advantage of this characteristic and milk it for all it is worth; witness Debbie Rennie's European nose-picking narrative at the tail end of her *Poetry in Motion* videotape, Bill Ennis' toilet music account in *Bill Ennis: Live at SMI!*, and Elinor Kraft's cruise banquet description in *Elinor Kraft: Live at SMI!*

Such rebelling, such twisting and squirming to evade control, and such jesting help make Deaf American literature an incredibly rich and multifaceted body of works. It is a multidimensional minority literature that trumpets "body as text" in the context of identity politics. It is uniquely bicultural, bilingual, bimodal—even trimodal. Many national literatures draw upon both oral and literary traditions, but no other literature has a visual-kinetic component that results in a visual literature or visuature. This visuature has properties so far outside what is usually considered linguistic and literary that only analogies with dance, graphic art, cinema, and performance can do it justice.

References

Bahan, Ben, and Sam Supalla. 1992. *ASL Literature Series*. Videocassette, 60 min. San Diego, Calif.: Dawn Pictures/DawnSignPress.

Bullard, Douglas. 1986. *Islay: A Novel*. Silver Spring, Md.: TJ Publishers.

A Deaf Family Diary. February–March 1994. Scripted Don Bangs, directed by Patrick Graybill, produced by SignRise Cultural Arts, Publick Playhouse, Cheverly, Md.

Ennis, Bill. 1991. "Nitty," in *Bill Ennis: Live at SMI!* Videocassette, 60 min. Burtonsville, Md.: Sign Media.

Glickman, Ken. 1993. *Deafology 101: Deaf Culture as Seen through the Eyes of a Deaf Humorist*. Videocassette, 60 min. Silver Spring, Md.: Deafinitely Yours Studio.

Kraft, Elinor. 1993. *Elinor Kraft: Live at SMI!* Videocassette, 60 min. Burtonsville, Md.: Sign Media.

Miller, Mary Beth. 1991. *Mary Beth Miller: Live at SMI!* Videocassette, 60 min. Burtonsville, Md.: Sign Media.

My Third Eye. 1971–72. Directed by J. Ranelli. Written and produced by National Theatre of the Deaf.

Peters, Cynthia. 2000. *Deaf American Literature: From Carnival to the Canon*. Washington, DC: Gallaudet University Press.

Rennie, Debbie. 1990. *Poetry in Motion: Original Works in ASL*. Videocassette, 60 min. Burtonsville, Md.: Sign Media.

Ryan, Stephen M. 1991. "Planet Way over Yonder," vol. 5 of *ASL Storytime*. Videocassette, 30 min. Produced by Department of Communication, Gallaudet University.

ASL Literacy in Early Childhood: ASL Poetry

ROBYN SANDFORD

We know that literature exposure and development in young children is critical for their literacy development in one or more languages. To date, there has been no research on the early American Sign Language (ASL) literacy development of young Deaf children. Through my experience working in the nursery/junior kindergarten classroom, I have noticed that the children pick up and express ASL poetry in a natural way from both formal teaching and informal interaction in the classroom. The children seem to enjoy this stress-free acquisition of ASL poetry and naturally expand their ASL vocabulary and grammar through this language play. Because there is no research or curricula on ASL poetry development in very young Deaf children to guide me as I work with my students, it is critical that I describe the ASL poetry genres that I present to them and describe the genres that they seem to acquire most readily as well as the stages of development that they go through. This will provide other teachers of literacy to Deaf children with needed information on how to address ASL poetry in our classrooms.

It will also assist us in developing an ASL poetry component for an ASL literature curriculum. Despite lack of research on the early ASL literacy development of young Deaf children, implications and recommendations from this study may encourage educators of literacy to increase their awareness of ASL poetry and may increase their motivation to explore ASL poetry with their young Deaf students in the classroom.

I introduce ASL poetry, research methodology, analysis, examples, findings, and implications/recommendations.

Introduction

To date there is no research on early ASL literacy development of young Deaf children. There is not enough information or research on ASL poetry in particular. Although it is not new among Deaf people, ASL literature is a new field of study according to Marlon Kuntze in *Telling Tales in ASL* (Fernandes 1997). Deaf schools are beginning to question curriculum design for introducing ASL poetry and teaching students to produce their own creative pieces. ASL poetry still tends to be overlooked for educational purposes, although it is listed as one of the ASL genres in ASL literature. According to Andrew

Byrne, a storytelling researcher, the ASL literature genres categories include poetry, stories, theater, narratives, success stories, fables, humor, legends, riddles, deaf rap (with rhythmic repetition), anecdotes, classifier stories, folklore/signlore, folktales, mystery, and romance. ASL literature is a body of stories, legends, poems, and other genres that have been passed down from one generation to the next by culturally Deaf people; it is conveyed in a visual-spatial dimension. ASL literature is unwritten language and therefore ASL literature is an "oral" (through the air) literature.

Lynn Jacobowitz states that ASL children's literature consists of manual form and shows morals, cultural values, beliefs, and traditions in stories, poems, folklore adapted for children, and other genres.

The definition of ASL poetry is a bit complicated. Marlon "Lon" Kuntze defined ASL poetry as a creative piece made up of carefully selected signs blended in artistic and aesthetically pleasing ways. ASL poetry is how the visual properties of signs are patterned. You can play with signs. Clayton Valli, a pioneer in ASL poetry research and an internationally known Deaf poet and expert in ASL poetry and ASL linguistics, identifies three poetic features in ASL poetry.

1. Rhyme:
   a. Handshape (HS) examples: numeral HS, alphabetical HS, worded HS, particular HS, closed HS, open HS, double HS, initialized HS;
   b. Movements: movement in contour, duration, size, hold emphasis;
   c. Locations: body, spatial, space level;
   d. Palm orientations: up, down, side-up;
   e. Nonmanual signals: eye gaze direction, eye gaze shift, eyebrow movement, mouth movement, head shift, body shift;
   f. Handedness: one hand, both hands, alternative hands.
2. Meter: lexical signs consist of hold and movement segments in sequence that can produce syllabic meter by using stress. Examples of stress are as follows:
   a. Hold emphasis: long pause, subtle pause, strong stop;
   b. Movement emphasis: alternating movement, repeated movement;
   c. Movement size: regular movement path, enlarged movement path, reduced movement path.
3. Rhythm: This implies the motion and arrangement of various feature poetics and has to do with counting.
   a. Rhymes;
   b. Handedness;
   c. Assimilation;
   d. Choice of a sign;
   e. Change of a sign;
   f. Creation of sign;
   g. Movement size;
   h. Movement duration.

Keep in mind that ASL poetry requires using poetic structures in ASL to create a grammatically cohesive work of art. Handshapes, movement, paths, space, and nonmanual signals (eye gaze, eyebrow movement, and body movement) could all be incorporated to demonstrate irony, emotion, point of view, and metaphor or to represent transition of time. This comment was made by Katherine DeLorenzo in "Poetry in Motion," *Gallaudet Today*, Fall 1999. Clayton Valli listed that ASL poetry has three poetic features. He exposed very young Deaf children to these features of ASL poetry when he visited the Learning Center for Deaf Children in Framingham, Massachusetts. He was thrown into water when they expected him to do ASL poetry in front of a very young audience (children as young as ages three and four, based on a grant from the Dewing Foundation that they had received). He invented the ASL poem *Cow and Rooster* for that occasion. *Cow and Rooster* has become very popular for very young children but like I said previously, there is still no research on ASL poetry development for children in the early childhood years.

Methodology

Ethnographic research methodology was used. Some ethnography studies research classroom interaction in the children's natural, cultural school environment. In simple terms, it examines a real-life school setting! Fourteen Deaf children were involved. They were chosen because I was their nursery and junior kindergarten teacher in a bilingual and bicultural program. It was a three-day/week program. Fourteen students included five nursery children at the age of three and nine junior kindergarteners at the age of four. Five children had Deaf parents, including one who had a Deaf father and hearing mother. Two of the nine children had Deaf siblings in the program. One of the children of Deaf parents had one younger Deaf sibling with Down syndrome. ASL poetry activities typically took place in the morning at approximately 9:15 a.m. Videotaping occurred three times per week over a nine-month period beginning in September 1997 and ending in June 1998.

Using field notes, I wrote almost everything right after taping each ASL poetry activity. I expressed my thoughts, my opinions, my insights, the children's actions, my successes, and my frustrations. I wrote what I saw. I used a notebook to organize, date, and record what occurred. I did not have to rely on memory of previous activities because it was all recorded.

To supplement this data, interviews were conducted with Deaf adults of Deaf children regarding ASL poetry and its functions. I will report about these in another presentation.

Consent forms were sent to parents for permission to use the videotaped data for research and educational purposes at conferences and for other professional development activities. Confidentiality is maintained in all written reports but cannot be maintained on videotape samples. Pseudonyms are used at all times.

Research team discussions were maintained throughout the study. It was a big asset along with team feedback and support. We met weekly for the first year and biweekly in the second year because of our increased confidence and experience as well as time-consuming teaching schedules that limited more frequent team meetings.

Analysis

To analyze the videotapes, I watched children's responses and expressions during ASL poetry activities on videotape several times. The research team watched the videotapes during team meetings as well. I did not know what to look for at first, and I made written notes if needed. After repeated viewings, I noticed patterns in the data. I read my field notes to see any parallel patterns.

Findings

After viewing the videotapes and reading my field notes, I found similar patterns emerge in this action research. I noticed patterns emerge concerning a variety of ASL poetry genres and made a chart for quick and easy reading. The patterns I found in my field notes are (1) motivation, (2) my approval, and (3) children's difficulty and frustrations with no success.

Summary, Implications, and Recommendations

Summary

I noticed that older children or children more highly skilled in ASL (according to those with lower ASL skills) were able to use ASL Number Story 1–10 as a result of their advanced organization skills, fine motor skills, marked and unmarked handshape development, memory skills, and higher concept skills.

Younger children were able to use one unmarked handshape story. For instance, unmarked handshapes 5, B, and C are easier to produce compared to the marked handshapes R, E, 7, and 8. Early unmarked handshape development is supported by Valli and Boyes-Braem in their studies of acquisition of handshapes in ASL among Deaf children of Deaf parents.

Both age groups continued to show their enjoyment and their willingness to learn. Both older and younger children were heavily exposed to ASL poetry, although fewer children used ASL poetry spontaneously.

Implications and Recommendations

For implications and recommendations, it is important that we professional educators in bilingual-bicultural programs allow ourselves to be open to feedback, to seek it, and to accept it as a part of our professional development rather than to view it as criticism, oppression, or a power struggle. We need to explore ASL poetry with our young students, to discuss our finding with our colleagues, and to make recommendations that are appropriate for three- to five-year-old youngsters.

1. An ASL curriculum is badly needed in provincial schools for Deaf students. I am not suggesting a Deaf studies curriculum, Deaf studies resources, or curricula adapted using ASL according to an English curriculum. ASL is a language for Deaf people, and so an ASL curriculum is needed for appropriate ASL instruction and use in the classroom.
2. Research is badly needed that applies to ASL poetry with young children. We need more research and documentation on specific aspects of ASL language development. The specific aspects of ASL requiring research are as follows:
    a. More research is needed on the seven unmarked handshapes. Which comes first in respective order? There is evidence on order, but which handshapes

come first and which are most useful? Which handshapes appear at which age? This research will help preschool teachers increase their knowledge and help them to prepare ASL literature/literacy units effectively in their preschool classrooms or home visiting programs.

b. More research is needed on ASL acquisition in Deaf children as early learners and late learners. In most preschool programs, children arrive in the programs with varying degrees of ASL skills. They learn together regardless of their ASL skill levels, and this impacts their acquisition of ASL literature.

c. More research and resources are needed on ASL poetry activities. There are plenty of resources for hearing preschool children learning English poetry and nursery rhymes. Is adapting this for Deaf children appropriate? Is this culturally sensitive?

d. More research is needed on ASL for a language arts curriculum for three- to five-year-old preschool Deaf children in a bilingual-bicultural program. To date there is no ASL curriculum for them specifically. We are currently developing an ASL curriculum for nursery school through twelfth grade in the Ontario Provincial Schools for Deaf children and field testing at the Ernest C. Drury School, Milton, Ontario, where I teach along with other provincial schools.

e. More research is needed on using specific ASL poetry features. For instance, we know that ABC stories are appropriate for older children (Sandford 2001), but what specific ages or specific grades are they appropriate for? It is important that all children be exposed to ABC stories. We need to categorize ASL poetry features for each grade and study the features we expect them to master at different ages. We need to apply this knowledge to the Ontario Curriculum.

f. More teacher training and/workshops are necessary regarding ASL literature curriculum. Presently in Deaf education there is much emphasis on reading and writing or on speech training for children with cochlear implants. No matter how wonderful the reading and writing programs, Deaf children still show struggles with their skills. We need to focus on their primary language (ASL) first—the language they have full access to without constraint. We can then proceed to the second language (English: reading and writing) using ASL literature programs as a foundation for reading and writing programs.

g. ASL literature/literacy education must be available not only for teachers but also for parents. Results from the second part of this study, my interview with parents, indicates a great need in this area.

h. More research is needed to see if ASL poetry helps children acquire ASL skills and English skills.

i. More research is needed on ASL handshape developmental order. There are an estimated 150 handshapes that need to be studied to determine the developmental order of acquisition. Do we put unmarked and marked handshapes in a specific ASL order for children to learn and recite? Can you imagine Deaf children having to memorize 150 handshapes?

j. More research is needed on the usage of ASL number systems for three- to five-year-old children. There is no ASL number system in current ASL developmental checklists. I have observed and studied children using and playing with ASL number stories 1–3, 1–5, and 1–10, but additional research is needed for support, reliability, and validity.

References

Bahan, B. 1992. ASL Literature: Inside the Story. In *Deaf Studies: What's Up*, 153–66. Washington, DC: Gallaudet University Press.

Baker-Shenk, C., and Dennis Cokely. 1980. *American Sign Language: A teacher's resource guide on grammar and culture*. Silver Spring, MD: T.J. Publishers.

Cummins, J. 1989. *Empowering minority students*. Sacramento, CA: California Association for Bilingual Education.

DawnSignPress. *Numbering in American Sign Language: Number signs for everyone*. 1998. San Diego, CA: DawnSignPress.

Fernandes, Jane K., E. Lynn Jacobowitz, and Marlon Kuntze. 1997. *Telling tales in ASL: From literature to literacy*. Videorecording.

Gibson, H., and A. Small. 1995. Reflections of ourselves: The Deaf community from both sides of the mirror. In *Signing On: Adopting a cultural perspective*, ed. D. Bobier. London, ON, Canada: McIntosh Gallery.

Halton District School Board. 1996. *The Halton Early Literacy Plan: Working together to support children's learning*. Halton Hills, Canada: Author.

Mahshie, S. N. 1995. *Educating Deaf children bilingually: With insights and applications from Sweden and Denmark*. Washington, DC: Gallaudet University, Precollege Programs.

Mounty, J. 1993. *Signed language development checklist*. Princeton, NJ: Educational Testing Service.

Ontario Ministry of Education and Training. 1999. *Teacher research in a bilingual/bicultural school for the Deaf students*. Bilingual Bicultural Education for Deaf Students monograph series no. 1. Toronto: Ontario Ministry of Education and Training.

Pettitto, L., and P. F. Marentetle. 1991. Babbling in the manual mode: Evidence for the ontogeny of language. *Science* 251:1492–96.

Sign Talk Development Project. 1995. *Discovering with words and signs: A resource guide for developing a bilingual bicultural preschool program for Deaf and hearing children*.Winnipeg, MB, Canada: Sign Talk Children's Centre.

Valli, C., and Ceil Lucas. 1995. *Linguistics of American Sign Language*, 2nd ed. Washington, DC: Gallaudet University Press.

Conceptual "Rhymes" in Sign Language Poetry

SARAH TAUB

The rich iconicity of American Sign Language (ASL) deeply influences the poetry that signers create (Taub, 2001). Poets make art from language by creating patterns of meaning (e.g., repeated images or metaphors) and patterns of form (e.g., repetition of phonetic material). In spoken languages, these levels are largely separate, but in sign languages, the two can interpenetrate. That is, the poet's concrete and metaphorical mental imagery can receive direct visual representation through the language's iconic lexical items and grammatical inflections. ASL's pervasive iconicity and the metaphorical and metonymic extensions of iconicity allow for merging of "rhyme schemes" and conceptual motifs. This strategy increases the cohesion and power of the poem. Iconicity does not detract from a language's capacity for abstract or poetic expression; instead, it provides an effective channel for that expression.

Let us start with a few words on sign language iconicity. Iconicity is a resemblance between linguistic form and meaning. For many years, sign languages were thought of as primitive because they had a great deal of iconicity; spoken languages were considered more "advanced" because most of their symbols were arbitrary. Indeed, much early work on sign languages was dedicated to showing that their iconicity was irrelevant to their linguistic structure. More recent work (e.g., Liddell, 1992, 1995; Taub, 2001; Wilcox, 2000; Wilcox, 1998) has embraced sign language iconicity. Taub (2001) and Liddell (1992) in particular have argued that sign language and spoken language iconicity are fully analogous; that languages are as iconic as they can be; and that sign languages have more iconicity than spoken languages only because the human conceptual system has many more visual, spatial, or kinesthetic images linked to concepts than it does auditory images.

Indeed, it is possible to give iconic representations to a large range of concepts through conceptual linkages such as metaphor and metonymy (Taub, 2001). For example, the ASL sign THINK-PENETRATE, which denotes successful communication despite difficulties, is both iconic and metaphorical. It depicts a long, thin object (a 1 handshape on the dominant hand) moving from the forehead to penetrate a barrier (a nondominant B). Each aspect of this image metaphorically represents something in the domain of communication: the thin object represents an idea, the forehead represents the locus of thought, and the barrier represents a difficulty in communication. Thus, iconic signs are not limited to concrete meanings.

Through a close analysis of Ella Mae Lentz's poem "Circle of Life," we discuss how ASL poets skillfully exploit their language's iconicity. Let us first survey the iconic resources of the language. Like most sign languages, ASL has two types of iconic signs. First, there is a productive system for describing objects' size, shape, and spatial location or movement; this system consists of iconic classifier handshapes (i.e., handshapes that denote a class of objects such as animates, round things, or long, thin things) plus movements and locations in space that correspond to the movements, locations, or shapes of the things described. Classifier descriptions represent particular events and incidents. Second, there are iconic lexical items that denote specific concepts, just as noniconic lexical items do; the iconic lexical items are often "frozen" versions of classifier descriptions.

Sign languages also make linguistic use of the space around the signer. First, classifier descriptions use signer space to set up representations of physical objects and their relative spatial locations and movements. Second, sign languages set up spatial locations that represent discourse referents, and pronouns and some verbs move to or from those locations to indicate those referents.

Iconicity has also made its way into ASL's grammar. Like many other sign languages, ASL has a complex system of verb inflections for temporal aspect. Most of these inflections are temporally iconic—that is, they involve a modification of the temporal characteristics of the verb that resembles the aspectual meaning they indicate. For example, repetitive aspect involves rapid repetition of the verb form with head nods; delayed-inceptive aspect (i.e., onset of event is delayed) involves a protraction of the initial part of the verb along with a finger-wiggle or tongue-waggle; and continuous aspect involves a repeated circular modulation of the verb's motion.

The poem "Circle of Life" was composed for the poet's brother's wedding; its main themes are *eternity*, *unity*, and *two becoming one*. Literary analysis of sign language poetry (Klima & Bellugi, 1979; Valli, 1994; Ornsby, 1995; Bauman, 1998) has treated the use of repetitive devices analogous to rhyme and alliteration (i.e., repetition of handshapes, locations, and movements), specially modified movements, and rhythm. This essay focuses on how metaphor and iconicity interweave with these poetic devices. The themes of eternity and unity are presented iconically through the use of circular signs, classifiers, and grammatical inflections; the theme of two becoming one is presented metaphorically through signs that overlap or join the two hands.

The poem can be separated into seven stanzas (Table 1); we focus on the stanzas with iconic imagery. The poem moves from a consideration of God and the eternal movements of celestial bodies to the specifics of two people growing up, meeting, and falling in love. A repetition of the celestial section firmly links their love and marriage to the eternal aspects of the universe.

The theme of *eternity as a circle* is introduced in stanza two and repeated in stanza six. These passages describe the eternal continuation of the turning of the earth, the passing of time, the rising and setting of the sun, and the yearly revolution of the earth around the sun. Every sign has a circular handshape or movement pattern. One sign, YES, presents the image of a nodding head, so its iconicity is irrelevant to the metaphor. The circular motion of WORLD and the circular handshapes of SUN and YEAR all represent

TABLE 1: Stanzas of "Circle of Life"

Stanza	Theme	Rhyme
1	God's plan	Flat B handshapes
2	Eternity	Circles
3	Transition to episode	B and 1 handshapes
4	Two people's history	Two balanced spaces, two-handed signs
5	Two becoming one	Two circles overlap
6	Eternity	Circles
7	Two becoming one	Two circles overlap

spherical celestial bodies; the poet emphasizes the circular shape and rotation of the earth with classifiers as well. SUN-RISE-AND-SET and YEAR also iconically represent the circular paths of celestial bodies. The notion of time has already been evoked by the motion of the planets, our original clocks, but it is made explicit with signs such as ERA and HOUR, both of which iconically depict circular motion on a clock face. Finally, the sign CONTINUE is given the inflection for continuous aspect, denoting continuation for eternity; this inflection, as mentioned previously, itself draws on the "circle = eternity" metaphor and consists of a repeated circular motion. These data are summarized in Table 2. We can see that the "eternal circle" imagery is introduced not merely on the semantic level, with concepts such as "sun" and "continue forever," but also on the visual level; moreover, the visual rhymes are not incidental to the conceptual pattern but integrated with it through iconicity. The tone is celestial, eternal, holy, undifferentiated.

The theme of *two people* is introduced in stanza four, with a description of the early life of the bride and groom. Though a few circle shapes are present (F classifiers, the

TABLE 2: Circular imagery in stanzas 2 and 6

Relation to theme	Sign	Type of circle	Image presented
None	YES	Fist handshape	Nodding head
Celestial body	WORLD	Movement	Spherical earth
Celestial body	CL:55	Curved handshapes	Spherical earth
Celestial body	SUN	Curved handshape	Spherical sun
Celestial body, time	CL:11	Movements	Earth spins on axis
Celestial body, time	SUN-RISE-AND-SET+	Curved handshape, circular movements	Sun rises and sets
Celestial bodies, time	YEAR	Fist handshapes, movements	Earth revolves around sun
Time	ERA	Circular movement	Motion of clock hands
Time	HOUR	Circular movement	Motion of clock hands
Time	CONTINUE$_{continuous}$	Circular movement	inflection for continuous aspect

Conceptual "Rhymes" in Sign Language Poetry

sign ENVISION, which creates a mental "sphere"), the imagery focuses on pairs or "twos," and every sign participates in the imagery. Table 3 summarizes the spatial and temporal devices used. The primary spatial device is that the poet sets up two balanced locations in signing space; the right location represents the groom, and the left represents the bride. F classifiers (a circle of thumb and index finger, with other fingers extended) are held at each location to represent each person, each name is finger spelled at the appropriate location, and pronouns are directed at the locations. We should note that the F is not a usual classifier for humans; the poet has gone out of her way to choose a form that incorporates a circle. Second, many two-handed signs are used, and a number of one-handed signs are articulated on both hands. Wherever possible, one hand is placed in each significant location; when this is not possible (i.e., when the sign must be articulated on the signer's body), the poet shifts her entire body first to the right and then to the left. There are several temporal devices as well: there are two phases of growing up—first to adolescence and then to adulthood; each phase consists of paired activities; and the entire section is introduced and concluded with two occurrences of the two-handed sign LIFE. Note that the two locations in space iconically represent the two people, and the two phases of growing up of course correspond to the two temporal stages of the couple's lives; the other instances of pairs are visual or rhythmic rhymes but do not iconically present "two-ness."

The fifth stanza integrates circle imagery with the pair imagery of stanza four, presenting the theme of *two becoming one*; this stanza describes how the couple meets

TABLE 3: Pair imagery in stanza four

Type of pair	Device	Image presented	Examples
Spatial	Two balanced spatial locations	Two people	Pronouns, classifiers, finger spelling articulated at those locations
Spatial	Two-handed signs with same handshape for both hands	None	LIFE, FAR, PLAY, FIGHT, LAUGH, CRY, SCHOOL
Spatial	One-handed signs articulated on both hands, one in each location	Two people	GROW-UP-TO-ADOLESCENCE, GROW-UP-TO-ADULTHOOD, GO-OFF
Spatial	Two-handed signs, if not body-anchored then articulated with one hand at each location	Two people	FAR, PLAY, FIGHT
Spatial, temporal	For pairs of body-anchored, two-handed signs, body tilts first to one location and next to the other	Two people	LEARN, EXPERIENCE
Temporal	Two phases of growing up	Two times	GROW-UP-TO-ADOLESCENCE, GROW-UP-TO-ADULTHOOD
Temporal	Paired, rhyming actions in each phase	None	PLAY and FIGHT, LAUGH and CRY, LEARN and EXPERIENCE
Temporal	Experiences framed by two occurrences of the sign LIFE	None	(see transcription)

TABLE 4: Stanza five: Physical closeness representing emotional intimacy

Type of sign	Level of closeness	Level of intimacy
F classifiers	Original locations (far apart)	Low
	Circling each other far apart	Low
	Touch	High
	Spring apart	Lower
	Overlap circles	Complete
ENGAGEMENT	Ring touches finger	Complete
MARRY	Hands clasp	Complete

and how they develop a marital love that should partake of eternity. The story is told almost completely through metaphorical classifiers. The poet begins with one F classifier in each person's space. The Fs then move out of their spaces, circling each other counterclockwise four times until at last they touch. They spring apart, with an averted gaze and head shake from the signer; touch again and spring apart with a second head shake; and finally overlap circles. The right F then encircles the left ring finger, in the sign meaning ENGAGEMENT, and at last the two hands clasp in the sign meaning MARRY. In this passage, distance between articulators metaphorically represents emotional intimacy between the two people. At first, they do not know each other. They meet and "connect," but call off the relationship more than once before establishing a permanent emotional bond. The two lexical signs that end the passage iconically present images related to marriage—engagement rings and handclasps—but we may note that the images also involve the joining of two items (hands and/or rings). At the end, the two have become one (Table 4).

After a repeat of circular imagery in stanza six, stanza seven briefly recapitulates the *two-becoming-one* theme: the F classifiers are presented in their original locations and once again labeled with the couple's names, and then the sign RELATIONSHIP (also meaning "bond" or "connection"), articulated with interlocked F handshapes, moves between those locations. The final sign is the two-handed CONTINUE, indicating a wish that the marriage would last. But this time the poet does not use the circular inflection for continuous aspect; instead, she moves the sign in an arc down and then forward. This motion may be simply an emphatic form. Alternately, it may draw on another well-known metaphorical/iconic device: the time line, where future time is represented as in front of the signer and past time is behind him or her; this modulation would emphasize that the continuation will extend into the future. In either case, we may note that the poet has abandoned her circular imagery. The shift to a forward motion emphasizes that though the marriage bond is divine and eternal, the couple face a future relationship specific to them alone. Their marriage will unfold in a particular time and place, unlike the endless, timeless circling of the planets and stars.

Let us review the ways in which each conceptual theme is presented. The first, *eternity as a circle*, is shown through simple rhymes with round shapes; through iconic lexical items that have images of round planets, orbits, and clock faces; through the iconic circular inflection for continuous aspect; and through classifier descriptions that represent planetary motions and movements of people. The second theme of *two people* is presented through the iconic designation of one area in space for each person; various other rhymes support the notion of "two." The third theme of *two becoming one* is shown through both iconic/metaphorical movements of F classifiers and iconic lexical items that depict closeness and hand-clasping. Iconicity of three distinct linguistic components—lexical items, classifiers, and aspectual inflections—contributes to the unified visual/conceptual imagery.

In conclusion, we may note that ASL supports highly sophisticated poetry. The major themes of the poem are presented simultaneously on both the conceptual level and the visual level, through iconic and metaphorical "conceptual rhymes." For "Circle of Life," the main conceptual rhymes are the circle as symbol of eternity and unity and the pair merging into one as symbol of marriage. The rhymes are presented through the fixed iconic imagery of lexical signs and grammatical inflections and through classifier descriptions that may be freely adapted to fit whatever image the signer has in mind. This technique allows conceptual motifs and rhyme schemes to merge completely. Scholars of an earlier time believed that the iconicity of sign languages limited signers to simple, concrete concepts. Nothing could be further than the truth; as we see from poems such as "Circle of Life," iconicity provides sign language with a highly effective channel for abstract and poetic thought.

References

Bauman, H.-D. L. (1998). American Sign Language as a medium for poetry: A comparative poetics of sign, speech and writing in twenty-century American poetry. Unpublished doctoral dissertation, SUNY Binghampton.

Klima, E., & Bellugi, U. (1979). *The signs of language*. Cambridge, MA: Harvard University Press.

Lakoff, G. (1992). The contemporary theory of metaphor. In A. Ortony (Ed.), *Metaphor and thought*, 2nd ed. Cambridge: Cambridge University Press.

Lakoff, G., & Johnson, M. (1980). *Metaphors we live by*. Chicago: University of Chicago Press.

Lakoff, G., & Turner, M. (1989). *More than cool reason: A field guide to poetic metaphor*. Chicago: University of Chicago Press.

Lentz, E. M. (1995). Circle of life. In *The treasure: Poems by Ella Mae Lentz*. VHS videotape. Berkeley, CA: In Motion Press.

Liddell, S. K. (1992). *Paths to lexical imagery*. Unpublished manuscript, Gallaudet University.

Liddell, S. K. (1995). Real, surrogate, and token space: Grammatical consequences in ASL. In K. Emmorey & J. S. Reilly (Eds.), *Language, gesture, and space*. Hillsdale, NJ: Lawrence Erlbaum Associates.

Ormsby, A. (1995). *The poetry and poetics of American Sign Language*. Unpublished doctoral dissertation, Stanford University.

Taub, S. F. (2001). *Language from the body: Iconicity and conceptual metaphor in American Sign Language*. Cambridge: Cambridge University Press.

Valli, C. (1994). *Poetics of American Sign Language poetry*. Unpublished doctoral dissertation, Union Institute.

Wilcox, P. P. (2000). *Metaphors in American Sign Language*. Washington, DC: Gallaudet University Press.

Wilcox, S. (1998). *Cognitive iconicity and signed language universals*. Paper presented to the Fourth Conference on Conceptual Structure, Discourse, and Language, 10–12 October, Atlanta, GA.

PART NINE

Recreation, Leisure, and Sport

The Role of Deaf Sport in Developing and Maintaining Deaf Identity in Great Britain

JORDAN EICKMAN

This essay is based on the provisional results of the latter two of three studies, named study 2 and study 3, performed for my doctoral dissertation, "The Role of Deaf Sport in Developing and Maintaining Deaf Identity," which focused on Great Britain (Eickman 2004).[1]

Study 2—Format, Method, Aims, and Research Questions

Study 2 consisted of a qualitative study, done in the form of a questionnaire survey based on Stewart (1991), of contemporary Deaf, nonculturally deaf (NCD), and hearing athletes, sport organizers, and teachers/coaches to determine their feelings and views on Deaf and general sport. The questionnaire survey utilized an opportunity sample and consisted of two slightly different versions (one each for deaf and hearing people). The aims of study 2 were to determine whether deaf respondents' cultural self-identification affected sporting behavior, their motivations for participating in sport activities, and their views on Deaf sport. Hearing athletes were used as a control group.

The research questions were as follows:

1. Are groups of deaf people with differing cultural self-identification involved in sport?
2. What is deaf people's involvement in sport? Do they play? Do they watch? Or do they do both activities?
3. Does cultural self-identification motivate and affect deaf people's involvement in Deaf sport and sport in general?
4. Does involvement in Deaf sport affect a deaf person's cultural self-identification?

---

1. This essay reflects my presentation at Deaf Way II. It also includes some clarifications drawn from my now-completed dissertation at the University of Bristol, United Kingdom (Eickman 2004), which incorporates virtually all this material and to which readers should refer for full coverage and citations on this topic.

Questionnaires' Content and Respondents

The questionnaires contained a wide variety of questions on sport including ones about playing sports in different situations and motivations for playing sports. Closed and open questions within the questionnaires gathered the following information about respondents: personal and sports background and cultural self-identification (for deaf respondents), importance of sports to them, extent of sports participation including sports played, playing partners, why they played sports, why they chose their sport playing partners, their identity's link to sports participation, their experiences with Deaf sports, attitudes about playing with Deaf and hearing athletes, reaction to Deaf and hard of hearing/oral athletic success, and views on the importance of Deaf sports to Deaf people (regarding the Deaflympics, Paralympics, and Deaf Sport organization) and on the present state of Deaf sports (its positive aspects and problems).

A total of fifty-four respondents, twenty-two deaf (fourteen classed as Deaf, eight as NCD, based on their response to a cultural self-identification question) and thirty-two hearing, returned questionnaires. Only those respondents who affirmed they played sports and indicated they grew up in the United Kingdom, by listing only British schools among schools attended, were included in the final report.

Study 2 Preliminary Results and Conclusions

Selected study 2 results from four areas (respondents' characteristics, their sports involvement, their motivations for sports involvement, and their views on Deaf sports) are shared here through the following twelve points:

1. Two predefined groups of deaf people, Deaf and NCD, involved in Deaf sports are investigated in this study. Deaf respondents tend to grow up with more contact with other deaf people and prefer communicating manually, including using British Sign Language (BSL). NCD respondents tend to use the oral method of communication and grow up with less contact with other deaf people, in a mainstreamed school setting. The amount of contact with other Deaf while growing up may play a large role in which identity a deaf child adopts even though self-rated hearing loss may also be a factor.
2. The type of identity, Deaf or NCD, a deaf person has seems to affect motivation for, participation in, and views on sports.
3. Deaf and NCD respondents play with both deaf and hearing partners and at all levels of sports. Deaf respondents seem to prefer Deaf partners. NCD respondents seem to feel more comfortable playing with hearing partners than Deaf respondents do. This may be due to communication barriers between signing Deaf respondents and nonsigning hearing partners.
4. Deaf respondents prefer football, a team sport that may present communication problems, as their competitive sports, unlike NCD people, who prefer various individual sports. This difference may arise from a Deaf desire to be on a Deaf team, and this is linked to cultural self-identification.
5. Deaf and NCD respondents appear to draw similar social benefits from Deaf sporting events that they do not at hearing sporting events, which are a source of different benefits to each group.

6. Deaf respondents seem to name socializing as the most positive and important thing about Deaf sport. It is a social, as well as sporting, activity where Deaf pride can be demonstrated. NCD respondents see participation opportunities in Deaf sport.
7. Sport is a place where deaf people can get recognition from hearing people and show that deaf people are capable of achieving the same success as hearing athletes. The Deaflympics seem to meet Deaf and NCD respondents' different needs for socializing and competition in a communication barrier–free milieu, hence its support from both groups.
8. Less than overwhelming Deaf support for the Deaflympics indicate a lack of satisfaction with British Deaf sport and suggest some Deaf respondents feel Paralympic participation can address the perceived inequality in treatment of Deaflympic and Paralympic athletes.
9. Deaf respondents seem to feel other Deaf people should be involved in organizing Deaf sporting events while this does not matter to NCD respondents. Communication and cultural understanding may explain this desire.
10. Deaf respondents indicate a link between the Deaf club and Deaf sports, which points to a connection between Deaf sports and the Deaf community.
11. Sporting success is viewed differently by both groups. Gaining recognition within Deaf sport is important to Deaf respondents, who also seem to support other Deaf successes more than oral/hard of hearing successes. It seems that to enjoy support from Deaf people, one has to be a member of the Deaf community. NCD respondents seem to support all deaf successes, regardless of the deaf athlete's cultural self-identification.
12. Both Deaf and NCD respondents seem to view organization as a problem in Deaf sports. Deaf respondents also seem to display concern over lack of participation today. On the other hand, NCD respondents view the future of Deaf sports as growing and having more success.

Three themes that stood out are attitudes toward communication modes, toward contact with other Deaf people, and toward playing with hearing people. Deaf and NCD respondents have different views regarding these three themes, which seem to have a part in motivating all the other differences in sport participatory behavior, motivations for sports, and views on Deaf sports.

Model

The aforementioned results led to a theoretical model linking Deaf identity and Deaf sport, which is tested in study 3. Figure 1 shows a diagram of this model, which is divided into two dimensions: degree of affiliation to the Deaf community (or strength of Deaf identity) and extent of sport participation. Based on their characteristics, deaf people are placed within this model.

The letters near the origin, in each quadrant, are names for the groups of people who fall in that quadrant. For example, Deaf people placed in group A would be more active in sports, either through watching, playing, organizing, or coaching, and identify

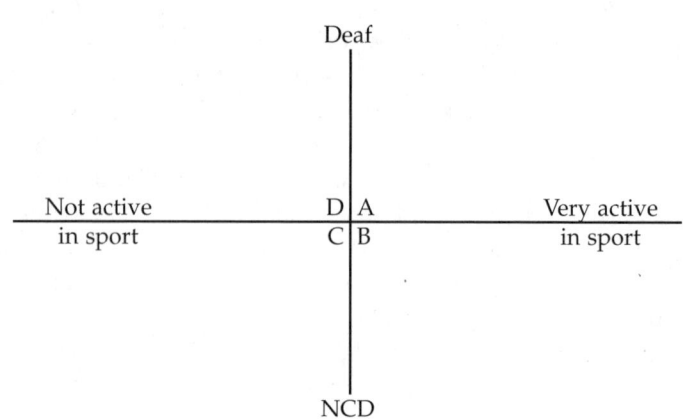

FIGURE 1: Model of Deaf identity and Deaf sports participation

more strongly with Deaf values and the Deaf community as the further to the top and right they are that quadrant.

The model has been constructed in this way based on the assumption that all deaf people have varying degrees of self-identification and affiliation with the Deaf community and interest and activity in sport. I have deduced what seem to be several premises and themes on how identity affects deaf sporting behavior from study 2. Classifying deaf sportspeople within the two dimensions defining self-identification with the Deaf community and degree of interest in sports acts as a guide for study 3's interviews. I hope that interviewing Deaf people with characteristics from each quadrant will lead to the induction of more underlying characteristics and factors involved with Deaf identity and a better understanding of how Deaf identity affects Deaf and NCD sporting behavior. The characteristics and points of view of both Deaf and NCD people who are neither active nor interested in sports will also help to frame the views of Deaf and NCD people who are interested and active in sports. This may be done through eliminating characteristics that do not affect sporting behavior as well as providing unique insight from people not involved with sports about Deaf sports, from NCD people about Deaf people, and vice versa. Characteristics, factors, and other data from study 3 interviews can be used to confirm or disconfirm the conclusions drawn from study 2 results and explore the role of Deaf sports in developing Deaf identity more fully. We hope this will lead to a greater understanding, clarification, and framing of the role of Deaf identity in Deaf sports and how Deaf sports affect both Deaf and NCD identities at the next, deeper, level.

Study 3—Format, Method, Aims, and Research Questions

Study 3 was a quantitative study, consisting of a set of in-depth semistructured ethnographical, personal interviews of Deaf and NCD people of differing interests in sports and self-identification with the Deaf community, which were loosely based on Spradley (1979). The interviews focused on how identity is self-constructed, the strength of identification with the Deaf community, how and why Deaf sports are or are not important, and how Deaf sports and social aspects affect them and their identity development. What each individual felt was involved in the process of moving from being NCD to culturally Deaf was of particular interest. The aim of Study 3 was to discover the underlying motives and factors influencing identity development in Deaf and NCD people, with particular attention to Deaf and NCD athletes. From this, it is possible to locate motives and factors that might be linked to Deaf sport participation.

The research questions were as follows:

1. Which steps might be involved in the Deaf identity development process?
2. How does participation in Deaf sports help move a deaf person along in the Deaf identity development process?
3. What factors influenced groups A–D members to develop the identity type unique to their respective group?
4. Is it possible for deaf members of groups B and C to "move upward" (see figure 1) into groups A and D, respectively, and become Deaf community members? If so, how?

Interviews' Content and Respondents

Question topics covered scholastic and educational experience, first and subsequent experiences with Deaf sports; self-identification; factors affecting self-identification; socialization process into the Deaf community; the roles of Deaf sports, Deaf clubs, and schools in the socialization process; perceived differences in old and young Deaf people's values; views on the mainstreaming trend and what it means to the Deaf community and Deaf sports; and communication and control issues within sports and Deaf sports.

Questions were adjusted appropriately for interviewees who had little or no interest in sport and for NCD interviewees. Thus, those interviewees could comment on the same topics and issues as the other sport-involved or Deaf interviewees did. For example, some NCD respondents were asked why they were not involved in the Deaf community, leading to insights about how they did not develop a Deaf identity, which resulted in them having a NCD identity.

The entire interview was conducted in sign language and videotaped with the interviewee's consent. Most interviews lasted between forty-five and ninety minutes. As the interviewee contributed additional material not directly covered by the questions but that was relevant to study 3's research aims, the interview shifted to explore that train of thought before returning to the next question on the list. Hence, each interview was unique, allowing for differences in interviewees' experiences and areas of knowledge to be reflected yet allowing information to be gathered on common topics for comparative purposes.

Not every question was asked in every interview because of time constraints and/or the interviewee's background and experience. For example, most group C and D members were not asked whether they preferred a Deaf or hearing manager (coach), because these groups contain interviewees who do not participate in sports. In these cases, this was a judgement call by the interviewer based on what was known about the interviewee, what was shared up to then during the interview, and whether the interviewee could contribute through answering a particular question.

Twenty-four deaf individuals were interviewed in twenty-one interviews. Each interview was conducted on a one-to-one basis, with the three exceptions: one interview each with two separate husband-wife pairs and a pair of deaf sport organizers. Interviewees were chosen for their suitability in representing one of the four identity type groups (A, B, C, or D) within the model of Deaf identity and Deaf sports participation (see figure 1).

Study 3 Preliminary Results

Interviewees were classified into groups A–D based on the following criteria:

> Group A: Showed a strong interest and active participation in sports and clearly identified themselves as Deaf.
> Group B: Showed a strong interest and active participation in sports and did not clearly identify themselves as Deaf.
> Group C: Showed little or no interest in sports and did not clearly identify themselves as Deaf.
> Group D: Showed little or no interest in sports and clearly identified themselves as Deaf.

Interview data indicated that some interviewees did not fit into groups A–D, and thus a group E was created with the following working definition:

Group E members do not clearly identify themselves as Deaf but do identify themselves to some degree with Deaf people, the Deaf community, and/or sign language. They may prefer signing to speech but may also choose to communicate orally with others, in particular hearing people. The level of interest and participation in sport is not affected by their identity transition. They may also admit they are in between a NCD and a Deaf identity. Figure 2 shows how group E fits in the theoretical model linking Deaf identity and Deaf sports.

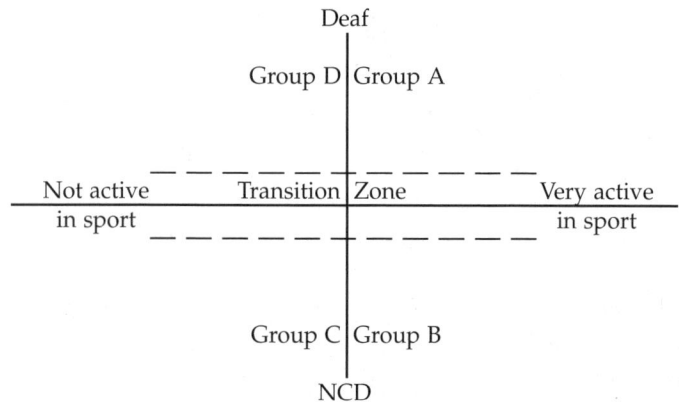

FIGURE 2: Position of group E in the model of Deaf identity and Deaf sports participation

Study 3 Preliminary Conclusions

We can give answers to each of study 3's research questions. The steps involved in the Deaf identity-development process are acceptance of one's deafness, learning BSL, using BSL, regularly and persistently mixing with Deaf people at Deaf community events to adopt Deaf values, and membership in the Deaf community and completion of an adult Deaf identity. Having contact with Deaf people, in particular Deaf role models, facilitates all those steps. They are sequential in nature; however, there are overlaps. For example, socializing at Deaf community events helps one learn and gives opportunities to use BSL.

The conditions needed for the Deaf identity-development process to take place are created by Deaf social spaces. Such spaces can be formed by Deaf clubs, Deaf schools (those having Deaf adult role models), Deaf sports, and other Deaf community activities. Creating a Deaf social space is how Deaf sports help move a deaf person along in the Deaf identity-development process.

What Deaf sports' Deaf social space offers are recreational and social opportunities where BSL is used and that Deaf people control. Oftentimes this social space is hearing free, allowing Deaf people to enjoy themselves in an environment where they do not feel threatened by hearing people or need to communicate by speech or other unnatural means. Deaf communication needs are met. Deaf people are in a position to control how their Deaf identity is shaped and expressed and ensure their Deaf identity needs are met. Also, the number of Deaf people that Deaf sport events attract is also a pulling factor. Social networking and information-sharing opportunities arise. All these benefits bolster and intensify Deaf identity. However, it is up to the deaf person to make the decision to attend, actively participate, and take advantage of what Deaf social spaces offer, including those Deaf sports-created spaces.

To complete the Deaf identity-development process, deaf people must successfully ingrain Deaf values and practices into themselves. The set of Deaf values and practices have been described and defined to the extent where Deaf people can distinguish between Deaf and NCD people. Many factors, other than Deaf sports, also come in play regarding whether a deaf person successfully completes the Deaf identity-development process. These factors come to the forefront by studying people whose characteristics fall within each of the four quadrants created by the two dimensions (groups A–D) or whose characteristics are in transition between quadrants (group E; see figure 2). The importance of these influencing factors is underlined by the fact that whether the Deaf identity-development process is completed ultimately determines the type of identity (Deaf or NCD) a deaf person develops.

The most important factors that influenced groups A–E members to develop the identity type unique to their respective group include the type of school, method of education and communication they were raised with, and how their family responded to their deafness. These factors are the ones that control whether deaf people have access to Deaf social spaces and thereby whether they have opportunities to develop their Deaf identity.

It is possible for group B and C members to "move upward" (see figure 2) into groups A and D, respectively, and become Deaf community members. This is achieved by successfully completing the Deaf identity-development process. There are two tracks to achieve this process. Deaf children whose introduction to the Deaf community is made early, usually in a deaf school or a Deaf family, are on the faster track. They benefit from being exposed to Deaf social space more frequently and at a younger age. They are able to develop their own network of Deaf friends, learn from older Deaf role models, and acquire BSL and Deaf cultural values while growing up. The slower track, usually taken by mainstreamed children or hard of hearing young adults, requires that the deaf people overcome the factors blocking them from Deaf social spaces. This takes more effort, time, and persistence. Regardless of which track an individual takes, all the steps of the Deaf identity process have to be successfully completed to reach a fully Deaf identity.

Deaf identity is and should be the normal state of being for deaf people. However, anti-Deaf identity factors such as oralism, hearing parents who have difficulty accepting their child's deafness, and medical views of deafness as a disability rather than a cultural identity cut deaf people off from Deaf social space. Contact with Deaf social space is important in the process of developing Deaf identity.

Deaf sport can take a role in developing Deaf identity in Britain to counter the effects of those anti-Deaf identity factors, the declining numbers of Deaf schools, and the declining importance of the Deaf club. However, ideally Deaf sports should be part of the "traditional route" of Deaf social spaces in Deaf identity development alongside Deaf schools and Deaf clubs. Today in Britain, Deaf sports are failing to provide adequate Deaf social spaces because of weak leadership in the Deaf sports structure, both at the national and club levels. Deaf sports also are competing with technological advances in communication devices, mainstreaming, and changes in society values toward a more integrated society that may lead individuals to have less interest in sports. All those forces have made the Deaf club weaker by shifting a primary Deaf social space from the Deaf club to the Deaf pub. These forces, by increasing the friction of distance, have shortened the critical distance that Deaf people are willing to travel for Deaf socialization. However, it is possible for Deaf sports with strong Deaf leadership to overcome these forces and provide a Deaf social space where Deaf identity development can occur.

Interviewees have said that Deaf sports are the best and fastest way into the Deaf community. Deaf sports and the Deaf social space encompass many benefits to many different kinds of Deaf and NCD people.

References

Eickman, Jordan. 2004. The role of deaf sport in developing Deaf identity. Ph.D. diss., University of Bristol.

Spradley, James P. 1979. *The ethnographic interview*. Fort Worth, TX: Harcourt Brace Jovanovich.

Stewart, David A. 1991. *Deaf sport: The impact of sports within the Deaf community*. Washington, DC: Gallaudet University Press.

Deaf Women and Sports in Nigeria: Problems and Prospects

ANTHONIA NGOZIKA EGUZOUWA

The United Nations statistics estimate that there are more than 10 million deaf people across the globe. Though the incidence of deafness is more pronounced among males than female, there is a growing general population of deaf women. Nigeria is assumed to harbor one of the largest deaf populations on the African continent, and from the statistics and records available, the population of deaf women in Nigeria is rising astronomically.

However, to come to terms with the reality of our present situation concerning deafness and deaf people in all ramifications, it is imperative to give a broad-based definition of who deaf people really are, and we ought be particularly cognizant of the fact that deaf women form an integral aspect of the broad-based definition.

Deaf People

To enhance our overall knowledge of who deaf people really are, this definition suffices: generally, deaf people are those in whom the sense of hearing is nonfunctional for the ordinary purposes of life. It could therefore be said that to be deaf is not to be able to hear. Deafness is a condition that can be total or partial.

However, going *pari passu* with this definition are a few salient characteristics associated with deaf people of which we must know to attune us to their temperaments, psychology, likes, dislikes, and general view of things and significant others around them.

Major Characteristics of Deaf Individuals

Characteristics of deaf individuals usually reflect the effect of hearing impairment or problems associated with deafness:

1. Social and personal adjustments: This mainly has to do with the social and personal adjustment of the affected individuals. This is connected with the communication problem deaf people usually have, which contributes to social

and behavior difficulties. Nonetheless, participating in sports and other recreational activities tend to ameliorate this problem.

2. Academic achievement: Academic difficulties are a by-product of hearing impairment. However, this is not surprising considering the poor language development and lack of auditory exposure to the environment, resulting from the handicap of deafness. Still, engaging in comprehensive sports activities enhances the deaf person's self-esteem and erases the toga of academic failure. Other areas affected by hearing impairment/deafness include social maturity and personality development.

Definition of Sports

Sports are defined as activities in which people compete in running, jumping, throwing, shooting, playing table tennis, and so forth. It also means an outdoor or indoor game(s), competition, or activity that has rules and needs bodily effort and skills. Sports generally have the positive effects of releasing tension; promoting overall physical fitness of the participants; providing release from stress; serving as an avenue to escape from despondency, frustration, and occasionally unemployment; and nowadays serving as a means of livelihood and likewise enhancing local and international cooperation among officials and actual participants.

Women in Sports

Over the years, sporting activities were essentially restricted to males; they were used by men as a means of developing combat skills, physical agility, and so forth. Women were merely spectators. Despite all the discrimination, restrictions, and bias against women in sports, women have now emerged as a force to be reckoned with in sports participation and sports administration. It is imperative to recognize the role of women in sports: educate a boy and you educate one man, but educate women and you educate the family and the society. Educating a woman will build a healthy, united, self-reliant, honest, and corruption-free society. Sports foster the virtues of personal integrity, self-discipline, honesty, industry, modesty, and sense of responsibility. Women can contribute immensely in the promotion of family culture and development of society through sports in Nigeria.

Aims and Objectives

1. To bring to fore the teeming population of deaf sportswomen in Nigeria.
2. To shed light on the problems encountered by Nigerian deaf women.
3. To sensitize the Nigerian sports administrators of the need to urgently support deaf sportswomen.
4. To increase awareness of deaf women's sports.
5. To instigate a revolution in deaf women athletes via electronic and print media.
6. To engender societal recognition for deaf women in sports in Nigeria.
7. To highlight the major problems hindering sports participation by Nigeria deaf women.

8. To shed light on the prospects of deaf women's sports in Nigeria and to highlight the way(s) forward.

Statement of the Problem

The real problems hindering the full-fledged participation of deaf women in the many available sports in Nigeria are numerous and multifaceted. Zealous as deaf women are in the country, these problems still persist and constantly constitute clogs in their achievements.

For our purposes, however, these problems are outlined here:

1. Parental opposition to the participation in sports by their deaf daughters/wards.
2. Financial problem(s) on the part of deaf women and their families.
3. Lack of societal encouragement of deaf women taking part in sports.
4. Lack of recognition of deaf women athletes generally by society, especially the sports ministry and sports administrators, although the trend is gradually being eroded.
5. Lack of competitions/games for the women who are lucky enough to be able to partake in some local and international competitions.
6. Government's apathy to the development of deaf sports in particular and disabled sports in general.
7. Lack of focus among deaf athletes women themselves.

Solutions

1. Parental support of the participation of their female wards in sports generally.
2. Promotion of awareness of the existence of deaf women's sports through electronic and print media.
3. Constant organization of practices for deaf women to put them in proper shape and physical condition for the task ahead.
4. Discovering hidden talent from all the nooks and crannies of the country.
5. Showing genuine interest in the growth and development of deaf women's sports in the whole county.
6. Societal recognition of deaf women's sports and support by corporate bodies and individual philanthropists.
7. Restructuring of the Nigerian Deaf Sports Federation (NDSF), and adequate funding to encourage deaf women.

The Way(s) Forward

Deaf people in general are beset by the problem of how to adequately assert themselves in their immediate environment and larger society. They face a lot of obstacles in their attempts to wriggle out of their disadvantaged status. Much as they try to make inroads in commerce, education, the sciences, agriculture, and other fields, they are always frustrated and grossly misunderstood by many.

However, sports are becoming the only creditable avenue of fully shedding of the mantle of underachievement. Therefore, concerted efforts must be made by

1. the Nigerian federal government to give full support to deaf women's sports;
2. the various state and local government councils;
3. corporate bodies and individual philanthropists; and
4. the parents of deaf women by endorsing their deaf wards to engage in sports.

The D/deaf Community, Leisure, and Public Recreation

GINA A. OLIVA

The term *leisure*, when used in everyday conversation, usually means "free time" or "relaxing and fun activities." Although these definitions are useful, they do not fully explain the important role leisure plays in our collective and individual lives. Most adults give little conscious thought to leisure either as a concept or as a critical element in their lives. In the Western world, adults may begin giving consideration to leisure when they are approaching retirement.

Because people give so little active thought to their leisure, they are sometimes surprised to find out that leisure studies is a field of academic study. Mainstream research on leisure includes studies of how people spend their time, what kind of recreation pursuits involve the greatest monetary expenditures, and how playgrounds can be made safer, to name only a few.

From this research, one can learn what motivates people to participate in certain forms of leisure. Why do people love skiing? Why are computer games so popular? Why do D/deaf people spend so much time socializing? One can also learn what factors people identify as preventing them from participating in certain leisure activities. These are called "constraints" to leisure. "I don't have enough time." "I can't afford it." "I don't have anyone to do that with." The most common constraints are time, money, and availability of people to join us in activities that we do not wish to do alone.

In America we "live for the weekend." We actually have a restaurant named after this phenomenon—T.G.I. Friday's (Thank God It's Friday). This phrase loudly proclaims that our jobs are a pain in the butt and weekends are a breath of fresh air.

It is commonly believed that people of particular kinds of employment (doctors, college professors, writers, professional athletes, movie stars, travel agents) "enjoy their work." However, even they look forward to weekends and vacations—to their leisure. For most of us, leisure is equally if not more important than work and family responsibilities, even though it occupies much less of our time.

Why do we look forward to our weekends? Leisure research explores the relationship between leisure choices and life satisfaction. In general, these studies show a consistent and overriding relationship between leisure satisfaction and life satisfaction (Driver and Brown 1986; Edginton et al. 1998). The goal of leisure practitioners and researchers, in a broad sense, is to enhance quality of life by understanding the effects our leisure opportunities and choices have on our lives, our communities, and our futures.

Leisure and Life Satisfaction

To assist our thinking about leisure and life satisfaction, it is helpful to review the classic work of Abraham Maslow (1943), whose ideas are still taught in basic psychology courses today. He identified a "hierarchy of needs" and postulated that the more basic needs must be met before a person will have the resources to pursue higher-level needs. These needs are sustenance (food and water), safety (shelter and protection), belongingness and love, esteem and achievement, and self-actualization. The first two needs are generally met through work; we use the money we earn to pay for food and shelter. The higher three needs can be met through work or leisure.

Belongingness and love needs are met through relationships with family, friends, and loved ones. Are we happy in our primary relationships, be they with spouse, significant other, children, or parents? What about our secondary relationships, our friends or family members with whom we are not as close? Healthy adults meet belongingness and love needs within leisure time, that is, at home and at places of leisure. The activity could be sitting on the deck, making cookies, going on a white water kayak trip, or taking a craft workshop together. Except for some solitary leisure pursuits, most such activities involve other people and conversation with these people.

What of the belongingness and love needs of D/deaf individuals? Let us first consider D/deaf children, their caregivers, and their peers. Are the D/deaf and hard of hearing children in an environment where these needs are met? Are they involved in leisure activities with individuals with whom they can easily and comfortably converse? For adults, the questions are the same. We must remember that shared conversation is as important as the activity itself.

The top two needs—esteem/achievement and self-actualization—can be met through work or leisure. One might have a sense of achievement from becoming a top executive, a full professor, or a dean or by winning a grant. Or, one might have a sense of achievement from running a marathon, swimming sixteen laps for the first time, or painting a prize-winning watercolor.

What about the achievement needs of D/deaf people? It is widely accepted that many D/deaf people are underemployed or even unemployed. This may be even more so in other countries, particularly developing countries. Thus, although some D/deaf people may meet their achievement and self-actualization needs through their employment, these may be the exception. For most D/deaf adults, as with most hearing adults, the higher level needs will be met only through individually satisfying leisure activities.

Csikszentmihalyi (1990), a psychologist who has focused his life work on the phenomenon of leisure, provides additional ideas for this discussion. He proposed that true, satisfactory, and effective leisure could be defined or determined by the extent to which an activity results in the subjective experience of "flow." He defined flow as a sense of high well being, and his studies demonstrated that this "flow feeling" would be experienced when an activity included several requisite elements. These elements are (a) the skills required for the activity must approximately match the doer's ability (not too easy, not too difficult), (b) the doer must experience complete concentration on the activity at hand, (c) the doer must have a sense of control over the activity, (d) the doer must experience a loss of self-consciousness, and (e) the doer must experience a "timelessness" (unawareness of the passage of time).

The concept of flow can be demonstrated using an example: hanging wallpaper. Many individuals would groan and fidget and say "not me, never!" However, some individuals would enjoy a wallpapering project. Why? If we apply the concept of flow, then the happy wallpaperer is one who knows how to do it and is sufficiently challenged by the number of corners, the type of pattern, and so forth. Also, the doer wants to do it (i.e., is not told by someone to do it). The doer has the time to do it at a leisurely, engrossing pace; maybe the doer hangs the wallpaper with a favorite CD playing or on a glorious day when the windows can be open and the air temperature is just perfect. That would be a flow experience, and according to Csikszentmihalyi and other leisure scholars, thus qualify as bona fide leisure for *that* person, but not for the person who says "not me, never!"

What of the many D/deaf persons involved in organizing recreational activities, such as banquets in the 1800s,[1] the Timberfests and bowling tournaments of today? Have they experienced flow while engaged in these planning activities? What about those involved in planning the many local D/deaf festivals? Do they enjoy and become engrossed in the process? Do D/deaf persons *attending* Timberfest or D/deaf festivals experience this flow phenomenon?

Serving on a volunteer committee or participating in a contest (such as Timberfest or a bowling tournament) may very well allow for all five criteria and thereby can produce true flow as Csikszentmihalyi and other leisure theorists define it. With such participation, D/deaf people could experience achievement, self-actualization, and enhanced life satisfaction.

Public Recreation

In any given town in the United States, there are tax-supported parks, community centers, swimming pools, arts centers, baseball fields, and other facilities designed for leisure. Managed by local jurisdictions, they offer programs, classes, festivals, and other structured leisure activities. According to a leading textbook, the goals of these agencies are to build awareness of leisure opportunities; support the transmission of cultural heritage; help individuals acquire skills, knowledge, and constructive attitudes; and promote fun, social interaction, psychological well-being, and creativity (Edginton et al., 1998). Through these facilities and programs, hearing individuals have many opportunities to meet their esteem/achievement and self-actualization needs. They can experience flow right in their own neighborhoods.

Numerous park and recreation agencies also offer programs geared to the special interests of local ethnic minority groups. Through these programs (workshops,

---

1. Bernice Mottez (1993) describes the banquets that were organized by the French D/deaf community during the nineteenth century. These were much anticipated, well-attended, and well-remembered events. They are an early example of the D/deaf communities propensity to organize their own recreation.

festivals, performances, etc.), minorities receive support for their culture, customs, and community.

"Inclusion" in Public Recreation

During the past few decades, park and recreation agencies have followed the "inclusion" trend in public education.[2] This philosophical position, rooted in the idea that people with disabilities should not be segregated from people without disabilities, drives several widespread practices in the public recreation and parks arena. College programs preparing park and recreation professionals teach these individuals that disabled persons (including D/deaf and hard of hearing persons) *want* to be included in general recreation programs with their "non-disabled peers." The emphasis is on learning to provide access or "inclusion services." Park and recreation professionals have been indoctrinated with the idea that integrated activities are inherently better than segregated activities. They have been trained to put a little box on their advertisements that says, "Interpreter provided with three days' notice."

The National Therapeutic Recreation Society (NTRS) has published a position statement on inclusion: "The purpose of the Position Statement on Inclusion is to encourage all providers of park, recreation, and leisure services to provide opportunities in settings where people of all abilities can recreate and interact together.... People are entitled to opportunities in the most inclusive settings" (NTRS Report 1997).

This position statement has greatly reinforced the widespread practice of interpreter provision for "regular recreation opportunities" as the main and often sole means of providing access for D/deaf individuals. However, the same position statement shows recognition of the social element in satisfactory leisure, acknowledging that adults have the right to choose when, where, and with whom they will spend their leisure time: "The social connection with one's peers plays a major role in his/her life satisfaction. The opportunity to choose is an important component in one's quality of life: individual choice will be respected.... Environments should be designed to encourage... choices and acceptance that allow for personal accomplishment in a cooperative context" (ibid.).

The NTRS position statement is hopeful but perhaps unrealistic with regards to the attainability of integration of signers and nonsigners: "properly fostered, inclusion will happen naturally. Over time, inclusion will occur with little effort and with the priceless reward of an enlightened community" (ibid.).

---

2. In 1975, P.L. 94-142 initiated a movement in America away from residential schools and programs for disabled children and adults and toward greater involvement in public schools. In the late years of the twentieth century, this movement became known as the "inclusion movement." U.S. legislation regarding education for children with disabilities uses the terminology "least restrictive environment" (LRE) to describe school environments where disabled children should be educated. It is popularly interpreted as that environment that is most "normal" and/or that includes nondisabled children; e.g., a neighborhood school. Thus, in the recreational setting, LRE would mean "with nondisabled persons" (e.g., in "normal" recreational programs).

Inclusion: The "Deaf Way"

In education, mandated "inclusion" has resulted in many isolated D/deaf and hard of hearing children. In recreation, however, regardless of the efforts of professional bodies such as NTRS, "inclusion" really cannot be mandated. Adults decide for themselves how, when, where, and with whom they will recreate. The "inclusion movement" in public recreation has not resulted in D/deaf people rushing to take advantage of opportunities for one simple reason. As our collective history tells us, D/deaf adults rarely chose to attend or participate in anything where they would be the only D/deaf person involved.

Although no hard evidence exists related to the frequency with which D/deaf people take advantage of public recreation, or the manner of their participation, anecdotal evidence suggests that D/deaf people do take advantage of opportunities that require little if any communication with nonsigners. They are likely to use a public pool or tennis court. They go to parks and attend festivals with their family and friends. Some enroll in mainstream fitness classes, although it seems that many drop out because of communication issues.

Traditionally, D/deaf people have organized all of their own recreational activities. National sports groups and the World Games for the D/deaf are the most elaborate of these organizing efforts. Thus, nonprofit groups such as the Montgomery County Association of the D/deaf (MCAD) and commercial enterprises such as D/deaf Expo plan, promote, and manage D/deaf festivals with little if any assistance from public recreation entities. Could parks and recreation agencies assist in these efforts? Could D/deaf leaders ask for and expect support for these cultural celebrations?

In Montgomery County, Maryland, D/deaf adults have been very active in providing the impetus for change in how parks and recreation agencies serve local D/deaf populations. The Maryland Deaf Festival is a shining example of grassroots efforts and provides data that can be shared with public parks and recreation to illustrate how greatly committed local Deaf residents are to their community. Further, several Deaf parents with Deaf children have decided that they want their children to have more recreational opportunities, that public recreation exists to serve them as well as everyone else, and that they have had some unique ideas as to how they want their children included. They have enrolled their children en masse in summer camp programs. Deaf fathers have volunteered to coach sport teams consisting of both D/deaf and hearing players.

In this manner, Deaf parents have been instrumental in creating new ways for D/deaf and hard of hearing children to be involved with and served by public recreation agencies. These examples demonstrate how the ingenuity of D/deaf adults, in the interests of their D/deaf children, can forge novel and exemplary approaches to "inclusion." Programs resulting from these innovations can truly meet the leisure needs of D/deaf children while simultaneously providing a rich leisure experience for neighboring hearing children. This model, developed by Deaf adults for D/deaf children, enables the tax-supported parks and recreation agency to exceed the status quo—"call us if you want an interpreter." It enables them to fulfill their obligation to provide socially meaningful leisure opportunities to all members of the greater community.

This phenomenon could be repeated in other parts of the United States and the world. Have other Deaf parents in other states done likewise for their children? Perhaps they have, but where is the documentation? Is it true, as we surmise, that D/deaf people are not actively taking advantage of the vast network of community resources for leisure opportunities—neither for themselves nor for their children? By not taking advantage of this network, are they missing opportunities to meet their belongingness and love, achievement, and self-actualization needs? Are they missing opportunities to experience flow? If we would like public recreation's stance on inclusion to change, we must be able to provide them with information and guidance. Deaf adults in their own localities can approach public recreation agencies to educate them as to the D/deaf community's needs and to offer themselves for collaborative efforts. Finally, Deaf adults who do this need to document and share their successes as well as challenges with others who are concerned with the well-being of D/deaf and hard of hearing children.

Imagine a world where the experiences of those Deaf children, whose Deaf fathers coached their sport teams made of up of both D/deaf and hearing children, could be had by all D/deaf and hard of hearing children all over the globe. Then D/deaf people would have the same opportunities for fulfilling leisure and life satisfaction as hearing people have—they would have more opportunities to experience flow. Hearing children and adults would have an opportunity to experience the Deaf community and its culture in a complimentary light.

Ferdinand Berthier had the right idea in 1840:

> Recently there were some unkind remarks made about our fraternal association. It was said that nothing would be more disastrous for the D/deaf-mute than to limit himself to only the company of other D/deaf-mutes. To regroup D/deaf-mutes into a separate nation, a special caste, would be to condemn them to a deplorable exclusion. Those who say such things have misunderstood what is in our hearts. Our spirits have never harbored such egoistic intentions of separatism. We have been rejected from the banquets of hearing-speaking people. They have wanted to suppress the language of D/deaf-mutes: that sublime universal language given to us by nature. And yet D/deaf-mutes have said to their speaking brothers "Come among us! Join us in our work and in our play; learn our language as we learn yours; let us form one people united by indivisible ties." My brothers, is that egotism? Is that isolation? Let our accusers with no conscience just dare again to raise their voices against us! (Mottez 1993)

References

Csikszentmihalyi, M. 1990. *Flow: The psychology of optimal experience.* New York: Harper Collins.

Driver, B., and P. Brown. 1986. Probable personal benefits of outdoor recreation. In *A literature review of the President's Commission on Americans Outdoors,* 63–70. Washington DC: U.S. Government Printing Office.

Edginton, C., D. Jordan, D. DeGraaf, and S. Edginton. 1998. *Leisure and life satisfaction: Foundational perspectives.* Boston: McGraw-Hill.

Maslow, A. H. 1943. A theory of human motivation. *Psychological Review* 50 (July): 370–96.

Mottez, B. 1993. The D/deaf-mute banquets and the birth of the D/deaf movement. In *D/deaf history unveiled: Interpretations from the new scholarship*, ed. J. V. Van Cleve. Washington, DC: Gallaudet University Press.

National Therapeutic Recreation Society. 1997. "Position statement on inclusion." Ashland, VA: NTRS/NRPA.

PART TEN

Sign Language and Interpreting

How to Be All Things to All People: ASK!

CAROLE LAZORISAK AND LYNNE EIGHINGER

Interpreters face the dilemma of having conflicting sets of expectations from the consumers they serve. Deaf consumers consider attitude the most important of the interpreter's characteristics. However, hearing consumers feel knowledge and skills are the most significant characteristics. Interpreters report feeling obligated to choose between these competing expectations to prevent their services as being perceived as less than satisfactory based on the type of consumer. Given this, interpreters are searching for a framework to help them assess the performance of an interpreted event by meeting the criteria defined by their consumer group. In this paper, we present several models for assessment.

Notably, the two consumer groups have differing cultures; they hold differing views and perspectives of values and norms. The most common issue that arises when people of different cultural and linguistic backgrounds communicate directly relates to their ability to deal with the differences and similarities of their cultural values, norms, and interests. As interpreters, we are at that interface, working with and between two groups of people with differing language and culture. Acculturated individuals are able to unite and combine norms, values, and interests to achieve a certain blending for a successful cultural and language discourse.

In the United States, cultural issues arise when an interpreter works with consumers who use either American Sign Language (ASL), the language of the Deaf population, or English, the language of the hearing population. One of the reasons for this is the perception of hearing people (the majority) that their cultural values, norms, and experiences are shared and followed by Deaf people (a minority group). Because of this, the challenge arises as interpreters feel pinched not only by the original conflicting expectations of two consumer groups but also by greater conflicting views of an entire culture and population. Charged with the task of managing communication events, it is incumbent on interpreters to understand not only the consumers' sets of expectations but also to understand how these play out in a given community at large and to resolve these dilemmas in ways that allow the goals to be reached.

To better understand today's challenges for interpreters, it is important to first consider the historical development of signed language interpreting as a profession. Clearly, we have seen a shift in its practitioners. In the profession's earliest stages, most interpreters had a high level of connection to deafness, which stemmed from their great personal involvement either as volunteers or as tradespeople. These interpreters were members of the Deaf community and, to greater or lesser degrees, subscribers to its values and norms; they had little formal or academic training in translation and interpretation. Over time, the profession grew with the passage of federal and state legislation, and a growing number of interpreters entered professional training as a conscious, academic choice, as a job with prospects for satisfying employment.

What we see today is that this profession has given rise to a new breed of interpreters with increased academic training but with only limited actual exposure to or interaction with Deaf people. Many interpreters-in-training report that in the course of their academic schooling, they had never even met a Deaf person, the consumer base they want to serve. If, in their businesses, interpreters subscribe to the saying "the customer is always right," interpreters enter this business doomed by conflicting expectations and lack of cultural experience because they are not deeply educated in the norms, values, and interests of this consumer group. In other words, they would find the goal of "the customer is always right" difficult to fulfill because they do not know what the Deaf culture considers to be "right."

As "what is right" and service expectations differ among Deaf and hearing consumers, the pyramid model of cultural relationships can be used to provide a framework for assessing the performance of interpreters. The pyramid model of cultural relationships combines the key three attributes: knowledge (K), skills (S), and attitudes (A).

Depending on the consumer group, the pyramid model of cultural relationships will be a KSA or ASK triangular structure, as illustrated in figures 1 and 2.

This tool—the pyramid model of cultural relationships—contains the same critical metrics but differs in prioritization and will be used by Deaf and hearing clients to evaluate an interpreter's services. Because they prioritize attitudes, the Deaf consumer uses the ASK structure whereas the hearing consumer uses the KSA structure. Therefore, interpreters must balance this as they provide a service to a specific audience.

Although the prioritization of these attributes changes given the consumer group, they are all critical because all three must be present in a successful interpreter. Knowledge (K) is the ability to recall information and apply it to the real world. Knowledge allows one to know what to do in a situation, as well as to know where, when, why, and how to do it. Skills (S) are processes and the things one does. Skills put knowledge into action or use; one must have the skill in order to do something. Attitude

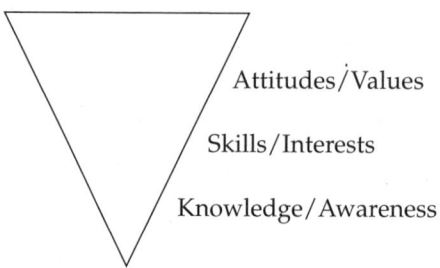

FIGURE 1: **Pyramid model of cultural relationships—ASK**

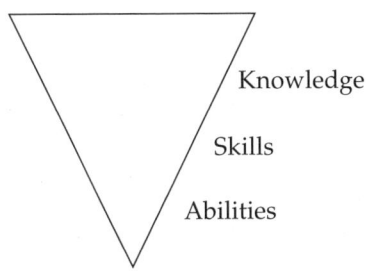

FIGURE 2: Pyramid model of cultural relationships—KSA

(A) implies choice—one chooses whether or not to do something. These terms are defined further as they relate specifically to this model.

The attitude component of the pyramid is important because the possession and use of feminist-relational values such as empowerment, cooperation, active listening, consensus building, commitment to social justice, and valuing experiences succinctly portray the intent of the term *attitude* (Eighinger & Karlin, 2001). To best meet the expectations of Deaf people, interpreters must keep close relationships with the Deaf community. A frequent and consistent response by Deaf consumers on the question of expectations and preferences for interpreter characteristics is that attitude is a primary requisite for success.

Deaf consumers of interpreting services place a high priority on the attitude aspect as exhibited in the ASK structure of the pyramid. Attitude and values expected and accepted by the Deaf community include patience, empathy, self-awareness, ability to work with differences, willingness to be open, a strong value system while maintaining open-mindedness and acceptance of other's values, and life experiences and struggles as well as life choices. It should also be noted that light humor is essential to the discourse process because it opens doors and enables open communication and interaction.

These contributing qualities enrich a person's use in the communication process and promote quality of discourse, interaction, and relationships. Patience and empathy requires a finely tuned, intuitive sensitivity to a diverse group. Empathy promotes unconditional openness and genuineness of a relationship, which usually leads to a positive outcome. Empathy can be described as transcendent respect for humanity. Self-awareness and ability to work with and within differences move participants from an initial connection to a relationship. The initial connection may last a few seconds to hours, but the more willing a person is to be open, the shorter the time span to create the relationship.

At the same time, the hearing consumer (who typically provides remuneration for services) must also have their expectations met and satisfied. Hearing customers typically gauge the employability (or contractibility) on tangible issues that are easily proven by documentation such as résumés, degrees and certification, and licensing cards. To sustain viable businesses, interpreters must be sensitive to satisfaction variables presented by these contracting customers and maintain tangible evidence of qualification to satisfy them.

Another level of the pyramid is skills. Defined skills of interpreters are the ability to gather information on individual language use, communication style, and overall context including, when needed, life experiences. Discerning communication styles and thought processes can be accomplished through observation and interaction. This requires active listening, which includes the ability to recognize and produce the language preferred by Deaf customers. In making appropriate communication choices, it is crucial that the interpreter be adaptable and use tools including different language modes as well as visual-gestural and oral systems in common use by Deaf people. Because Deaf people "code switch" depending on their perception of their hearing partner and of the communication event, interpreters must be flexible. Hearing people primarily use auditory linguistic modes and have great difficulty adapting to the visual-gestural modes used by Deaf people.

The knowledge component of the pyramid relates to knowledge of cultural groups. Knowledge should include understanding human development, cultural experiences and perspectives, cultural and social behaviors, and issues of cultural similarities and differences. This includes the willingness to do ongoing readings, research, observations, interactions with diverse groups, and assessment of personal progress in expanding knowledge of specific areas or topics.

Because interpreters serve more than one consumer at a time, as they act as a liaison between hearing and Deaf people and must balance their needs and expectations. The pyramid model contributes to an interpreter's ability to foster relationships between Deaf and hearing individuals. These attitudes, skills, and knowledge can be acquired through interaction, sharing, and observing language and cultural differences and thus enhance one's professional demeanor in working with diversity.

Another tool used to evaluate interpreters' performance is the two-dimensional customer service model. Customer service has two primary dimensions: the first is the procedural dimension consisting of established systems and procedures to deliver products and/or services; the second is a personal dimension related to how service personnel, interpreters, interact with their customers through their attitudes, behaviors, and communication skills. (See figure 3.)

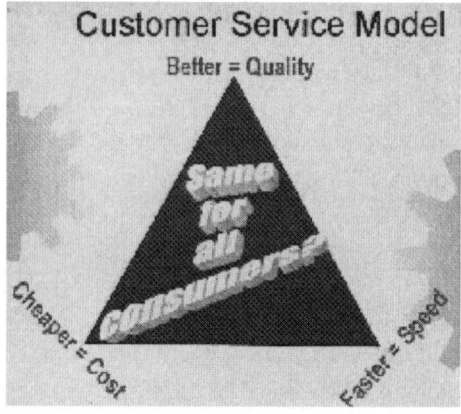

FIGURE 3: Two-dimensional customer service model

This two-dimensional framework clearly demarcates customer service priorities. Interpreters, while providing a human service, must also focus on the procedural aspects of providing that service and working with established systems and procedures. The provision and attention to the procedural dimension typically is a focus on the hiring entity's satisfaction. Unfortunately, as many Deaf people can attest, these customers control the ability of interpreters (or the referral agencies contracting them) to maintain their livelihood and to sustain a living wage. This provides a powerful incentive to interpreters to consider the satisfaction of this side of the triangle as a priority. For this reason, interpreters place a strong emphasis on the procedural aspect of their service provision. Herein lies the internal discord that interpreters express after discovering the chasm that exists between customer expectations: having entered the field because of a motivation to provide a human service (to the Deaf community), they realize the need to, understandably, maintain employability in the marketplace for which they are frequently unprepared.

In business relationships, providing things "better, faster, and cheaper" is the way to ensure customer attraction and retention. In some ways, the better, faster, cheaper mantra of business can benefit both sets of consumers (hearing and deaf). However, more often than not, Deaf consumers are not served by these concepts.

To provide a "better" service requires interpreters to maintain a commitment to lifelong learning and professional development to the benefit of all consumers. However, this professional development should investigate and address the entire service, including sociological, psychological, cognitive, and physical aspects of the service provision. A majority of pre- and in-service training focuses on aspects related to ASL to the exclusion of these other aspects, which might not be as visible, of the interpreting process. In training programs, students focus on earning a living, and this becomes the priority. There is little time to understand and explain the vulnerable nature of the interpreted event to ensure that the goals of all consumers are met. This lack of a research base has led to the lack of a national standard, which undermines the profession of interpreting and the subsequent provision of services.

Providing faster service has implications of serving both consumers, yet, in reality, it can adversely affect one side of the triad: the Deaf consumer. Faster service can mean cutting response time to requests for interpreting service but can and does relate to the provision of the interpreting service. Anecdotal evidence suggests that interpreters feel rushed by outside influences that do not permit them to provide a thorough and in-depth attention to all of the communication partners' goals. Interpreters trying to, as mentioned previously, provide a service that allows them to build and maintain a relationship with the customer (the paying customer and/or the interpreter referral agency) can overtly and covertly circumvent the goals of the event in an effort to align themselves with the goal to provide the service as fast as possible.

The last aspect of providing a service that is attractive to customers involves pricing. This is a double-edged sword, and one that cannot easily be defined as an adverse effect or benefit to either customer group. The following facts must first be acknowledged: (1) The community needs interpreters. The issue of civil rights has been one this country (the United States) and others have supported, sought, and even fought for on the battlefield, in the halls of government, and in the courts. (2) Interpreters must earn a living wage. In the absence of this, they will seek other avenues of support. (3) Conversely, many interpreters working with the most vulnerable in our society, our children, earn at or below a living wage and can be considered among our nation's working poor. This discipline within the interpreting field attracts recent graduates who are, by the nature of the market, willing to accept work at a lower wage in order to receive experience that will progress them up the economic ladder. (4) Hearing customers, required by law to provide communication accessibility and focused on profit ratios, in turn to satisfy their own stakeholders view the provision of interpreting services to a low-incidence population as an unnecessary expense. (5) Interpreter referral agencies also must be concerned about their stakeholders and cannot ignore a focus on profit. Fiscal decisions are made to increase profits by decreasing overhead, which often includes taking advantage of the aforementioned commodity phenomenon: utilizing interpreters with lower levels of education, credentials, and experience in order to increase profits.

Currently, the pricing issue is a priority relating only to the interaction and negotiation with the hearing consumer side of the triad. Deaf consumers frequently are directly and indirectly penalized because of the pricing structure established by independent interpreters and interpreter referral agencies. Services are denied, delayed, or substandard as a result of the decisions made related to the pricing of interpreting services. As mentioned previously, it is a double-edged sword. Interpreters and agencies must earn a living wage and have, heretofore, been defensive and hesitant in discussing issues of a reasonable rate with Deaf consumers who are, albeit often indirectly, affected by decisions made related to pricing.

The second dimension of customer service is the personal dimension. This personal dimension and attitudinal efforts are not intentionally reserved for the interaction with and between the interpreter and the Deaf consumer; it is more often than not the case. In dealing with hearing customers, the priority is ensuring the procedural dimension is satisfied not by design but by default. Herein is the issue: interpreters' focus has been on developing knowledge, skills, and abilities and professional development primarily in the area of performance skills, almost to the exclusion of attitudinal and behavioral skills. Subsequently, there is a dearth in knowledge of how to maximize and capitalize on these personal skills to enhance the relationships and benefits to all consumers.

As has been written many times, no one person possesses a monocultural background. Each person possesses primary and secondary cultural characteristics. Primary characteristics such as ethnicity and age cannot be altered, whereas secondary characteristics such as socioeconomic status and religion, although not casually changed, can be altered throughout the course of a person's life. Additionally, all are exposed to hereditary and environmental influences that mold and influence worldviews and affect communication events, especially interlingual communication. As can be seen, every person is a unique combination of primary and secondary cultural characteristics, which clearly challenges the traditional scope of considering people as either monocultural or even bicultural.

Based on the nature of deafness and its minority culture and language status, there may be a tendency for hearing people to treat Deaf people differently out of fear, ignorance, and/or prejudice. However, once exposed to the similarities and differences of culture, values, norms, and language discourses, hearing interpreters become more aware and better equipped to work and communicate with a rich, culturally and ethnically diverse consumer population. One of the significant contributors to this success is the ability to make a paradigm shift from having a monoculture/monolingual orientation to a multicultural/multilingual orientation. For this paradigm shift to happen, immersion in the new culture and ample time to absorb the cultural experience are paramount.

ASK is a model that can be used for this paradigm shift to occur. Applying the ASK structure of the pyramid of cultural relationships to daily interactions and activities to welcome and celebrate diversity allows one to become acculturated and on the way to becoming respected and accepted by a new cultural community.

References

Eighinger, L., & Karlin, B. (2001). *A feminist-relational approach: A social construct to event management*. Retrieved from http://www.signs-of-development.org/website/Letters.htm.

Eighinger, L. (2002). *Salary comparison matrix*. Retrieved from http://www.signs-of-development.org/Data/Salary.htm.

Padden, C., & Humphries, T. (1988). *Deaf in America: Voices from a culture*. Cambridge, MA: Harvard University Press.

LaBelle, T., & Ward, C. (1994). *Multiculturalism and education: Diversity and its impact on schools and society*. New York: State University of New York Press.

Lazorisak, C. (2000). *The pyramid model of multicultural relationships*. Retrieved from http://signs-of-development.org/Data/ASK.pdf.

Moll, L. (Ed.). (1990). *Vygotsky and education: Instructional implications and applications of sociohistorical psychology*. Cambridge, UK: Cambridge University Press.

Variation in Sign Languages: Methodological Issues and Research Findings

CEIL LUCAS, ROBERT BAYLEY, RUTH REED, ROB HOOPES, STEVEN COLLINS, AND KAREN PETRONIO

Sociolinguistic research on signed languages, although still in its infancy, has produced a considerable body of knowledge over the past twenty years, providing unique insight into the complex structures and uses of signed languages throughout the world. As with spoken languages, sociolinguistic inquiry has described and explained linguistic phenomena of signed languages that cannot be accounted for by formal linguistic inquiry. In particular, the variable use of linguistic forms (e.g., phonological, morphological, lexical, and syntactic variables) can seldom be fully explained without reference to social factors such as gender, age, and social class and without reference to the context of language use. In addition, sociolinguistic methodology is particularly suited to describing systematic differences between two or more varieties of a signed language.

In this essay, we examine the research issues and methodological choices that confront researchers who study sociolinguistic phenomena in signed languages by discussing the methodologies and findings of three recent studies of variation in American Sign Language (ASL): Hoopes' (1998) study of the complex patterning and linguistic functioning of pinky extension as it variably occurs within the lect of a single native signer; Collins and Petronio's (1998) study comparing and contrasting the Deaf-Blind variety of ASL with "standard" ASL; and Lucas, Bayley, and Valli's (2001) study of the distribution of phonological variables across sociolinguistic and geographic factors (sex, age, race, economic class, and geographic region in the United States). These studies vary markedly in their goals and methods and, therefore, help to illustrate the research issues and methodologies available for investigating sociolinguistic phenomena in signed languages.

An expanded version of this essay appears in Dively, et al. (2001) under the title "Analyzing Variation in Sign Languages: Theoretical and Methodological Issues."

Three Studies: Methods

Confirming a Variable: The Pinky Extension Study

The pinky extension (PE) study relies on data from a single individual's conversational signing to examine patterned variation in the PE variable (Hoopes 1998). Sociolinguistic variables do not vary only from one signer to another. The variation we see in ASL signing in Deaf communities does not result from one signer using one variant and another signer using a different variant. Rather, a single speaker/signer ordinarily uses two or more variants of a single variable, even within the same conversation. Signing with one's pinky extended on some signs has been anecdotally discussed as a possible phonological variable. Signs such as THINK, WONDER, and TOLERATE (the latter two illustrated in figure 1) can be signed either with the fourth finger closed or fully extended.

The goals of Hoopes' (1998) study were to determine whether PE showed patterned variation that correlated with phonological, syntactic, or discourse constraints

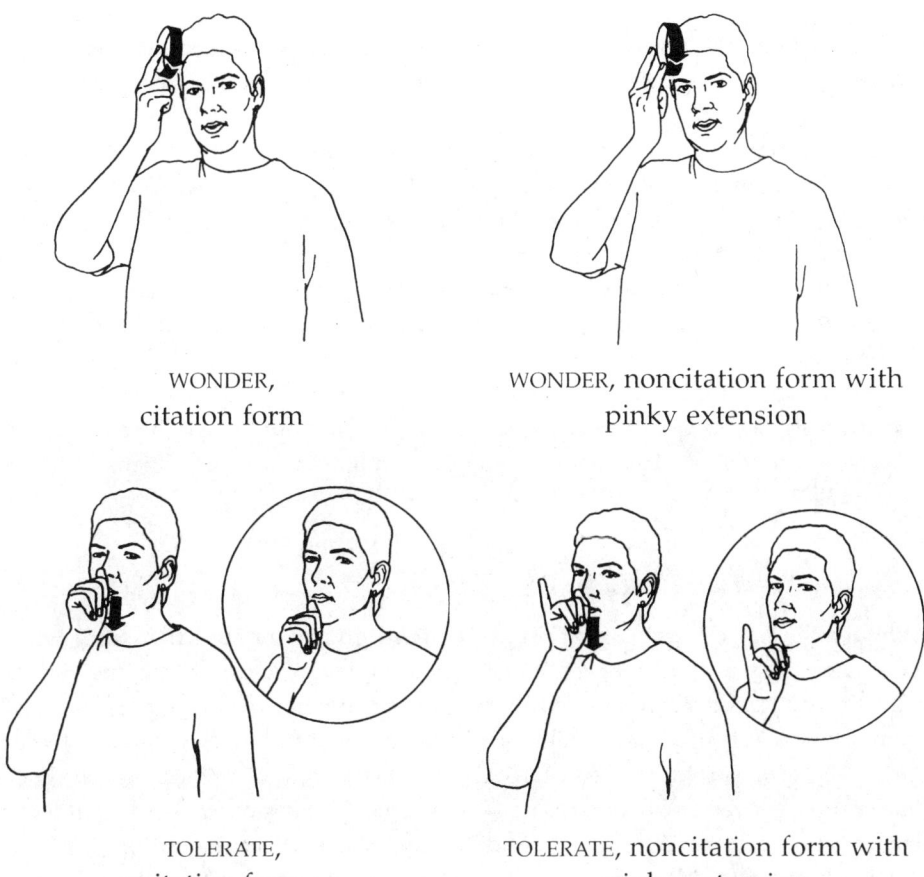

WONDER, citation form

WONDER, noncitation form with pinky extension

TOLERATE, citation form

TOLERATE, noncitation form with pinky extension

FIGURE 1. Citation and noncitation forms of WONDER and TOLERATE. Reproduced by permission from Dively et al. 2001, 148.

and to consider functional explanations for these correlations. The PE study set out to describe this potential variable as part of one individual's signing style and to discuss possible constraints on the individual's use of PE.

The signer for the PE study was a 55-year-old European American Deaf woman. She was deafened in infancy and was the only Deaf member of her immediate family. She attended a residential school and Gallaudet College. She was videotaped in conversation over four separate sessions, each one to two hours long, for a total of seven hours of conversational data. Her conversational partners varied in how well she knew them (one was a long-time friend, another a recent acquaintance) and in whether they were hearing or Deaf.

One hundred occurrences of PE were extracted from the videotaped data for analysis. Each of these occurrences was coded for the following linguistic and social factor groups: (1) preceding handshape, (2) following handshape in which PE occurs, (3) discourse topic, (4) handshape of PE sign, (5) syntactic category of the PE sign, (6) level of intimacy between informant and conversational partner.

Hoopes also coded a subset of these occurrences for prosodic features, which involved timing the duration of the tokens by the number of frames each lasted. These durations were averaged and compared with the duration of tokens of the same lexemes, without PE. The constraints that were investigated for this subset of tokens included the duration of the sign, whether there was a preceding or following pause, and repetition of the sign.

Some potential occurrences were excluded from the pool of PE tokens. Occurrences of PE in finger spelling were excluded because it was assumed that PE in these cases resulted from processes other than those that could cause PE in lexical signs. Also excluded were instances of "lexicalized" PE, in which case the non-PE variant and the PE variant would not co-occur in the signing of one individual. Lastly, signs in which PE did not occur over the full production of the sign were not included in the set of tokens.

The analysis of the full 100 tokens, not including the prosodic analysis, consisted of comparing percentages of tokens in each of the subgroupings of the constraints. In the prosodic analysis, Hoopes compared the average duration of the signs with and without PE.

Identifying Variables: The Tactile ASL Study

Although the ASL of sighted Deaf people has been studied for more than forty years, the signing of Deaf-Blind people is a new subject of linguistic research. In their study of Tactile ASL, Collins and Petronio (1998) set out to describe changes in signing that occur when ASL is used in a tactile rather than a visual mode. The goal was to describe the particular variety of ASL used in the Deaf-Blind community when Deaf-Blind people converse with other Deaf-Blind people. Collins and Petronio considered that variation between sighted ASL and Tactile ASL could occur at all levels of linguistic structure. In this level, however, we focus on phonological variation.

To collect representative samples of Deaf-Blind conversation, Collins and Petronio used two sets of conversational data, one more informal, one more formal. Informal data were collected at a party attended by eleven Deaf-Blind people. The more for-

TABLE 1. Questions Addressed by the Tactile ASL Study

Level of Linguistic Structure	Questions
Phonology	In Tactile ASL, the receiver's hand is placed on the signer's hand. Does this physical difference in the mode of communication result in changes in any of the sign parameters, handshape, movement, location, and orientation?
Morphology	Deaf-Blind people are unable to see the nonmanual adverbs and adjectives that accompany many lexical verbs and adjectives. How are these morphemes conveyed in Tactile ASL?
Syntax	Word order in questions in visual ASL varies. What word orders occur in questions in Tactile ASL?
Discourse	The back-channel feedback given by addressees in visual ASL is inaccessible to Deaf-Blind people. What type of back-channeling in Tactile ASL replaces the headnods, headtilts, and facial expressions of back-channeling in visual ASL?

mal data came from conversations between three pairs of Deaf-Blind people, all using Tactile ASL to tell stories to each other. The fourteen signers in the second data set had all been born deaf, knew and used ASL prior to becoming legally blind, became blind as a result of Usher Syndrome I, and regularly socialized with Deaf-Blind adults who used Tactile ASL. Tactile ASL can be received with one or both hands. To limit the possible variation that could occur even within Tactile ASL, only one-handed conversations were used to describe the variety.

Research questions specific to each level of linguistic structure were formulated. These questions are given in table 1. All of these questions are focused on describing differences between visual and tactile ASL. The videotaped conversations were examined for evidence of structures or strategies that do not occur in visual ASL.

Broad Quantitative Description: Sociolinguistic Variation in ASL

The goal of Lucas, Bayley, and Valli's 2001 study was to provide the basis for a description of phonological, morphosyntactic, and lexical variation in ASL. One of the variables, a set of three variants of the sign DEAF, is reported on here. The sign DEAF has many possible forms, but occurrences of only three of these forms were extracted from the videotapes. In citation form (+cf),[1] the sign begins just below the ear and ends near the corner of the mouth. A second variant begins at the corner of the mouth and moves upward to the ear. This variant is called the "chin-to-ear" variant. The third variant considered here, the "contact-cheek" variant, simply contacts the lower cheek. These variants were compared using a statistical program that requires many examples of the variation as input but that allows the researcher to investigate the effects of many potential constraints at the same time. In this section, we first discuss the benefits and requirements of this kind of quantitative analysis. Then, we describe

---

1. Citation form (+cf) is the form of a sign as it would appear in a sign language dictionary or as it might be taught in a sign language class. Noncitation form (–cf) is the form of a sign as it might occur in everyday conversation, a variant of the +cf form. Of course, citation forms occur in everyday conversation as well.

TABLE 2. Demographic Characteristics of Informants in Sociolinguistic Variation in the ASL Study

Race and Socio-economic status	African American		Euro-American	
	Middle Class	Working Class	Middle Class	Working Class
Age	15–25	15–25	15–25	15–25
	26–54	26–54	26–54	26–54
	55+	55+	55+	55+

how data were collected and how occurrences of the variants of DEAF were extracted from the videotaped data.

The goal of the quantitative study of language variation is to understand linguistic phenomena and their relationship to social structure. We want to be able to understand, for example, the direction of linguistic change or the relationship between the form and the syntactic function of a class of signs. We also want to be able to test hypotheses about the relationships between different linguistic and social constraints, to compare alternative analyses, and to create models that allow us to make predictions (Guy 1993, 235). Percentages of occurrence or nonoccurrence of particular variants cannot account for many possible simultaneous influences on variation, both linguistic and social. To accomplish the goals of the study, Lucas et al. needed to use statistical procedures that could model simultaneously relationships among the many contextual factors that promote or inhibit use of a particular variant. In linguistics, the programs known as VARBRUL have been used most extensively for this type of modeling because they have been deliberately designed to handle the kind of data obtained in studies of variation. They also provide heuristic tools, which allow the investigator to reanalyze the data easily as hypotheses are modified.[2]

Videotaped data for this study were collected during 1994 and 1995 at seven sites located in different regions of the United States: Boston, Massachusetts; Frederick, Maryland; Staunton, Virginia; New Orleans, Louisiana; Kansas City, Missouri/Olathe, Kansas; Fremont, California; and Bellingham, Washington. All sites have thriving communities of ASL users. Six groups of Deaf ASL signers, all white, participated in Staunton, Frederick, and Bellingham. Six white groups and five African American groups participated in Boston, Fremont, Kansas City/Olathe, and New Orleans. In total, 207 signers participated. Their social and demographic characteristics are summarized in table 2.

Working-class participants were defined as those whose education did not extend past high school and who were working in blue-collar jobs. Middle-class participants had completed college and were working in professional positions. The age group divisions were designed to correlate roughly with changes in the language policies

---

2. The statistical bases for the VARBRUL programs are set out in Sankoff (1988), and the procedures for using the software are explained in Young and Bayley (1996) and in the documentation that accompanies the programs. The present study used GoldVarb for the Macintosh (Rand and Sankoff 1990). Space does not permit a full explanation of the steps involved in a multivariate analysis with VARBRUL here. The topic is discussed in detail in the literature on the subject (e.g., Bayley 2002; Guy 1993; Sankoff 1988; Young and Bayley 1996).

TABLE 3. Coding Scheme for Linguistic Concerns on DEAF

Linguistic Constraint	Specific Location
Grammatical function of DEAF	noun
	adjective
	predicate adjective
	compund
Location of the preceding segment	high (at ear or above)
	middle (between ear and chin)
	low (chin or below)
	pause
Genre of text in which DEAF occurs	conversation
	narrative

in Deaf education over the past ninety years. Older participants had purely oral instruction, the middle group was in school during the period of Total Communication, and the younger participants began school at the beginning of the return to the use of ASL in the classroom.

The videotaped data collection sessions consisted of three parts: conversation, sociolinguistic interview, and lexical variation elicitation. All tokens of the three variants of DEAF, a total of 1,618 occurrences, were extracted from this videotaped database for coding for multivariate analysis. Each token was entered into the statistical database along with its values for social and linguistic factors. The social factors coded were the following: region, age (fifteen to twenty-five, twenty-six to fifty-four, older than fifty-five), gender, ethnicity (African America, white), class (working, middle), and language background (native ASL, other). The linguistic factors coded were designed to provide a follow-up to Lucas' (1995) study, which found that the grammatical function of the sign was the most significant constraint on the form of DEAF. Table 3 gives the coding scheme for the linguistic constraints.

Once coding was complete and the data were entered, VARBRUL estimated the factor values (or probabilities) for each contextual factor specified (e.g., the handshape of the preceding segment or the social class to which a signer belonged). The program provided a numerical measure of the strength of each factor's influence, relative to other factors in the same group, on the occurrence of the linguistic variable under investigation. VARBRUL factor values range between 0 and 1.00. A factor value, or weight, between .50 and 1.00 indicates that the factor favors use of a variant relative to other factors in the same group. For example, in the results reported in the following section, compounds (e.g., DEAF CULTURE), with a factor value of .66, favor use of –cf forms. A value between 0 and .50 indicates that the factor disfavors a variant. Thus, in the same results, predicate adjectives, with a factor value of .37, disfavor use of –cf forms of DEAF. The output also includes an input probability, a measure of the overall tendency of signers to use a particular variant. In the results, the input value for –cf forms of DEAF is .743. This value reflects the fact that –cf forms were far more common in the data than +cf forms. Of 1,618 tokens analyzed, 1,118, or 69 percent, were –cf. Finally, the program provides several measures of goodness of fit between the model and the data (see Young and Bayley 1996, 272–73).

These are the methodologies of the three studies, each designed with different goals in mind, though linked in the goal of describing variable linguistic structure as it is situated in the use of ASL in Deaf communities in the United States. Table 4 summarizes the goals and methodologies of the three studies.

Findings

This section summarizes the more important findings of the three studies that have provided the data for our discussion of the methods of variationist linguistics and their applications for signed languages. The details of the studies are available in Hoopes (1998), Collins and Petronio (1998) and Lucas, Bayley, and Valli (2001).

Pinky Extension

Hoopes (1998) analyzed the occurrence of a single phonological variable—PE—in the signing of a single individual. Prior to this study, it had been observed (by Lucas and others) that some signers extend their pinky during particular signs, contrary to the citation forms of these signs.

Hoopes sought to determine whether the occurrence of PE was indeed a variable and, if so, whether the frequency of occurrence correlated with any linguistic or social factors. One goal of sociolinguistic inquiry is to correlate social and economic factors (e.g., sex, age, race, education) with the frequency at which a variable occurs in a given signer's or speaker's language use. To accomplish this goal, tokens must be collected from language users in each sociolinguistic category under analysis. Why, then, would Hoopes undertake to study a single signer?

The primary reason is that this was a pilot study to determine if PE varied at all. Because our understanding of the structure of ASL is still emerging, it is often difficult at the outset of a sociolinguistic study to know whether the linguistic form under analysis is indeed variable. In this case, it was entirely possible that the occurrence of PE was subject to a categorical, as opposed to a variable, rule. Before a larger study was undertaken, it was necessary to determine if PE was in fact variable, and, if so, whether it could be correlated with any linguistic or social constraints.

The findings indicated that the frequency of occurrence of PE upon signs did, in fact, vary and that the frequency of occurrence correlated with linguistic factors (handshape and syntactic category) and the one social factor analyzed (degree of social distance). The most intriguing finding, however, was that PE tended to co-occur with prosodic features of emphatic stress. Specifically, it tended to occur (1) with lexemes used repeatedly within a discourse topic, (2) before pauses, and (3) with lexemes lengthened to almost twice their usual duration. This suggests that PE is itself a prosodic feature of ASL that adds emphatic stress or focus to the sign with which it co-occurs. It is quite analogous to stress in spoken language as indicated by a stronger signal as a result of greater articulatory effort.

It should be noted that sociolinguistic methodology was crucial to this last finding, that is, that PE played a prosodic function in the signer's lect. Prosody has largely been ignored by linguists working within the Chomskyan framework, with its tendency toward categoricity. Prosody tends not to be subject to categorical rules. However, as

TABLE 4. Summary of Goals and Methodologies of the Three Studies

Goals and Methods	Study 1 Pinky Extension (PE)	Study 2 Tactile ASL	Study 3 Sociolinguistic Variation in ASL
Research questions	Is PE a sociolinguistic variable? What linguistic constraints possibly condition PE?	How does Tactile ASL differ from visual ASL in its morphology, syntax, and discourse structure?	What are the linguistic and social factors that condition use of three variants of DEAF? Which of these constraints are strongest?
Informants	1 Deaf woman, an ASL user	14 Deaf-Blind ASL and Tactile ASL users	207 Deaf ASL users
Videotaping procedures	4 conversations lasting from 1 to 2 hours each	Conversations at a party lasting 4 hours (11 participants); Storytelling sessions (6 participants, paired)	Groups of 2 to 6 participants in three situations, Conversations in the group; Interview with the researcher; Responding to questions on lexical variants
Videotape analysis	Extracted 100 occurrences of PE. Compared timing of a subset of these occurrences with tokens of non-PE signs	Developed specific questions about linguistic structure. Extracted examples of each type of structure from conversations. Generalized over examples to a statement about variant structure.	Watched videotapes for signers using DEAF. Glossed each occurrence of DEAF with information about constraints in a text database.
Methods of analysis	Coded each instance of PE for linguistics and social constraints. Compared percentages of PE and non-PE in different environments. Compared prosodic features. Suggested constraints that may condition PE.	Compared structures in Tactile ASL with parallel structures in visual ASL.	Coded each token for linguistic and social constraints. Entered coded tokens into VARBRUL. Used VARBRUL probabilities to find relevant and irrelevant constraints. Suggested variable linguistic rules that are part of the grammar of ASL.

Hoopes' study shows, when one searches for factors that constrain but do not absolutely determine the occurrence of a linguistic form, the patterning of prosodic features emerges.

Tactile ASL

Collins and Petronio (1998) focused on differences and similarities in the phonological form of signs used in visual and Tactile ASL and examined handshape, location, movement, and orientation.

Early studies of visual ASL sought minimal pairs to determine the distinctive parts of signs. Minimal pairs were interpreted as providing evidence for three parameters: handshape, movement, and location. For instance, the signs DONKEY and HORSE use the same location and movement but differ in handshape; MOTHER and FATHER use the same handshape and movement but differ in location; and SICK and TO-BECOME-SICK use the same handshape and location but differ in movement. Battison (1978) later identified a fourth parameter, orientation, based on pairs such as CHILDREN and THINGS. These two signs have identical handshape, movement, and location. However, they differ in the palm orientation: the palm of the hand faces upward for THINGS but toward the floor for CHILDREN. Using these four parameters, signs in the Tactile ASL data were examined to see if there were any phonological differences between the tactile and visual versions of the same sign.

Collins and Petronio found that the handshape parameter was unaffected by whether the sign was in the tactile or visual mode. The other three parameters (movement, orientation, and location) displayed the same type of variation because of the phonological assimilation that occurs in visual ASL. However, although the same forms of variation occurred in Tactile ASL, this variation was sometimes due to (1) the receiver's hand being on the signer's hand and (2) the necessary physical proximity of the tactile signer and receiver. As a result of the physical closeness, the Tactile ASL signing space was generally smaller than that used in visual ASL. This smaller space usually results in smaller movement paths in signs. In addition, because the signer's and receiver's hands are in contact, the signing space shifted to the area where the hands were in contact; correspondingly, the location of signs articulated in neutral space also shifted to this area. The orientation parameter showed some variation that resulted from modifications the signer made to better accommodate the receiver. One change, unique to Tactile ASL, occurred with signs that include body contact. In addition to the signer's hand moving toward the body part, the body part often moved toward the hand in Tactile ASL. This adaptation allowed the receiver to maintain more conformable tactile contact with the signer.

The variation, adaptations, and changes that Collins and Petronio describe are examples of linguistic change that has occurred and is continuing in the U.S. Deaf-Blind community. In the past several years, in addition to an expansion of the American Association of the Deaf-Blind, many state chapters of this organization have grown in membership. Deaf-Blind people are increasing their contact with other Deaf-Blind people. The opportunity for Deaf-Blind people to get together and form communities has resulted in sociolinguistic changes in ASL as Deaf-Blind people modify the language to meet their needs. From a linguistic viewpoint, Tactile ASL provides us with a unique opportunity to witness the linguistic changes ASL is undergoing as the Deaf-Blind community adapts the language to a tactile mode.

Variation in the Form of DEAF

Lucas, Nayley, and Valli's 2001 study focused on a number of sociolinguistic variables, among them variation in the form of the sign DEAF (fig. 2). To examine the constraints on this variable, the researchers performed multivariate analysis of 1,618 tokens using VARBRUL. The results indicated that variation in the form of DEAF is systematic and conditioned by multiple linguistic and social factors, including grammatical function, the location of the following segment, discourse genre, signer's age, and signer's region. The results strongly confirmed the earlier finding of Lucas (1995), which showed that the grammatical function of DEAF, rather than the features of the preceding or following sign, is the main linguistic constraint on variation (see Lucas and Bayley 2005 for more detailed discussion). In this section, we focus on the role of the grammatical category because the results for this factor suggest that variation in ASL operates at a much more abstract level than has previously been documented. We also briefly review the main results for age and geographical region.

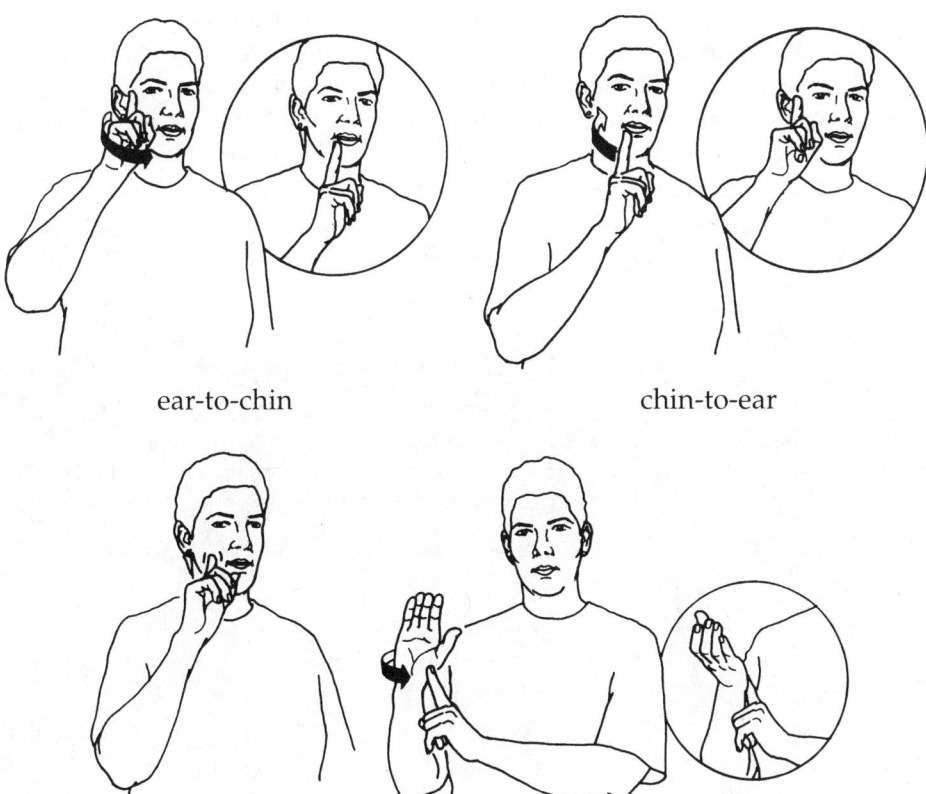

FIGURE 2. The three variants of DEAF analyzed in the sociolinguistic variation study. Reprinted by permission from Dively et al. 2001, 151.

Lucas, Bayley, and Valli examined three separate variants of DEAF: the citation form, the chin-to-ear variant, and the contact-cheek variant. Although the three variants might logically be related to one another in a number of different ways, on the basis of what is known about the history of ASL as well as observations of processes governing ASL compound formation (see Lucas, Bayley, and Valli 2001 for details), the researchers in this study hypothesized that the variants were related to one another as follows: the citation or underlying form is ear-to-chin. In the first stage, this form variably undergoes metathesis and surfaces as chin-to-ear. In the second stage, the metathesized form undergoes deletion of the first element and surfaces as contact-cheek, a process that is especially common in compounds (e.g., DEAF^CULTURE). This model of the processes underlying variation in the form of DEAF necessitated two separate quantitative analyses: 1) + cf versus –cf, including both chin-to-ear and contact-cheek; 2) chin-to-ear versus contact-cheek. Note that citation forms were eliminated from the second analysis because only forms that have undergone metathesis are eligible for deletion of the first element.

The results of both analyses for the grammatical category factor group are shown in table 5. For each analysis, the table includes the following information: the application value, or value of the dependent variable at which the "rule" is said to apply, the VARBRUL weight or factor value, the percentage of "rule" applications, and the number of tokens of each factor. The table also includes the input value, the overall percentage of application, and the number of tokens in each analysis.

The results of the first analysis show that compounds favor (p = .66) and predicate adjectives disfavor –cf (p = .37). Nouns and adjectives, the majority of tokens, are close to .50 and form the neutral reference point (p = .515). The results of the second analysis, which excluded +cf tokens, show that compounds very strongly favor one –cf variant, contact-cheek (p = .85). The results also show that adjectives and predicate adjectives that have undergone metathesis are unlikely to undergo deletion. Finally, as in the first analysis of +cf versus –cf, the value for nouns (p = .49) is close to .50, which again serves as the neutral reference point.

TABLE 5. Influence of Grammatical Category on Choice of a Form of DEAF

Analysis	Factor	VARBRUL weight	%	N
Analysis 1: +cf vs. –cf (application value: –cf)	Noun, adj.	.515	71	1063
	Predicate adj.	.370	58	361
	Compound	.660	81	194
	TOTAL/input	.743	69	1618
Analysis 2: chin-to-ear vs. contact-cheek (application vakyeL cibtact-cheek)	Noun	.490	17	411
	Adjective	.403	10	191
	Predicate adj.	.338	12	299
	Compound	.850	56	151
	TOTAL/input	.142	20	1052

An obvious question arises as the interpretation of these results. Why should the grammatical category to which DEAF belongs have such a large effect on signers' choices among the three variants, whereas other factors, such as the location of the following segment, have no significant effect? One possibility is that the grammatical constraints are a synchronic reflex of a change in progress that originates in compounds and then spreads to nouns and adjectives and finally to predicates. A change from ear-to-chin to chin-to-ear, beginning with compounds, a grammatical class that is most subject to change, is arguably a shift in the direction of greater ease of production. Such a change would conform to Kroch's (1978) model of change from below, which, at least in the case of consonants, tends to greater ease of articulation. This explanation is supported by the fact that there exist a number of ASL signs that move from chin-to-ear in their citation form. Only two of these, however, clearly allow metathesis. They are HEAD and MOTHER^FATHER ("parents").[3] Metathesis is not allowed by other common signs with a phonological structure like DEAF, consisting of a hold, a movement, and a hold (e.g., INDAN, HOME, YESTERDAY). The fact that metathesis is not allowed by most signs whose citation form is chin-to-ear (i.e., signs that move up) while it is allowed by DEAF (where the citation form moves down) suggests that chin-to-ear movement is the less marked sequence. DEAF, then, may be undergoing a change from a more marked to a less marked form, which is characterized by greater ease of production.

As we have noted, in addition to identifying significant linguistic constraints on DEAF, Lucas, Bayley, and Valli also found significant social and geographic constraints. Although social class, gender, and language background proved not to be statistically significant, both age and region were highly significant. In conducting their analyses, Lucas, Bayley, and Valli considered each age group within a region as a separate factor to investigate whether ASL was changing in the same way across the country or whether the direction of change differed from region to region. The results showed interregional differences, which the researchers suspect are related to changes in deaf education policies in particular areas and to the complex relationships of residential schools to one another. However, in the analysis of +cf versus –cf forms of DEAF, one dominant pattern emerged, which was shared by four sites: Virginia, Louisiana, California, and Washington state. In each of these sites, both the youngest and the oldest signers were more likely to use –cf forms of DEAF than signers aged twenty-six to fifty-five. This dominant pattern is illustrated in figure 3.

To sum up, Lucas, Bayley, and Valli have shown that variation in the form of DEAF, like variation in spoken language forms, is constrained by multiple linguistic and social factors. Although much remains to be done, particularly in understanding the complex relationship of age and region to signers' choice of a variant of DEAF, the study illustrates the contribution that variationist linguistics can make to sign language research.

Conclusions

The methodologies and findings from the three distinct studies described here demonstrate the range of variation within a signed language and the diversity of approaches

---

3. There is some question as to whether HOME permits metathesis. Liddell and Johnson (1989) claim that it does, but there is disagreement among Deaf informants whether it does.

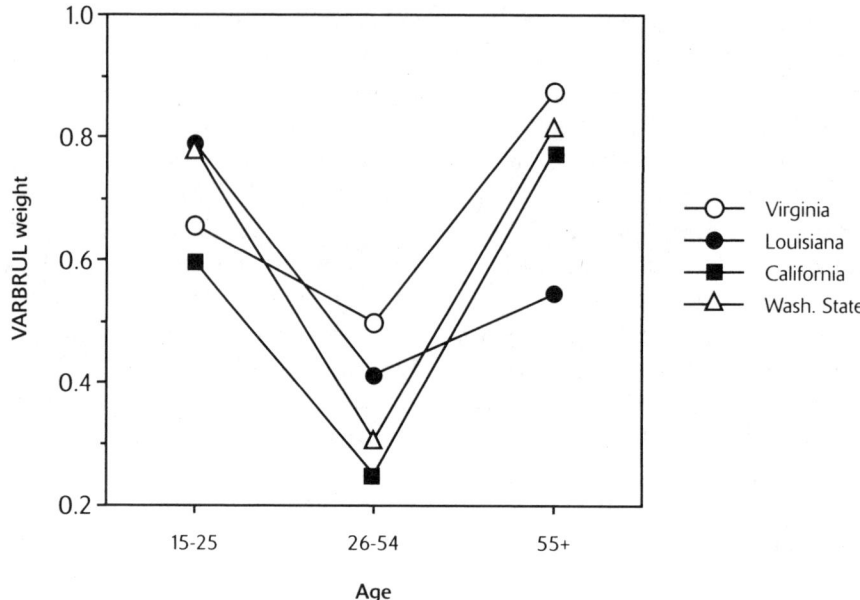

FIGURE 3. The dominant pattern of VARBRUL factor values for noncitation forms of DEAF by age and region

available for studying this variation. Systematic variation is characteristic of all natural languages. Studies such as those discussed here provide additional evidence that signed languages function in the same way as all human languages. At the same time, studies of variation in signed language illustrate the contributions research in signed languages can make to our understanding of the basic properties of all languages, whether spoken or signed. Finally, studies such as those described here demonstrate that variation is not a result of a signer's mistakes, or "lazy signing." Rather, it is an inherent property of the language itself. Just as there is more than one way to be Deaf, there is more than one way to sign DEAF.

References

Battison, Robbin. 1978. *Lexical borrowing in American Sign Language: Phonological and morphological restricting*. Silver Spring, Md.: Linstok Press.

Bayley, Robert. 2002. The quantitative paradigm. In *The handbook of language variation and change*, ed. J. K. Chambers, Peter Trudgill, and Natalie Schilling-Estes, 117–41. Oxford: Blackwell.

Collins, Steven, and Karen Petronio. 1998. What happens in Tactile ASL? In *Pinky extension and eye gaze: Language use in Deaf communities*, ed. Ceil Lucas, 18–37. Washington, DC: Gallaudet University Press.

Dively, Valerie, Melanie Metzger, Sarah Taub, and Anne Marie Baer, eds. 2001. *Signed languages: Discoveries from international research*. Washington, DC: Gallaudet University Press.

Guy, Gregory R. 1993. The quantitative analysis of linguistic variation. In *American dialect research*, ed. Dennis R. Preston, 223–24. Amsterdam: John Benjamins.

Hoopes, Rob. 1998. A preliminary examination of pinky extension: Suggestions regarding its occurrence, constraints, and function. In *Pinky extension and eye gaze: Language use in Deaf communities*, ed. Ceil Lucas, 3–17. Washington, DC: Gallaudet University Press.

Kroch, Anthony. 1978. Toward a theory of social dialect variation. *Language in Society* 7: 17–36.
Liddell, Scott K., and Robert E. Johnson. 1989. American Sign Language: The phonological base. *Sign Language Studies* 64: 195–278.
Lucas, Ceil. 1995. Sociolinguistic variation in ASL: The case of DEAF. *Sociolinguistics in Deaf communities*, ed. Ceil Lucas, 3–25. Washington, DC: Gallaudet University Press.
Lucas, Ceil, and Robert Bayley. 2005. Variation in ASL: The role of grammatical function. *Sign Language Studies* 6: 38–75.
Lucas, Ceil, Robert Bayley, and Ceil Valli. 2001. *Sociolinguistic variation in American Sign Language*. Washington, DC: Gallaudet University Press.
Rand, David, and David Sankoff. 1990. *GoldVarb: A variable rule application for the Macintosh (version 2)*. Montreal: Centre de recherches mathématiques, Université de Montréal.
Sankoff, D. 1988. Variable rules. In *Sociolinguistics: An international handbook of the science of language and society*, vol. 2, ed. Ulrich Ammon, Norbert Dittmar, and Klaus J. Mattheier, 984–97. Berlin: Mouton de Gruyter.
Young, Richard, and Robert Bayley. 1996. VARBRUL analysis for second language acquisition research. In *Second language acquisition and linguistic variation*, ed. Robert Bayley and Dennis R. Preston, 253–306. Amsterdam: John Benjamins.

Linguistic Development and Deaf Identity in Rural Rio Grande do Sul, Brazil

RICARDO VIANNA MARTINS

I present results that come from a series of interventions we did that began in 1999 in an area of villages where the population varies between twenty-five thousand and thirty thousand inhabitants. The main goal of those projects was to improve deaf people's knowledge of the Brazilian Sign Language (LIBRAS) in these small country villages. Even though they are not far from the capital (between thirty and sixty miles), deaf people there have almost no sign language.

We found deaf students in those villages with many years of schooling who are still illiterates. Many of them did not even know how to sign their entire name. Often they are not in school but in APAE (institutes for mentally handicapped people).

Like the students, the teachers had the same level of LIBRAS—almost nothing. Those teachers do not realize the subjective, social, and the cultural meaning of sign language for deaf people.

The teachers are aware of their lack of training and its impact on their development and the future perspectives of their pedagogic work. For many of these teachers, for example, the last unique courses they had were in the eighties. In those towns where deaf people are not numerous, many deaf people do not discern between deaf and hearing people. They are not in a position that permits them to reject, accept, or negotiate with their rights to drive, drink, have a boyfriend (if the deaf person is a girl, the control is harder), and have children (sterilization is in mind of some mothers who do not "want to have a grandchild with the same problem").

In those towns, because they have no language, deaf people are put in an asymmetric and inferior position to negotiate their rights and desires with their family, the school, and the community in generally. Without a sign language, deaf people of smaller villages do not have any chance of getting out of this cycle of dependency: they are outside both a deaf and hearing community.

Any person, deaf or hearing, accesses a human community through language. His or her constitution is made of symbols, most of them words. In an identification process, if there are no symbols, and particularly words, there is no subject. The person is actually empty. He or she is not actually there.

The Beginning

Our study is actually a series of projects. It started in Charqueadas (a village with 28,000 inhabitants, forty miles out of Porto Alegre) in 1999 with a project named "Deafness: Education and Citizenship" that had a concept of bilingual education.

Even if we conceptualize sign language as a "natural" language, it is not available for deaf people without instruction, which would also happen with acoustic languages for hearing people. Everyone, to acquire language, needs to learn from other speakers. That is why it takes a deaf adult, who usually learn LIBRAS in a city, to break a long cycle of alienation from language by introducing LIBRAS. That is why our first step was to hire a deaf teacher.

The alienation goes far beyond the language. In a family, according to Goldfeld (1997), because they usually do not know how to sign, the interaction of family members and deaf children is reduced to a minimum.

The interaction between children and a deaf teacher will not only make possible the students' language development but also increase the teachers' abilities in LIBRAS, who usually receive only a few notions of sign language. An intense and constant contact with LIBRAS permits students and teachers to share some knowledge. Otherwise, we see poor relationships between students and teachers.

The presence of a deaf teacher comes also to subvert, to a great extent, the stereotype of deafness, which is very close to a mental handicap. Deaf people are usually treated as disabled and dependent with no job opportunities or opportunities for jobs that require no skills. A deaf teacher opens a new perspective never dreamed of by these people. It is possible for them to drive, go to a university, travel, have a family, and have autonomy.

Visiting the villages around Charqueadas, we found the same conditions. Then we started to propose to them our pilot project, now with an extra goal: create a network between those villages. At the same time that we improved the sign language for deaf people and their teachers, we also did workshops to discuss and give goals for deaf education. Putting all these people in contact, promoting same cultural activities (parties, meetings, and travel), created an unexpected synergy between deaf people that helped them to acquire LIBRAS quickly. Once the students have learned a new word or concept, they immediately transmit it to the others and to their teacher in a dynamic that was not limited to a classroom.

This project, like other bilingual projects in Latin America that work with Spanish and native languages (López, 1997), is possible in the long run. The maturity of these kinds of projects arrives after years of hard work, after native speakers become teachers, when they arrive in a sociolinguistic reflection of the situation they share. This kind of task means not only to teach a language, but also to essentially change the minds of the people charged with education, which is often the hardest part of the work.

The Project

In synthesis, the project has the following characteristics:

1. Immediate goal: the dissemination of LIBRAS in the villages close to Porto Alegre.

2. Motive: the small numbers of deaf people in these communities who do not travel, have contact with other deaf people, or have any autonomy because they lack a language.
3. Methodology: the backbone of our project is the deaf teacher. The deaf teacher will effectively transmit the sign language to the deaf students. Once the students acquire a language, it does not leave them and it will be easier to transmit it to a community (family, hearing teachers, friends). The teacher's presence, as we said before, will give a new perspective to the students.
4. Evaluation: we will use "Instrumento de Avaliação de proficiência da LSB" (IAPLSB) (Quadros, 2000) to evaluate the linguistic development over the course of a year where the students have contact with a deaf teacher two days per week.

Evaluation involves showing a short film to a student, two or three times, and immediately asking the student to retell the story. We film that narrative and then evaluate four points: The use of space referents, the use of verbal concordance, the use of classifiers (adjectives), and the use of nonmanual expressions (such as facial expressions).

The linguistic development process starts with the first contacts with the deaf teacher. Crain and Lillo-Martin (1999) claim that there are no significant differences between learning an oral language and learning a sign language. In their universal grammar hypothesis, these authors point out that the form and the time of acquisition are the same for a wide variety of languages around the globe, including sign languages.

The interest in linguistic evaluation is to bring objective data, which are always more economical and punctual. Then we do not have only an impression, which is too subjective, but useful information that can be easily used and comprehended. Besides, we know that in deaf education matters we have almost no data, and certainly none for the countryside.

Primarily Results

The final report of this project must be done in July 2002. We are now doing the latest linguistic evaluation and interviews. Based on preliminary results of IAPLSB, we can objectively say that at the beginning of the project (April and May 2001) students had low average scores (0–0.27) for their use of space referents, verbal concordance, classifiers (adjectives), and nonmanual expressions, on a scale of 0, no use, and 1, skilful use. That means that the students had no knowledge of LIBRAS. They were communicating only by mimicking, not with a sign language.

On the other hand, students in Charqueadas, which has had a deaf teacher since the beginning of 1999, averaged 0.86 in textual production. (See table 1.)

Specifically, in Charqueadas, where we did the closest and more extensive work, we observed significant changes in body attitude, facial expression, and social attitude. Students went from apathy to participation, from inaccessibility to approachability, from loneliness to companionship. These changes were due to a presence of a deaf teacher. More than teaching LIBRAS, he gave them the possibility of new

TABLE 1 Average and Standard Deviation of IAPLSB

Town	No. students	Average	Standard Deviation
1 Charqueadas	4	0.86	0.14
2 B	12	0.27	0.25
3 C	6	0.25	0.16
4 D	6	0.00	0.00
5 E	6	0.29	0.29
6 F	14	0.14	0.16

Data obtained between April and May 2001.
All the students are more than twelve years old.

options for interaction and, essentially, new possibilities of identification (symbolic and imaginary).

To conclude, having a language, such as sign language, will permit deaf students to allow them to be a master not just a slave of a sign.

References

Crain, S., & Lillo-Martin, D. (1999). *An introduction to linguistic theory and language acquisition.* Oxford, MA: Blackwell.
Goldfeld, M. (1997). *A Criança surda.* São Paulo: Plexus.
López, L. E. (1997, April). La diversidad étnica, cultural y lingüística latinoamericana y los recurso humanos que la educacíon requiere. *Revista Iberoamericana de Educación.* Retrieved on August 22, 2006, from http://www.oei.org.co/oeivirt/rie13a03.htm
Quadros, R. (1997). *Educação de surdos—a aquisição da linguagem.* Porto Alegre: Artes Médicas.
———. (2001). Instrumento de avaliação de proficiência da LSB. *Relatório final técnico-científico.* Bolsa recém-doutor, UFRGS, Pós-Graduação em Educação.

The Role of the U.S. Court Interpreter in the New Millennium

CARLA M. MATHERS

In some quarters of this country, there is a movement afoot to create a monolingual society through the establishment of English-only statutes. Nevertheless, the United States boasts a long history of respecting the multilingual needs of litigants by providing language interpreters in legal cases. Many of the law cases reported in the United States suffer from challenges to the interpretation, or lack thereof, of non-English speaking litigants who use spoken-language interpreters. Deaf litigants can benefit from these decisions by analogy, though in certain cases, Deaf litigants have more rights to language access than do non-English-speaking litigants. For example, the Americans with Disabilities Act provides Deaf Americans with the right to reasonable accommodations in diverse spheres of the legal system that are not, at the time of this writing, in effect on behalf of non-English-speaking litigants.

In the criminal law arena, the rights to language access for both Deaf and other non-English speakers are more ingrained and established than in the pursuit of private disputes brought before the civil legal system. In the criminal justice system, the state has brought its considerable power to focus upon an individual with the result that one's liberty can be lost. As a check on the tremendous power of the state, the framers of the Constitution devised the Bill of Rights to protect the individual liberties of citizens from abuse by the ubiquitous power of the state. The state, by virtue of having the means to strip citizens of their life and liberty, is constrained by the concepts in the first ten amendments to ensure circumspection in the exercise of its weighty power.

The Sixth Amendment guarantees that a trial will be conducted fairly to the accused. The amendment is designed to counteract the power disparity between the resources of the government and the vulnerability of the individual. The Sixth Amendment reads: "In all criminal prosecutions, the accused shall enjoy the right to a speedy and public trial, to be informed of the nature and cause of the accusation, to be confronted with the witnesses against him, to have compulsory process for obtaining witnesses in his favor, and to have assistance of counsel for his defense."[1]

---

1. Amendment VI, U.S. Constitution.

United States ex rel. Negron v. New York[2] is the seminal case applying the Sixth Amendment to the context of a non-English-speaking defendant. In that case, Mr. Negron sat through his prosecution for murder without the benefit of language interpretation. The Confrontation Clause of the Sixth Amendment provides that the defendant has a right to be confronted with the witnesses against him. As a result, though physically present, Mr. Negron was not linguistically present and unable to confront the English-speaking witnesses against him.

In addition to Mr. Negron's confrontation rights being violated, it is arguable that other important constitutional rights such as his right to effective assistance of counsel, to be present at trial, to due process, and to equal protection were compromised because of the lack of meaningful access to the proceedings. The *Negron* court eloquently explained Mr. Negron's dilemma as "as a matter of simple humaneness, Negron deserved more than to sit in total incomprehension as the trial proceeded. . . . Particularly inappropriate in this nation where many languages are spoken is a callousness to the crippling language handicap of a newcomer to its shores, whose life and freedom the state by its criminal processes chooses to put in jeopardy."[3] In *U.S. v. Carrion*,[4] the duty to provide an interpreter was insightfully described as "the right to an interpreter rests most fundamentally, however, on the notion that no defendant should face the Kafkaesque specter of an incomprehensible ritual which may terminate in punishment." Indeed, the *Negron* court likened the trial without an interpreter to an "adjudication [that] loses its character as a reasoned interaction . . . and becomes an invective against an insensible object."[5]

With the right to an interpreter being solidly placed upon constitutional grounding, courts began to refine the contours of the number, type, and duties of the court interpreter. One of the earliest commentaries on court interpreters divided the roles for spoken-language interpreters into three functions. According to Chang and Araujo, an interpreter may work with a non-English-speaking witness to perform the function of *witness* interpreting; an interpreter may translate communications between a non-English-speaking party and a client to perform the function of *party* interpreting (also called defense interpreting); and an interpreter may translate the proceedings and discussion by the judge, opposing counsel, or others for a party during the proceeding to perform the function of *proceedings* interpreting (Chang & Araujo, 1975).

If one followed this theoretical model, in any case in which there were non-English-speaking parties and witnesses, there would be at least three interpreters corresponding to each function. In reality, at least in the spoken-language interpreting context, one interpreter (or one team of interpreters) sits at counsel table with the party and the client and performs the functions of the proceedings and the party interpreting. A second interpreter (or set of interpreters if they are to work in teams) is brought in only to perform witness interpreting for non-English-speaking witnesses.

The logic is not complicated. According to the foremost treatise on federal practice and procedure, two interpreters are necessary because of the constitutional

---

2. 434 F.2d 386 (2nd Cir. 1970).
3. *Negron*, 434 F.2d at 390.
4. 488 F.2d 12, 14 (1st Cir. 1970).
5. *Negron*, 434 F.2d at 389.

underpinnings involved in a criminal trial (Wright & Miller, 2001). Wright and Miller clarify,

> During the time an interpreter is translating questions and witness testimony, she cannot translate attorney-client communications or the proceedings. Of course, the interruption in party or proceeding translation might be brief and could be at least partially remedied after the testimony is completed. But the importance of the policies at stake is said to require uninterrupted service. Similar thinking lies behind other state court decisions on two related points. Thus several courts have held that a proceedings interpreter must be appointed even though defense counsel has the language ability to translate the proceedings for his client. Other decisions conclude that separate party interpreters must be appointed where there is more than one defendant.[6]

Sign-language interpreters also perform the functions of party interpreting, proceedings interpreting, and witness interpreting. Likewise, sign-language interpreters only provide two (or two teams if the interpreters are working together) of interpreters to perform the three functions. Unlike spoken-language interpreters, who collapse the function of proceedings interpreting and party interpreting, sign-language interpreters collapse the function of proceedings interpreting and witness interpreting. A second interpreter is retained to sit at counsel table and interpret private conversations between the deaf client and the attorney. In addition, the table interpreter interprets all of the pretrial attorney-client conversations in the law office. The table interpreter functions in the capacity as a resource to the team on interpretation issues: she is involved in the case to that extent.

There are two major rationales for this division of labor: First of all, as a matter of simple physical placement, sign-language interpreters stand in the well of the courtroom facing the deaf party or facing the deaf witness. Spoken-language interpreters whisper interpret from the table where the non-English speaker is seated or stand unobtrusively next to a non-English-speaking witness on the witness stand. Hence, it is a matter of physical ease for the spoken-language interpreter to alternate between the party and the proceedings functions. As long as no non-English-speaking witnesses are present, there is no disruption to the proceedings. If a non-English-speaking witness is present, a second interpreter team is retained.

In the case of sign-language interpreters, when counsel does not sign and seeks to speak privately with the deaf client during a proceeding, it is disruptive to have the interpreter leave the well area of the courtroom or leave the witness-interpreting role and huddle at the table for a private conference. Some cases permit the defendant to unilaterally stop the proceedings and call the interpreter over for the private conference with counsel. This is known as *borrowing the interpreter* to perform the function of party interpreting. However, at least one state has said this violates the defendant's constitutional rights because it may inhibit the person's ability to speak with counsel. The deaf person might feel like he or she is disrupting the proceedings by unilaterally interrupting the proceedings for a conference. There is a fear that the

---

6. *Ibid.*

judge or the jury will view this behavior as obstructionist. This arrangement presents a situation in which the defendant's ability to exercise his or her Sixth Amendment right to counsel may be chilled.

The same result holds true when the there is a codefendant case and the codefendants are forced to share an interpreter for the proceedings and for private conversations. A feeling of mistrust in seeing the interpreter that the defendant has used for private conversations now interpret private conversations with a codefendant or other hostile party might very well chill the defendant's ability to consult with counsel, thereby infringing on his or her constitutional rights.

These measures are highly controversial and not the standard practice at the time of this writing, though as more and more interpreters become educated, the bar becomes educated as well. There is a move to raise the standard of practice from what might be considered constitutionally borderline to that of best practices. Best practices dictate that defendants should not feel as if their comments will be relayed through the same mechanism that the adverse party's are channeled. Interpreters play a large part in this education process. As a result of conferences that bring together sign-language court interpreters, conferences nationally and internationally that bring together deaf community members, and conferences that bring together members of the bar, this education process has begun and will continue. The result, in the long run, will be a more equitable legal system for the people of the community who rely upon sign language interpreters for access to justice.

References

Chang, W. B. C., & Araujo, M. U. (1975). Interpreters for the defense: Due process for the non-English speaking defendant. *California Law Review* 63, 801–823.

U.S. v. Carrion, 488 F.2d 12, 14 (1st Cir. 1970).

United States ex rel. Negron v. New York, 434 F.2d 386 (2nd Cir. 1970).

Wright, C. A., & Miller, A. (2001). *Federal practice and procedure: Evidence* § 6056. (Eagen, MN: West Group Minnesota.

Narratives in Tactile Sign Language

JOHANNA MESCH

In visual signing, eye gaze movement and head movement are used as perspective markers. However, many people who have Usher syndrome 1 use tactile sign language. What do they do when they describe something without nonmanual marking of perspective? For example, a deaf-blind signer describes a skiing trip involving three people. The signer does not use gaze directions or head movements for each person in the narrative. Will the signer use only hand movements for marking of perspective so the deaf-blind receiver gets a good idea of what happened in the story?

About Tactile Conversation

The material for this study consists of two videotaped dyads from my earlier research on deaf-blind conversations (Mesch 1998, 2001). The participants were born deaf or became deaf at an early age and experienced deteriorating vision as they got older. They use Swedish Sign Language as their first language, although in tactile mode they communicate by touching each other's hands.

Hand positions in the conversations between two deaf-blind signers are used in monologue position or dialogue position (Mesch 1998, 2001). Monologue position is where A executes signs with both hands under B's hands. In dialogue position, A and B both have their hands in different places in contact with each other. A has his right hand under B's left hand and his left hand on top of B's right hand.

In the conversations between deaf-blind people, the position chosen is the one that is best suited to the situation: monologue or dialogue position. Monologue position is usually used in situations involving an interpreter but also in conversations between deaf-blind people where one conversational partner is the receiver for most of the time. Dialogue position is used most often in everyday conversations between deaf-blind people (fig. 1). A receiver can also use one hand during a signer's narrative (his other hand is in rest position but can use it to help understand some signs if it is needed for receiving these signs). Some examples, which are from conversations in dialogue position, are given later.

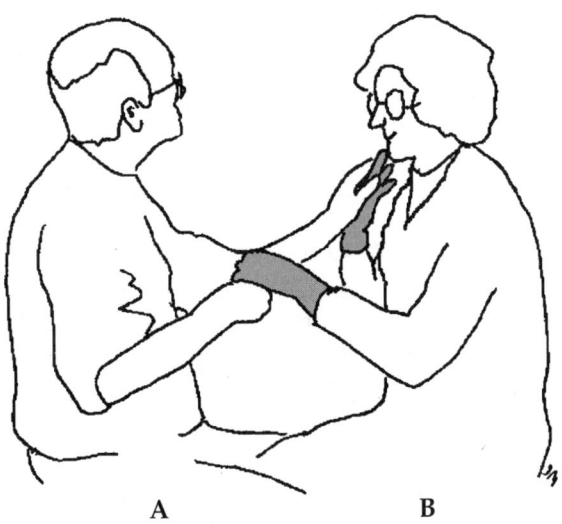

FIGURE 1. Dialogue position

Reference in Narratives

In visual sign language, the signers usually have a rich reference system, for example, topographic and representational spaces (see, for example, Bahan and Supalla 1995). Signing space is used for the perspective markers referring to people or things in a narrative. A signer may use different locations/directions in signing space to represent referents, that is, use different loci (cf. Engberg-Pedersen 1993). A change of perspective from the narrator to another person is reflected through noun phrases and motion and location verbs (Ahlgren and Bergman 1994, about Swedish Sign Language). Bahan and Supalla (1995) show the role of eye gaze as one of the nonmanual behaviors in an ASL narrative. These include a change in eye gaze, a pause, a blink, or a head nod.

Introducing Topics

Everyday conversations, in the conversations of deaf-blind people as well, are often completely unplanned, and the topics of conversation vary from one conversation to the next but also within the conversation. Deaf-blind people introduce topics and give accounts of their own experiences to each other by using different perspectives. Topics can include their own experiences or those of other people.

In example 1, the signer requests feedback by executing the sign CONGRESS at the beginning of the utterance with an extended duration. Acceptance of a topic is needed from a receiver. After feedback from the receiver, the signer continues with the topic.

Example 1
{
   A   FIRST WORLD CONGRESS-dur(.) (b:YES-tap) CONFERENCE
          DEAF-BLIND KNOW DEAF/BLIND FROM BELGIUM BELGIUM
          B-E-L-G-I-U-M

B BELGIUM Y-E-S
A AGREE, TACTILE-SIGN-LANGUAGE NOT
A The first world congress (b:yes) conference, for deaf-blind people. You know? There was a deaf-blind person from Belgium B-e-l-g-i-u-m.
B Belgium yes.
A That's right. He didn't use tactile sign language.

Establishing a topic in a narrative entails presenting a background with some lexical signs for referents. This introductory procedure helps a deaf-blind receiver know what a signer is talking about and where the referents are located as WE-TWO-r in example 2. A signer can also initiate a topic through a question, as in example 2.

Example 2
B WHAT PERF (.) WHAT DURING EASTER INDEX-adr-dur
A INDEX-c YES POSS-c GRANDMA WE-TWO-r CAR TO
D-U-R-A-S-A-S (B:YES) BEFORE LUNCH TELEPHONE
THERE-fl CHECK EXIST ENOUGH SNOW . . .
B What did you do for Easter?
A My grandma and I drove to Durasas (b:YES). Before lunch we called there to check if there was enough snow . . .

The use of constructed dialogues, which can include thoughts, appears in narratives. Deaf-blind narrators use signs for the referents instead of pronominal pointings and determiner nominal phrase. Some of these signs have the locus markers.

Signers first use some signs for the participant or spelling for new information. They will refer to them by signing noun phrases for one referent or two/three referents and by using a motion and location verb.

Receivers also can feel hand movements as the "voices" of actors when a narrator changes his or her quality of hand movements to reveal something about the character of the person who is saying something or acting.

Referring to Participants

Signers can tell about their own experiences of the trip, about their own life experiences, or about the experiences of others. In example 3, the signer tells about his meeting with young teenagers at a conference. Manual marking of perspective (forward-left) is used for CHILDREN and manual marking of perspective (forward-right) is used for interpreter SIGN-fr and for himself READ-fr when the deaf-blind man is signing with his interpreter. The name of a referent may be signed and/or spelled out. Pronominal pointing is used somewhat, mostly INDEX-c or INDEX-adr.

Example 3
A INDEX-c UNDERSTAND FIRST CAUSE CAUSE CHILDREN-fl LOOK-AT
INDEX-c INTERPRETER SIGN-fr READ-fr CHILDREN-fl LOOK-AT
WONDER WHAT INTERPRETER EXPLAIN-fl HANDS
TACTILE-SIGN-LANGUAGE CLEAR FINE FUNCTION WELL
A I understand. Because children were looking at me and the interpreter signed and I read. They looked at us and wondered what it was. The interpreter

explained that it was tactile communication. They understood right away. That was nice.

Change of perspective

Here are some signs for MAN with a prepositional sign IN-forward-left (I-fl) and INDEX-C in example 4, which work as perspective markers. The question-word W-H-A-T (in example 4) is considered to be a thought. After signing the spelled sign W-H-A-T, the signer uses the verb SAY-THANKS-fl with the perspective marker (forward-left) and goes back to her thought, GOOD. This expresses the thought of the signer and the reply to the person running the lift through manual marking of perspective and hand movements as the "voices" of the actors.

Example 4
A   MAN I-fl WORK "LET-GO" NEED NOT "LET-GO" FREE
    (b: YES-tap) INDEX-C W-H-A-T SAY-THANKS-fl GOOD
    poly-GO-LIFT poly-GO-DOWNHILL-SKIING-up-down
    REPEAT poly-GO-fl PAY NEG "LET-GO" x2 INDEX-C REPEAT   GOODx2
    poly-GO-LIFT BE FIVE SIX TIME GO-ROUND
B   HOW-MANY HOW-MANY SAY INDEX-adr HOW-MANY TIME
A   FIVE OR SIX TIMES GO-ROUND-UP FREE BUT NOT
    POSS-C GUY PAY

A   The guy running the lift waved me by and thought I didn't have to pay. I was surprised and thanked him and took the lift up. I didn't have to pay the next time either but could continue to go for free. I went up the ski lift for free five six times.
B   How many how many did you say, how many times?
A   Five or six times for free, but my guy had to pay.

This analytical work has provided me with many insights into how referents are located spatially without nonmanual features. As shown in example 5, the signer would signal the perspective changes to the receiver what is happening in the story.

Example 5
MAN IN-fl WORK "LET-GO" NEED NOT "LET-GO" FREE
Referent-------dialogue----------------------

INDEX-C   W-H-A-T SAY-THANKS-fl GOOD
Referent   thought---dialogue------- thought

poly-GO-LIFT poly-GO-DOWNHILL-SKIING-up-down
action-------------------------------------

Conclusions

It has been very interesting and instructive for me to analyze the conversations of deaf-blind people in tactile sign language, giving special attention to the referential framework.

To refer to people or things without gaze directions is one of the problem areas for a deaf-blind. Some deaf-blind people have eliminated problems by using markers other than eye contact, gaze directions, and head movements. They use more signs for nouns, name signs, or spell noun phrases for the referents. Marking for perspective is usually done for two or sometimes also three participants. These noun phrases and motion/location verbs can be located left-forward, right-forward, or without locus from the point of view of a participant.

The introduction of topics is used very carefully for checking with a receiver what a signer is talking about. It has been interesting to analyze in greater detail how deaf-blind people start and end a topic, but this article is only a preliminary study. Changing topics, as well as ending a topic, requires cooperation with the other conversational participant, as does closing a topic, which I intend to study in more detail.

References

Ahlgren, Inger, and Brita Bergman. 1994. Reference in narratives. In *Perspectives on sign language structure: Papers from the Fifth International Symposium on Sign Language Research*, vol. 1, ed. Inger Ahlgren, Brita Bergman, and Mary Brennan. Durham, UK: Isla.

Bahan, Ben, and Sam Supalla. 1995. Line segmentation and narrative structure: A study of eye gaze behavior in ASL. In *Language, gesture and space*, ed. K. Emmorey and J. Reilly. Hillsdale, NJ: Lawrence Erlbaum Associates.

Engberg-Pedersen, Elisabeth. 1993. *Space in Danish Sign Language: The semantics and morfohosyntax of the use of space in a visual language*. International Studies on Sign Language and Communication of the Deaf, vol. 19. Hamburg, Germany: Signum-Verlag.

Mesch, Johanna. 1998. *Teckenspråk i taktil form—turtagning och frågor i dövblindas samtal på teckenspråk* (Tactile Sign Language: Turn taking and questions in conversations of deaf-blind people in sign language). PhD diss., Stockholm University, Department of Linguistics.

Mesch, Johanna. 2001. *Tactile Swedish Sign Language—turn taking and questions in signed conversations of deaf-blind people*. International Studies on Sign Language, vol. 38. Hamburg, Germany: Signum-Verlag.

Appendix 1: NOTATION CONVENTIONS

INDEX-adr	Place-deictic reference to the addressee
SIGN-f	Locus marker indicating directions and positions relative to the signer: front of signer.
-c	near or in contact with the signer's body.
-l	left
-fl	front-left
-fr	front-right
-r	right
poly-SIGN	Indicates a polymorhous (modified) or polysynthetic sign
-dur	Very short delay
(b: YES-tap)	Remark with feedback
(.)	Short pause

PART ELEVEN
Technology

Genetics: A Future Peril Facing the Global Deaf Community

JOSEPH J. MURRAY

In the summer of 2001, I had the privilege of meeting the founder of the Porto Association of Deaf People, located in northern Portugal. I asked him, a living piece of Deaf history, what he thought was the biggest change in the Deaf community over the past fifty years. He thought for a moment and then replied, "Many of today's Deaf people go around wearing hearing aids," he signed, "and the quality of their signs has degraded, with more oral components and awkwardly produced signs." His reminiscences were tinged with an element of sadness, as he went on to describe to me a world before hearing aids were invented and Deaf people who came to the Deaf club used what he considered a better form of their national signed language.

My conversation with this man made me think about what today's Deaf youth will find in our community fifty years down the road. The major change in his time was hearing aids, which obviously parallel the major technological attempt to cure deafness in our time: cochlear implants. Although cochlear implants are having an impact on the current Deaf community, I believe there is something else that we as a community have overlooked until now. I contend that the major future peril facing our global Deaf community is the rise of genetic science and the social discourse surrounding this science. A thriving specialty of genetic science—researching hereditary deafness—exists today. The ultimate outcome of this research is to identify, treat, and eventually reduce the incidence of hereditary deafness. If one follows this research program to its logical conclusion, the aim is to eliminate hereditary deafness, and thus most Deaf people, from humanity. This is the future peril facing our up-and-coming generation of young Deaf leaders.

In this essay, I consider the genetics question in light of the Deaf community's previous battles against biotechnology. The first parallel that occurred to me, cochlear implants, is an obvious example of the biotechnological intervention that the genetics revolution is leading us toward. Reviewing the Deaf community's tactics in the cochlear implant debate can allow us to better prepare for the coming debate over Deaf people and genetics. The implantation of Deaf children at ever-younger ages is a fact in most developed and some developing countries. When cochlear implants first emerged, they were vehemently opposed by members of the Deaf community and their representative bodies. Many Deaf leaders and organizations drew a firm line in the sand and advanced powerful arguments against the implantation of children younger than eighteen years old. For one, they charged, experimental medical devices should not be implanted into children, especially because there was no research into the long-term consequences of implantation. Also, a Deaf child with a cochlear implant is still deaf and would still need to know sign language. And, because Deaf people form a unique cultural community with its own language and culture, Deaf leaders came out against the very idea of a surgical operation to "fix" a cultural condition. Today, this firm line in the sand has now been blurred by the facts on the ground. Large numbers of Deaf children are being implanted at ever-earlier ages; in some schools implanted Deaf children are the norm. Today, the standard line among most national associations of Deaf people is that it is fruitless to oppose the spread of cochlear implants among young children, even among babies. Instead of working against implantation, they say, we need to work with medical professionals to advance the Deaf point of view and ensure, above all, that Deaf children are still allowed to use sign language. For better or worse, cochlear implants are no longer actively opposed by organizations of Deaf people. The earlier arguments about cultural integrity and opposing experimentation on children have largely disappeared. Instead, a so-called realistic position of accommodation in the hopes of preserving at least some access to Deaf culture and signed languages for Deaf children is now the norm. Opposition has changed to accommodation.

The research that is taking place in genetic science will have profound implications for the survival of Deaf people in the twenty-first century. This science is actively working toward the technical ability to largely eliminate hereditary deafness from humanity. There is an explicit parallel here to the debate we underwent with cochlear implants, but the consequences of the genetics debate are far more serious. Deaf associations and Deaf individuals rightfully decried the use of cochlear implants on young Deaf children, but the fact is that these children will most likely join the Deaf community upon adulthood.[1] If past experience with oral educational methods is any indication, those cochlear-implanted Deaf children who grow up without an education in their native national signed language will be linguistically stunted compared to their sign-language-using peers. In this light, cochlear implants are a serious threat to what we already have accomplished in the past three decades with the recognition of signed languages across the world and the growth of bilingual-bicultural educational programs. Widespread cochlear implantation attached to an oralist pedagogical program will diminish the Deaf community's current cultural renaissance. The accomodationist stance Deaf organizations have adopted in regards to cochlear implants means the Deaf community will be reduced to its traditional fallback position of rehabilitating "oral failures." However, if Deaf organizations decide to adopt an accomodationist stance on genetic research aimed at eliminating deafness, it will not simply stunt our community's development, it will mean the end of the Deaf community as it now exists.

Advances in genetic testing techniques have made it possible for medical professionals to conduct prenatal testing for a variety of genetic diseases, including some

---

1. Harlan Lane notes many professionals report an "adolescent rejection" phenomenon wherein implanted children are no longer willing to use their implants. Harlan Lane, *The Mask of Benevolence: Disabling the Deaf Community* (New York: Alfred A. Knopf, 1992), 228–29.

forms of hereditary deafness. Although there are more than four hundred different forms of hereditary deafness, one particular form, connexin 26, may account for one-third of existing hereditary childhood deafness.[2] Prenatal genetic counseling is now becoming more widely available around the world, and the battery of standard tests includes a test for connexin 26. Parents who find their fetus carries a disease or disability are given the option of aborting that fetus. Today, genetic tests are given only to those individuals who seem likely to have children genetically different from a previously defined physical norm. However, scientists are working on computer-chip-based tests that would be able to easily and cheaply identify a number of genetic differences. Although today's options are crude—abortion or birth—future options may include fetal genetic engineering that could eliminate deafness in the womb.

These developments are taking place in an era where biotechnology and bodily manipulation are already becoming seen as normal. Today, a broad unspoken agreement exists on the idea of constant refinement of oneself and one's body to conform to the needs of larger society. The manipulation of one's body to ensure success is not seen as unnatural but as a necessary means of survival in the modern world. Take cell phones, for instance. Seeing people walking around with wires out of their ears talking into disembodied air is now commonplace. These phones are visually similar to cochlear implants. In Korea, some parents are opting to give their children tongue surgery to facilitate their pronunciation of English. With fluent English, one parent explained, their child could succeed in the global marketplace.[3] In China, one can undergo height-enhancement surgery.[4] During this surgery a person's shinbones are sawed in half and then affixed with metal braces. A dial is attached to the leg, leading down to the braces. A twist of the dial every now and then spurs bone growth in the break, thus adding a few inches of height onto otherwise short individuals. Enhanced height facilitates meeting a mate; getting a secure, well-paying position; and generally enjoying success in life. Cochlear implant surgery can be best understood in this light—as a means for hearing parents to ensure their Deaf children succeed in the global marketplace.

In this new era, diversity can be redefined to mean not respect *for* difference but ability to succeed *in spite of* difference. Thus, one can be Chinese or Korean or American but still manage a multinational company with tall stature and fluent spoken English. One upside to this is that this is part of the argument Deaf people have been making for decades. Deaf people, as the saying goes, can do anything but hear. Yet, most hearing people do not understand this. The ability to succeed in society is predicated on integration into society at its lowest common physical denominator. Thus physical difference—however small— from a defined norm becomes something to be repaired as quickly as possible.

This bodes ill for Deaf people in the genetics debate, but it also explains why we did not succeed in the cochlear implant debate. The Deaf response to the cochlear implant debate failed for two reasons. First, we are out of tune with a society intent on manipulating individual bodies for participation in mass society. Second, we came too late to stop cochlear implantation before it became an established part of the

2. Kathleen S. Arnos, "Genetics and Deafness," *Sign Language Studies* 2, no. 2 (2002): 159.
3. Barbara Demik, "Some in S. Korea Opt for a Trim When English Trips the Tongue," *Los Angeles Times*, 31 March 2002.
4. Craig S. Smith, "Risking Limbs for Height, and Success, in China," *New York Times*, 5 May 2002.

corporate biomedical establishment and ended up fighting an after-the-fact battle. Instead of holding onto our line in the sand, we ended up conceding and compromising, hoping to salvage the best we can for the next generation of Deaf people.

With genetic testing, we face a new challenge. It is still early enough to influence how larger society views the manipulation and elimination of genetic difference. However, before we can do so, we as a community need to decide what our response will be. Do we see deafness as something future generations would do well to live without? Some of us do, some of us do not. We need to have a serious discussion among ourselves about whether we will concede or draw a line in the sand. We need to discuss what it means to be Deaf, and what is it that is so valuable about being Deaf that it is worthy of a place in the future of humanity.

Whatever our response, it is important to keep in mind the vast majority of hearing people do not share our opinion that "it is dandy to be Deaf," to quote Deaf leader Roslyn Rosen. Media coverage of a case where two Deaf American women hoped to conceive a Deaf child shows there is widespread opposition to the idea of Deaf people trying to conceive deaf children.[5] Two Deaf American women, hoping for a Deaf child, picked a Deaf man from a multigenerational Deaf family as their sperm donor. An American newspaper reporter followed the women throughout their pregnancy and childbirth, up to the first medical consultation that confirmed their child was indeed Deaf, much to their joy. For many Deaf people, having a Deaf child is indeed a joyous occasion. The original article was disseminated by the global media with the Deaf couple inaccurately portrayed as an extreme example of selfish parents undergoing genetic manipulation to create a Deaf child. It is important to note that this was not a case of genetic manipulation: the parents did not undertake any genetic engineering; they merely chose a donor in the hopes of maximizing the chances of having a Deaf child. The final outcome was by no means assured. What is so frightening about this case is that it is not just about this one couple; a large number of Deaf couples do want Deaf children, and public reaction to this case shows there is little or no support for this sentiment in society at large nor among genetic counselors, of whom a large majority would refuse to allow Deaf parents to abort a hearing fetus.[6] Hearing parents may, of course, abort a deaf fetus. This case has the potential to define deafness and genetic testing to society at large, and we need to address this issue head on. Why should society allow Deaf people to try to have Deaf children? How can we convince society that hearing parents should not automatically destroy their deaf embryos or abort their deaf fetuses?

It should be emphasized that currently there is no movement among geneticists to restrict the reproductive rights of Deaf people or people with disabilities,[7] nor does any government currently mandate the elimination of fetuses with deafness or a disability. My concern is not with existing mandates or restrictions but with what may come in the future. The case of the Deaf sperm donor and the furor it aroused show how little support is out there in general society for the perpetuation of Deaf people

---

5. Liza Mundy, "A World of Their Own," *Washington Post*, 31 March 2002.

6. This is, of course, a hypothetical scenario advanced by ethicists as an interesting philosophical question. As of the time of this talk, there have not been any reports of this form of abortion actually being requested. Dorothy C. Wertz, "Drawing Lines: Notes for Policymakers," in *Prenatal Testing and Disability Rights*, ed. Erik Parens and Adrienne Asch (Washington, D.C.: Georgetown University Press, 2000), 265.

7. Kathleen S. Arnos, "Genetics and Deafness," 155.

in future generations. In the twentieth century, Deaf people underwent sterilization and forced abortions because they were Deaf and the state did not want them to have Deaf children, complaining that Deaf people were a financial drain on social resources.[8] Future attempts to restrict the reproductive freedom of Deaf people will likely not start in as blunt a manner as a formal prohibition of pregnancies that may lead to Deaf children. Rather, there could come a series of measures from government regulation of private industry, explained as being for the common good. There are already restrictions in place prohibiting those with hereditary deafness from donating to sperm banks. The next step could conceivably be a requirement that those who want artificial insemination must receive donor sperm only from these banks, ostensibly for public health reasons. Once genetic screening becomes more widespread, health insurance companies may assign a higher policy premium to children whose parents elect not to go through with prenatal genetic screening, on the grounds that insurance companies need to prepare for unknown health risks. If fetal genetic engineering becomes a reality, the elimination of hereditary deafness and other forms of genetic diversity may become commonplace. In this context, the birth of a deaf child would be understood by society as something easily avertable and the choice to have a deaf child as being a personal preference. The costs of social accommodations to Deaf people will become increasingly important, with Deaf people being seen as incurring unnecessary social expense. There may come a time when Deaf people will be ruled to have no legal right to telephone relay, sign language interpreting services, and language-appropriate schools, because their deafness was a lifestyle choice by their parents and not a disability society feels obligated to accommodate.

Deaf people urgently need to enter into a dialogue with one another on how we will approach this future peril: where will we draw the line in the sand when it comes to genetics? There are a number of questions we need to consider. Do we oppose all elective abortions because prospective parents have the right to abort deaf fetuses? Do we come out against prenatal genetic testing for deafness? How do we respond to genetic research, not only into hereditary deafness, but all genetic research? What about gene therapies that attempt to cure adult-onset deafness? Do we accept this but not fetal genetic treatments for deafness? These are just a few of the questions we need to address to present a coherent argument to the general public.

Then there is the question of tactics. How do we bring our views to the attention of policy makers? At some point, others will try to obliterate whatever line we draw. What do we do then? Again, the cochlear implant debate gives us a hint of what to expect. At the risk of oversimplification, one can say the cochlear implant debate was largely dominated by Deaf organizations, Deaf leaders, and proponents of a cultural view of Deaf people on one side and medical professionals and proponents of a medical approach on the other. In this debate, leaders of Deaf organizations were considered radical for advocating more research into cochlear implants or for suggesting culturally Deaf people did not need cochlear implants. However, the Deaf community actually had very few true radicals when compared to other civil rights debates, such as the fight against apartheid in South Africa, the U.S. civil rights movement, or the global movement for women's suffrage. We had no militants and only a few

---

8. See Horst Biesold, *Crying Hands: Eugenics and Deaf People in Nazi Germany* (Washington, D.C.: Gallaudet University Press, 1999).

sporadic nonviolent protests against cochlear implants. Martin Luther King Jr. was considered a radical when he first came to prominence in the fight against segregation; by the time more radical groups and leaders such as Malcom X came along, King became to be seen as someone even the U.S. president could negotiate with. The presence of other groups agitating for civil rights in more active ways enabled leaders such as King to negotiate with policy makers.

What the Deaf community needs in the genetics debate is a range of voices—that of researchers, that of representative organizations of Deaf people, and that of a peaceful nonviolent movement drawing attention to the fact that Deaf people are facing a threat to their very existence. It is this latter movement in which Deaf youth can play a special role. Their time and energy can attract public attention to Deaf people's views on genetics and shift the stamp of "radical" away from Deaf associations. Genetic research on deafness can be found in a few easily identifiable research centers, providing Deaf youth with logical sites for peaceful nonviolent actions, which can bring our concerns to public attention. We should not have to fight this fight alone. Tens of thousands of hearing people learn and research and use our signed languages. Does their commitment exist to supporting our activism in favor of the unborn members of our community? A number of religions oppose the genetic manipulation of humans. Does their commitment extend to actively protecting the right of Deaf individuals to exist? How about among ourselves? Do we all agree that Deaf people ought to exist in the future? If so, why? We need to find new arguments for this new challenge.

I leave you not with a solution, but with a brief glimpse of a situation we will certainly face in our lifetimes. Fifty years from now, will our community have Deaf youth to whom we can pass on our heritage? The answer is entirely in your hands.

Making Ourselves Heard: The Promise of No-Barriers Communication

RAYMOND J. OGLETHORPE

Thirteen years ago Deaf Way, the first Deaf Way conference, helped pave the way for self-advocacy and working with technologists and business to make known the needs of the disability community. Here we are again at this amazing conference, thirteen years later, reflecting on our accomplishments and continuing our collaboration. Much progress has been made but much is still to come. We are writing an important book together.

I recently paid a visit to one of our community sites on America Online (AOL), where individuals of the deaf and hard of hearing community regularly gather. Right there, as if somehow this has been planned, was a special feature about making friends online. This is the first posting I saw from a young woman who cannot hear. She said, "I've made more friends online than in the real world. In the real world I am different. In the online, I am me." To me, that is the unbelievable promise of no-barriers communication and freedom to be exactly who you are. That freedom has been a long time coming. There are many new exciting developments that will help people who are deaf or hard of hearing and people who cannot see realize their ambitions. Before I touch on the latest technical wizardry, here is a little history. Forgive me, because at heart I am still a technologist.

Let us start with the Internet, which is what I know best. The communications phenomenon got its start back in the 1960s as the brainchild of America's defense industry. It was primarily the tool of academics and civil servants until a couple of guys named Cerf and Kahn figured out how to link commuters of different protocols and operating systems together with a protocol called TCP/IP. That stands for transmission control protocol/Internet work protocol. You may be interested to know that Vint Cerf is a good friend of mine. Then came the World Wide Web (WWW), which brought the concept of multimedia to the Internet. It also helped to format this vast pool of knowledge on the Internet into organized layers of files, which could be transferred with ease from computer to computer. But all of this would have just been interesting conversation at academic gatherings if clever people, in Europe and in the New World, had not invented browser technology. That is what made it possible for early enthusiasts to actually find the information they were looking for. All of this would not have been of interest to you if companies such as Prodigy, CompuServe, and eventually AOL had not come along in the 1980s and brought the power of the Internet to consumers in an easy-to-use, feature-rich environment.

This led to an unbelievable proliferation of affordable and usable computers on desks and kitchen counters. We still have to deal with the obstacle called the digital divide. However, recent news has been very encouraging. The *Washington Post* last week reported that the gaps in the Internet access among urban and rural Internet users, ethnic groups, and people with varying levels of education is shrinking. By the way, according to the most recent U.S. commerce survey, 54 percent of the total population of America had access to the Internet last year. That is an unbelievable statistic considering where we started back in 1989. The same survey reveals that 62 percent of Americans who are deaf and hard of hearing now have access to the Internet. Internationally, according to the Nielsen net ratings, the number of people with Internet access at home grew by 16 percent from April 2001 to April 2002 to reach an astonishing 422.4 million home users in twenty-one countries, which illustrates the leap in the Internet's international appeal.

At the time of the first Deaf Way, there were no signs of the Web. For this Deaf Way II conference, most transactions from around the world were handled online. With the net, new communications methods have helped level the playing field. I am referring to the big three that mean so much to the audience. They are fax, e-mail, and my personal favorite, instant messaging. The fax machine has actually been around since before World War II. Newspapers used it to transmit photographs. It was not until the 1980s that the fax moved out toward greater public use. For people who are deaf and hard of hearing, faxes were the first step to independent and reasonably immediate communication with the hearing world and with each other. E-mail was invented in the 1970s, and its adoption rate has pretty much followed the curve of the Internet. It freed us from delivery services and it definitely sped things up, but not as much as instant messaging (IM), which is real time, two-way communication, whether the individuals on either end can hear or not. On AOL, IM works like this: Each member keeps a list of family members, friends, and business associates in a list called a buddy list. Whenever one of your buddies signs on, your computer lets you know and allows you to talk and type messages directly with him.

Telecommunications is making history, too. In this arena, wireless communications is absolutely big news, which is pretty amazing, considering wireless did not get off the ground until 1983. At first members of the deaf and hard of hearing community could not afford to stray too far from their text telephone (TTY) and fax machines. Then you had to stay close to your PC. Now none of us are tethered to anything any longer. Wireless took the last barrier to real-time communications by adding mobility. In the United States today, wireless transmission is now available in about 70 percent of the land area, which includes roughly 96 percent of the U.S. population. There ought to be somebody in that large crowd for everyone here to talk with. So now these little devices give you power. These devices are text-messaging devices, also known as pagers such as Wyndtell, Blackberry, and AOL mobile communicator. A lot of you I know have firsthand knowledge of these devices. Judy Harkins, professor of communication studies at Gallaudet University, said pagers are very, very commonplace and very much loved.

The benefits of this potent technology mix are just now becoming clear.

Privacy. Different situations will always require different kinds of communication. Instant messages, e-mail, and text-driven wireless devices reduce reliance on others to translate content for people who are deaf and hard of hearing. How many of these messages could or would you want to share with a third party?

Independence. No-barriers communication gives you control, all day, every day, or as we say in the technology business, 24/7. You can get in touch with whomever you want, whenever you want. Here are two stories from students right here in the Washington, D.C., area. The first involves the everyday mistake that we all make: getting locked out of our car. In this case, instead of trying to find a TTY, the young woman simply sent an instant message for help. The next case involves a fellow who got lost. He sent an instant message to his brother for directions, and he was on his way in no time. Of course, we cannot forget the tragic events of September 11, 2001. When information was so critical to all of us, when all other tools were inaccessible or inoperable, it was instant messaging that connected us to our associates and loved ones.

In the not-too-distant future, mobile access to the Internet will allow you to handle transactions that might not be as easy to take on in the brick-and-mortar world. For instance, you can do shopping and banking, make travel arrangements, and obtain information. With appropriately designed technology, people who are hard of hearing or blind have direct, unfiltered, and immediate access to the same information as everybody else, including news, directions, weather, and stock quotations.

Fluent conversation. No-barriers communication means you do not have to reduce what you say to small components that can be easily translated. What you say is not subject to wrong interpretation. You do not have to leave out the interesting parts to speed things up. Your communication can be spontaneous. It can be more effective. And it can be very, very satisfying.

Of course, the industry still has much to do to make all these devices as convenient and functional as possible. There is much rich content on the net that cannot yet be delivered on a small three-inch display device powered by little, itsy-bitsy memory. And interoperability must be taken into account. For AOL this requires a careful balance between completely open architecture, which anybody can write to and those who will accommodate the high levels of functionality, and security, privacy, safeguards that our members have come to expect. However, for your part, you need to stay informed on the issues that affect product development and make your requirements known, not just to AOL but also to all significant players who may influence positive outcomes. So, what are we going to do with all this new power? One of the things I have learned in the past years in implementing accessible technology is that it is just not something you want to do, but we do it because it is good business. It is like the cut in the curb that was designed to help people in wheelchairs navigate the city streets. Now, everybody who has wheels uses these cuts in the curb, including cyclists, rollerbladers, and people pushing strollers. So many newly minted technologies turn out to benefit not just the targeted audience, but everybody as well. Here are a few of the latest. Let us start with literacy tools. In this country, as my daughter so eloquently said, we take education for granted. But for children with disabilities, just getting through school can be a significant challenge. I learned on the

Gallaudet Web site that children who are deaf or hard of hearing are twice as likely to drop out of high school and half as likely to complete college. That makes literacy a prime candidate for no-barriers communication. The example I am about to share with you, by the way, is not from AOL. So far as I am able, I am trying to represent communication technology as a whole.

One really good example of technology that builds word power is the cornerstones project developed by WGBH National Center for Accessible Media (NCAM). The cornerstones goal is to help elementary students with hearing disabilities develop an in-depth understanding of the meaning of words. The curriculum is based on stories from the popular PBS series *Between the Lions*. Each story is complemented by signed versions. What is new is that each story has a hypertext edition, where students reading on computers can click on a word to learn its definition and see visuals that really convey the meaning. The first field test show that children using these tools are able to learn twice as many words as they did with more conventional techniques.

Now, let us look at the captions. A picture may be worth a thousand words, but sometimes a few words are worth more than all the pictures together. That is where captioning comes in. People who are deaf or hard of hearing rely upon captions in the classroom, at the movies, on television, and you guessed it, on the Internet. First, the classroom: you may be surprised to find out that 94 percent of teachers use video as a regular instructional tool during the academic year. However, not all students are ready for standard captions. For that reason, new edited captions are being made available to present content at a slower pace with simpler vocabulary. To see it in action, tune in to *Arthur*, another popular children's show on PBS. Second, the movies: here NCAM is in action again, developing a totally new captioning system for theaters called rear windows. A text display at the back of the theater shows reverse captions. They are reflected facing up on clear acrylic panels attached to the patron's seat. It actually looks like the captions are superimposed on the movie screen. So there go two barriers to your enjoyment of movies. One, you do not have to wait for special captioned screenings, and two, you get to sit wherever you want. It is quite new. Rear window is only available in about 100 IMAX and conventional theaters and at Disney theme parks. My guess the number of theaters offering rear window will multiply in the coming months and years. Third, captions on TV: in 1972, when captioning first made a debut on American television, only half an hour of programming per week was accessible to deaf and hard of hearing viewers. Today, that number is closer to 2,000 hours per week plus an addition of nearly 3,000 commercial spots.

The news here about captioning revolves around the transition from analog to digital technology. To mainstream viewers, digital means high-quality images. To deaf and hard of hearing people, digital means additional capacity. Digital transmission allows multiple caption streams to be delivered at the same time, theoretically up to sixty-four channels for each program. That should be either enough to satisfy or confuse anybody. Standard captions, edited captions, and multiple foreign languages can all be broadcast simultaneously. Beyond that, you will be able to have, and here is that magic word again, control over the look and feel of your captions, everything from font, type size, color, and placement of the captions on the screen.

Speaking of screens, what about captioning on the computer? In this age of increasing bandwidth, video is all the rage on the Internet. The latest advances involve software tools that allow captions, subtitles, and audio descriptions to be applied to digital multimedia, whether originally produced for the online environment or reproduced from other applications. If you go to the NCAM Web site, you can check out their latest offerings. It is a Java-based windows and Mac-friendly application called MAGpie (Media Access Generator). It is easy enough for schoolchildren to learn, and it is priced for everybody to afford. Essentially, it is free.

In the meantime, did you notice how cleverly I slipped in those words, "digital" and "bandwidth"? That means I am getting closer to the concept that represents the next wave of communications development, convergence. These days, the lines that separated methods of high-tech communications and traditional roles of communication devices are becoming very blurred. From your computer, you can talk on the phone or send a fax. From almost any organizer device, you can get your calendar and e-mail. From your television, you can access the Internet and send instant messages. From your phone or pager, you can pick up your e-mail. I think you can still even page somebody from your pager. You get the picture. That trend to unite communications functions and delivery methods is called convergence. We are going to get more exquisitely useful gadgets. Combined with the high-bandwidth transmission of cable and digital subscriber line (DSL) technology, convergence is leading the establishment of whole new kinds of networks in the not-too-distant future.

Let us talk about the home network. Imagine, with all your necessities, television, computers, personal digital assistants (PDAs), phone service, and—let's get wild here, your digital camera, your home-security station, your Sony PlayStation—all hooked up to a simple network managed from a single set-top box. What could you do? Well, doorbell alerts could show up on your television screen. Graphical television guides could be translated from your set-top box to a Braille note, which is a PDA for the blind. You could talk on the phone or send a fax from any computer. Sign languages sent via e-mail could appear on your television screen. Think this is Star Trek stuff? Folks, it is beginning to happen right now. Right now, about half of all broadband households have two or more personal computers. And get this: about 25 percent of today's broadband households are already installing a home network.

In fact, paving the way for the networked digital household and dealing with the roster accessibility issues is major focus of a number of companies, including AOL, today. Now I share with you some of the ways AOL as a company is acknowledging and responding to our members with specific needs. To begin with, we have engaged not one but three groups of incredibly experienced and knowledgeable advisors. One is NCAM, which I mentioned before. For three years, AOL has been a member of the NCAM business partners program. NCAM works with us developing solutions for accessible online services and content. Right now we are jointly implementing a new tool called CIRT. It is a sophisticated authoring program that allows us to repurpose video captions for the Internet. You should see tremendous use of this as we capitalize on the video assets of the AOL Time-Warner Enterprises. We also have the Accessibility Advisory Council, made up of sixteen leaders who represent the disability community across the board. They make recommendations to us during the development of new devices, services, and online content. They also advise us on policy issues that inform the work we do. AOL also benefits by working with people at I-CAN who help provide content to AOL sites to disability community.

Our messages are crafted not only by and for external uses of advocates and members but also for our employees. I have nearly seventeen thousand people who work for me all over the world on full-time projects. It is a big challenge to focus them all on the same performance criteria, and so we have inaugurated a continuous company-wide accessibility awareness program, called New Sensation. The New Sensation program features a technologist's tool kit, special coverage in employee online areas, and an awards program that recognizes sensational work in this area. This spring, the awards went to people who made screen readers an integral part of AOL 7.0 and to the team that revitalized our community area for people with special needs. Here is another posting that would not have been possible without their work. It is from a young mother looking for support as she raises her twin sons, who both have hearing loss. That message had been posted for just a few minutes before she got her answer. It says, "There is deafness chat Tuesday nights 9:00 to 10:00 p.m. in the AOL disabilities Cafe. You can find this information by going to keyword: Chat, schedule, lifestyles, and disabilities. Hope to see you there."

I started this talk by referring to the super class of pagers that have become standard equipment for people who are deaf or hard of hearing. Well, this past year, AOL has devoted resources to make the mobile communicator affordable to obtain. In fact, we did a pilot program right down the street at Gallaudet University and in concert with the university's Technology Access Program. You remember the anecdotes about the student locked out of the car and driver who lost his way? Guess what? The mobile communicator was used every day to solve those problems. A faculty member—you know how reserved they can usually be—claimed the pilot program went like gangbusters. That is just the way we at AOL want to keep it going. AOL is committed to accelerate the implementation of accessible technology supported by regular communication from you. If some part of the AOL service is inaccessible to you, we need to hear about it. If you think an AOL communications device needs more accessible design, we need to hear about it. If there is content you would like to see on AOL, we need to hear about that, too. If by some chance you do not inform yourselves, I know somebody who will. She is my daughter, Kimberly. Every time an AOL service is updated, every time a new product is launched, Kimberly is on the phone to her old man delivering an evaluation. Because of people like you, my daughter, Kim, and others in the accessibility community, barriers large and small have been removed during the past year and the thirteen years since Deaf Way I, to make AOL more accessible. That is what can happen when we make ourselves heard.

The Dilemma of Pediatric Cochlear Implants

JOHN B. CHRISTIANSEN AND
IRENE W. LEIGH

During the last few decades of the twentieth century, the topic of cochlear implants (CIs) emerged as one of the most divisive issues among deaf and hard of hearing people, educators, parents of deaf children, and others concerned about the welfare and future of deaf people and the deaf community. The controversy is most intense when considering the issue of CIs for children who are often too young to decide if this technology is something they want for themselves.

What makes this process a very emotional experience for many parents is the fact that the vast majority of parents who have deaf children are themselves hearing. Moreover, most of these parents have little, if any, contact with deaf people and little knowledge or understanding of deafness before learning that their child is deaf. Thus, they find themselves in a situation with which they have no experience or knowledge on which to rely when they need to start making decisions about how to socialize and educate their child.

What Is a Cochlear Implant (CI)?

Many deaf people have a sensorineural hearing loss. This essentially means that the microscopic hair cells in the cochlea are unable to stimulate the auditory nerve endings that are located in the inner ear. The auditory nerve, which connects the cochlea to the cortex of the brain, is thus unable to transmit sounds to the brain. A CI is designed to do the job of the hair cells and stimulate the auditory nerve fibers in the cochlea. Implants do not restore normal hearing, although they usually do better than hearing aids in enabling severely to profoundly deaf people to perceive sounds.

Generally, candidates for a CI should be twelve to eighteen months old or older, should have a severe to profound bilateral sensorineural hearing loss, and should receive little or no benefit from hearing aids. For a pediatric implant, both the child's

---

For more information about many of the issues discussed in this paper, see John B. Christiansen and Irene W. Leigh, *Cochlear Implants in Children: Ethics and Choices*. Washington, D.C.: Gallaudet University Press, 2002 (reprinted with a new afterword in 2005).

parents and, when appropriate, the child should be highly motivated to develop speaking and listening skills.[1]

The Preimplant Deaf Child[2]

Many parents of deaf children have a difficult time determining whether their child is deaf, although infant hearing screening in many, if not most, hospitals is rapidly changing this. Part of the reason is that most hearing parents are not expecting a deaf baby and are not sure how much a child normally hears in the first year of life. The problem is sometimes compounded by insensitive audiologists and pediatricians who do not always provide parents with the information they need to determine if their child is deaf. For example, we interviewed a mother of a ten-year-old boy who was implanted when he was six years old. This mother recalled: "We took our 5 month old son to the pediatrician and asked about his hearing. The pediatrician snapped his fingers in front of [our son's] face and [our son] blinked. . . . [The pediatrician] did not think there was a problem with [our son's] hearing. And, not wanting to believe that there was, we continued on [for several more months]."

Following the diagnosis of their child's deafness, many parents are understandably quite upset. One parent we interviewed said: "I think the worst thing I had to deal with in my life was finding out [that my child was deaf]. It was almost like a part of you dies." After parents accepted or became resigned to the fact that their child was deaf, they began searching for "solutions." One parent we interviewed said: "The scariest part of it is that you don't know what you're supposed to do next. And no one's telling you; there is no road map." In general, parents were starving for information, and help from other parents of deaf children was frequently seen as most useful, as were early intervention programs.

Communication was very important to parents before the implant. Hearing aids and learning to sign were common first steps taken by many parents (about one-half of the children in the GRI study used some signing before getting the implant). As one parent said: "Even though I am a big fan of cochlear implants, I think cochlear implants are absolutely wonderful, [our daughter] was able to gain a language very young and very fast with her sign language."

Many parents wanted their child to develop spoken language if possible, even if they initially used some form of sign communication with their child. Indeed, one of

---

1. CIs have been available for about forty years, although the vast majority of people who have received a CI have been implanted during the past ten years. Although most of those who received an implant prior to 1990 were adults, currently a little more than half of the implant surgeries performed around the world are done on deaf children. At the time of Deaf Way II in 2002, approximately thirty-five to forty thousand people worldwide had received a CI. According to information available on the Web sites of the three major CI companies, as of 2005 approximately ninety thousand children and adults had received a CI. It is not known how many people continue to use the device, although, presumably, most of them do use it, at least to some extent.

2. The discussion in this and subsequent sections of this essay is largely based on research conducted in 1999. One study was conducted by the Gallaudet Research Institute (GRI) in the spring of 1999. A twelve-page questionnaire was distributed to 1,841 parents of children with CIs around the United States; 439 of these questionnaires were returned (a 24-percent response rate). In addition to this research, in the summer and fall of 1999, the authors conducted fifty-six interviews with parents of sixty-two children with implants (and one without) in fifteen states and Australia. The parents in all of the families we talked with, except one, were hearing. In both studies, the sample was clearly biased in favor of implants because of the difficulty in recruiting parents with negative experiences.

the most important reasons why many parents find CIs attractive is because they believe it will lead to the development of better spoken language for their deaf child.

Although many parents we talked with found implants attractive, most of them did *not* jump into the decision to get the device for their child. Many parents went through a lot of soul searching before deciding to go ahead. In addition to the opportunity to learn spoken language, parents reported a variety of reasons for getting the implant, such as safety and the chance for their child to have more "options" in the future.

As parents think about whether an implant might be appropriate for their son or daughter, they usually have a good amount of contact with a CI center. One might surmise that the center would strongly encourage parents to get an implant for their child. However, most of the parents of children with implants that we talked with reported that the CI center did not pressure them into getting an implant.

While parents are trying to decide whether to get an implant for their child, they may have some contact with the deaf community. Often, this contact is not pleasant. As one parent we interviewed said: "When we spoke to the deaf community about the CI . . . certain members of the deaf community . . . their feelings were so angry and so hurtful. I mean, we were called child abusers . . . and butchers."

The question of when to implant is another issue that is of great concern to parents. Many parents feel that "the earlier, the better," because early exposure to spoken language would presumably make it easier for the child to develop spoken language himself or herself. Recent research suggests that there is some validity to this assumption, and, indeed, children are routinely implanted at an increasingly early age.

The Postimplant Deaf Child

After deciding that a CI is appropriate for their child, parents continue to confront conundrums, especially in the areas of communication and education. It may surprise some readers to learn that many parents have no strong objection to signing after implantation, and many children with CIs do in fact sign after getting the implant, both at home and at school. Many parents feel that signing is a vital part of their child's communication needs (along with speech and listening therapy). As one parent said: "I can never see [my implanted daughter] not being dependent on an interpreter. If she's in a big auditorium with people, or even if she's sitting in the front row . . . to catch all of it, she's gonna need sign language." It may also appear somewhat surprising that many parents of children with implants still see their child as deaf after getting an implant.

Many of the parents we talked with said they would probably be disappointed but would nevertheless accept their child's decision if the child stopped using the implant later, especially after the child turned eighteen. One father said: "We were even told by the child psychologist that the day may come when he tells us he hates us for having done this to him . . . and, well, I hope that doesn't happen, but if it does, then, gee, I'm sorry, we did what we thought was best. You don't want it, don't use it."

One important area where parents have to make a decision after implantation is the type of educational setting that would be appropriate for their child. Our research indicates that parents enrolled their children in many different types of programs (oral

TABLE 1. Support Services for Implanted Children

Support services	Percent of children receiving this service
Sign language interpreting	40
Teacher aide in the classroom	37
Resource room help	28
Media captioning (closed/real time)	24
Itinerant teacher support	22
Remedial work/tutoring	17
Classroom amplification	16
Personal assistive device	15
Oral interpreter	13

and signing), both preimplant and postimplant. Many children with implants are mainstreamed with hearing students, but virtually all of these children continue to require services of some type. Moreover, parents often have to fight for these services, which are important because 59 percent of children are judged by their parents to be behind their hearing peers in reading and 37 percent in math (according to the GRI study).

Some of the special support services that implanted children receive in school are listed in table 1 (from the GRI study).

Because the percentages add up to considerably more than 100 percent, it is obvious that many children use a number of services in school postimplant. Few children with CIs are able to thrive in school with no support services at all.

Because many parents assert that their implanted child is still deaf after getting the implant, it is important to stress that many children with CIs are not isolated from their deaf peers. The GRI study found that about one-third of the implanted children had only deaf classmates, one-third had only hearing classmates, and one-third had both deaf and hearing classmates.

Most of the parents who talked with us about their child's personality noted stability or improvement in social relationships postimplant. Very few parents noted psychological difficulties after implantation. When difficulties occurred, these were related to being implanted during adolescence, particularly when this was not a completely voluntary decision. (It should be noted, however, that most of the adolescent CI users we interviewed—and who got their implant during adolescence—wanted it and were happy with it.)

Given the fact that the initial decision regarding implantation is very nerve-wracking for many parents, it is important to note that most parents of children with implants are generally pleased with the results, and 62 percent (from the GRI study) wish they could have implanted their child earlier because they felt it would have better facilitated spoken language development. After the first year with the CI, 54 percent said they were very satisfied with their child's progress; at the time we interviewed them (usually several years postimplant), 67 percent said they were very satisfied.

However, not all parents are satisfied. The mother of a boy implanted when he was a teenager said that the implant: "Failed to meet my expectations." Father: "Mine, too." Interviewer: "What exactly did you expect?" Mother: "I expected him to grow to love it like he liked his hearing aids, and being better than the hearing aids. . . ." Father: "I expected he would have speech, improved speech, more speech." Interviewer: "Is there any way that it met your expectations?" Father: "Just that it brought his hearing up to a mild to moderate loss from a profound [loss]." Mother: "But, just because he can hear the sounds does not mean that he understands."

The Deaf Community and Cochlear Implants

After the implant, relations with the deaf community are an important part of the decision-making process faced by many parents, especially because many children with implants sign, are likely to have nonimplanted deaf friends, and frequently interact with others who are part of the deaf community. As noted previously, a number of parents of deaf children had some contact with people in the deaf community during the time they were considering implantation. In many cases this contact was not pleasant because, until recently, there was fairly strong opposition to pediatric implants by many culturally deaf people.

In an important sense, a position paper on CIs issued by the National Association of the Deaf in October 2000 most likely makes it easier for parents to decide to get a CI for their child: changing views in the deaf community, as reflected in the position paper, suggest that implantation will not irrevocably cut off the implanted child from the cultural deaf community. Rather, there seems to be a growing sentiment within the broader deaf community, as well as at Gallaudet University, to embrace, rather than reject, children and adolescents with implants. The 2000 NAD position paper reads, in part: "The NAD recognizes the rights of parents to make informed choices for their . . . children, respects their choice to use cochlear implants and all other assistive devices, and strongly supports the development of the whole child and of language and literacy" (NAD, 2001). This is a far cry from a 1991 position paper on cochlear implants that stated that the NAD "deplores the decision of the Food and Drug Administration [to approve implantation in children aged two to seventeen] which was unsound scientifically, procedurally, and ethically" (NAD, 1991).[3]

In an attempt to access the changing climate at Gallaudet University, we distributed a questionnaire to a sample of faculty, staff, students, and alumni in the spring of 2000. One of the statements on the questionnaire asked whether "Gallaudet University should do more to encourage students with cochlear implants to attend." Among those who responded, 59 percent agreed, 23 percent disagreed, and 17 percent expressed no opinion. Most of the deaf (54 percent), hearing (71 percent), and hard of hearing (65 percent) respondents agreed with the statement. Another statement in the questionnaire asked: "Faculty and staff should be encouraged to sign with voice whenever possible in order to make the University more 'user friendly' for students who use voice communication more than sign, as many cochlear implant users

---

3. Another example of the changing climate was the establishment of a CI center at Gallaudet University in 2000. One of the purposes of this center is to educate children with implants in an educational setting that emphasizes both visual and auditory learning.

do." In this case, 51 percent of the sample disagreed whereas 34 percent agreed and 15 percent did not know. In comparison to hearing (31 percent) and hard of hearing (24 percent) respondents who disagreed, a much higher proportion of deaf respondents disagreed (63 percent). Thus, although there may still be resistance in some areas to making accommodations for students with implants, the trend seems to be moving in the direction of inclusiveness rather than exclusiveness.

One reason some people have opposed pediatric implants was because it was thought that widespread implantation could lead to the "death of deafness." It is becoming increasingly apparent that this will not happen, especially in those areas of the world where medical resources are scarce and where adequate support services are not available. However, it is also becoming increasingly apparent that there is widespread sentiment, especially among parents of children with implants, that their children are still deaf and, as noted, still need a number of support services, especially in school. Many children are clearly benefiting from the CI, but there is no guarantee. CIs do not work by themselves, and intensive habilitation is required.

Conclusion

Parents of deaf children are frequently confronted with the need to make choices about issues they may have seldom thought about before learning of their child's hearing loss. These choices include communication styles, educational settings, and, of course, whether to get a CI for their child. Reasonably objective advice and information may be difficult to come by, not only because parents are new to the field and may find it difficult to evaluate the quality of the information, but also because the information itself may be presented in a way that implies there is only one "obvious" or "correct" way to proceed, whether that way be to implant or not to implant, to sign or not to sign, and so on.

It is somewhat ironic, perhaps, that the dilemma of pediatric CIs may be becoming easier for parents (and others) to resolve as it becomes increasingly clear that there are at least as many things that unite people in the different "camps" in the CI debate as there are that divide them. It is important to remember that implantation does not inevitably separate a young child from the deaf community or from deaf friends, that implantation does not mean a child will never learn to sign, and that implantation does not mean that in classroom settings an child will no longer require support services.

It is certainly true that implantation will probably make it easier for a deaf child to acquire spoken language, but it is also true that many deaf people who do not use spoken language are leading very successful and productive lives.[4] What is most important, perhaps, is that we recognize that there are many different avenues to success and that early identification of hearing loss, early communication between the deaf child and his or her parents and family, and a lot of hard work on everyone's part are some of the things that will continue to foster the common ground in the debate about the appropriateness of pediatric CIs.

---

4. It is important to keep in mind that fluency in a written language is not the same thing as fluency in a spoken language. Indeed, illiteracy is a major social problem in many places around the world, including the United States. Reading and writing are skills that must be learned, and they are skills that can be acquired more or less independently of one's ability to hear.

References

National Association of the Deaf (NAD). (1991). Report of the task force on childhood cochlear implants. *NAD Broadcaster; 13*, 1–2, 6–7.

National Association of the Deaf (NAD). (2001). NAD position statement on cochlear implants. *NAD Broadcaster; 23*, 14–15.

The Impact of Genetics Research on the Deaf Community

JANE DILLEHAY AND KATHLEEN ARNOS

We discuss recent developments in genetics and the future effects of this research on the deaf community, including genetic technology and its implications for the deaf community. The more knowledge that members of the deaf community have about genetic issues, the better the community is prepared to deal with the developing issues arising from genetics research.

The Human Genome Project was established in 1990 by the U.S. government with $250 million to support scientists from six different countries in developing genetic maps of all the human chromosomes. A genome is a complete set of the DNA in a cell. DNA is the chemical that carries all of the information and instructions for making an organism and helping it to function. A particular sequence of DNA is called a gene. Each gene carries information to construct or operate some feature of the human body, whether it is deafness, blood type, or some other characteristic. All the genes are carried in structures called chromosomes.

The Human Genome Project analyzes the DNA sequence to see how genes are constructed and where they are located on the chromosomes. The human genome contains forty-six chromosomes and approximately 3 billion base pairs of DNA. Surprisingly, there are only about thirty thousand genes in humans. Researchers had expected there to be many more, given that humans are the most intelligent animal on the planet. There are some species of plants that have more genes than humans and some species of animals, such as the mouse, that have about the same number of genes as humans.

One goal of the Genome Project is to develop genetic maps of human DNA; another important goal is to address the ethical, legal, and social implications of genetic technology. Although the Human Genome Project has already led to better diagnosis and treatment of many diseases, information about human DNA can create concerns related to confidentiality and privacy of genetic information, genetic discrimination,

---

This presentation occurred in the summer of 2002. Since that time, several new developments have occurred. Scientists at the University of Michigan have used gene therapy to grow new auditory hair cells in adult guinea pigs, a discovery that could lead to new treatments for human deafness and age-related hearing loss. A fertility clinic in Melbourne, Australia, used a genetic test to screen out embryos that carried a gene for deafness, an example of preselecting embryos to eliminate a non-life-threatening trait.

and reproductive options. Suppose someone's genetic makeup indicates that they may contract an illness later on in life. What implications would this have for health and life insurance or even possibly employment?

Many people have misconceptions about genetics. Unfortunately, many of the people who make legal and social policy are not always well informed on the issue either. After twelve years of research through the Human Genome Project, knowledge about the human DNA sequence is about 90 percent complete. The entire project will be finished in the summer of 2002. With increasing knowledge of human DNA, researchers are gaining the ability to look for specific things, for example, genes that play a role in breast cancer, heart disease, or Alzheimer's disease. In trying to isolate those genes, researchers are looking for a way to identify people at risk and to prevent these diseases from occurring. This is one example of the power of the information coming out of the Genome Project.

Research has shown that genetic factors account for 50 to 60 percent of people who are born deaf or who have early-onset deafness. There are four hundred different types of hereditary deafness, and so there are many genes that can cause deafness. In the past few years, researchers have mapped more than eighty of the four hundred different genes for deafness. That means that the location of the gene on the chromosome is known as well as the DNA sequence for that specific gene.

Most of the four hundred hereditary types of deafness are inherited in a recessive pattern. This means that a deaf or hard of hearing person must have the same gene variation from both parents, that is, two copies of the same gene, one from the mother and one from the father. In some cases, it may be possible to develop a genetic test for that gene. Using technologies from the Genome Project, techniques have been developed to examine specific genes to determine if there are variations associated with specific traits. For example, with a genetic test, it is sometimes possible for two deaf or hard of hearing people to better understand what type of genetic deafness they might have and what their chances may be for hearing or deaf children.

Connexin 26 is a specific gene for deafness that is very common in developed countries. This gene was first identified in 1997. In the United States and in European countries, 30 to 40 percent of all deaf people have this particular gene as the cause of their deafness. The connexin 26 gene is located on chromosome number 13. The inheritance pattern associated with this gene is called autosomal recessive, meaning in most situations the parents are hearing and carry one altered copy of this gene on one of their chromosomes (they are carriers of a deaf gene). If a child inherits two copies of this gene for deafness, the child is deaf or hard of hearing. In most situations, the parents never know that they are carriers before they have children. With each pregnancy, there is a one in four, or 25 percent, chance for those parents to have a deaf child. These parents may have one deaf child or several deaf children.

Because the connexin 26 gene is a common cause of deafness, it is fairly common for two deaf people, both of whom have connexin 26 deafness, to meet and have children together. All the children of such a couple will be deaf. This is an example of how genetic information can be very empowering. Knowledge about the inheritance of connexin 26 deafness can give people who have that type of deafness the power to choose whether they have deaf or hearing children, simply by their choice of partner. As more deaf and hard of hearing people learn about testing for this particular gene, and as more deaf babies are tested for this shortly after they are born, more will be learned about the choices that deaf and hearing parents will make based on the genetic information that is available to them.

People who want to know if they have connexin 26 as the cause of their deafness can be tested. There are many genetic centers in the United States and Europe where testing is available, and this service is offered at Gallaudet University. In one situation, a hearing couple with one deaf child requested prenatal testing on their second child to determine if that child would be deaf or hearing. Will this be more common in the future? The technology will allow both hearing parents and deaf parents to use these tests for this purpose. In the distant future, maybe years from now, gene therapy or drug-based therapies may have an impact on the deaf community.

It is hard to predict the impact of genetic technologies. These technologies will certainly have an impact on the diagnosis and treatment of common conditions such as cancer and heart disease as well as other rare genetic diseases. Will there be an impact on the deaf community in the future? Genetics information is very powerful and will allow both deaf and hearing people to make choices about future children. However, as with other genetic conditions, sometimes society as a whole, and in this case hearing society as a whole, may put pressure on deaf and hard of hearing individuals to make specific choices that may be choices that deaf and hard of hearing people do not want for their children. Health insurance companies and employers who pay for health insurance often try to dictate what choices people can make and what testing they can become involved in and force them to make certain choices. The good news is that the Human Genome Project has paid much attention to this area, and many states and the U.S. government have developed specific laws to protect individual people and their rights to make choices, whether that be a choice that society would support or not. Laws at the state and federal level are in place to prevent genetic discrimination.

The genetics programs at Gallaudet University and the Medical College of Virginia conducted a survey in 1999 to find out the attitudes of deaf and hard of hearing people about genetics technology. More than 300 people participated in this survey, including 62 members of the National Association of the Deaf, 126 deaf Gallaudet students, and 131 members of the Self Help for Hard of Hearing organization. These people identified themselves as deaf (40 percent), hard of hearing (42 percent), late deafened (7 percent), or hearing (11 percent). Thirty percent responded that they were bicultural and equally comfortable in the deaf and hearing communities. About 24 percent considered themselves part of the deaf community, and 46 percent part of the hearing community. The survey participants were asked to respond to this situation: "Suppose you or your partner were pregnant. Would you want a test to find out if the baby would be deaf, hard of hearing, or hearing before it was born?" Of the culturally deaf respondents, the vast majority (more than 65 percent) said they would *not* be interested in such a test (known as prenatal diagnosis). Of the bicultural respondents, about 50 percent said they would not be interested. For those who identified with hearing culture, about 30 percent said they would not be interested. Finally, respondents were asked why they would be interested in a prenatal diagnosis. The majority of people indicated that they would be interested in prenatal diagnosis to prepare for the needs of their child, to prepare for the language needs of their child, and to avoid medical tests for that child after the child was born. About 8 percent of the group said that they would consider abortion of a deaf baby. This group included individuals who identified with hearing culture and with deaf culture as well. About 3 percent said that they would consider abortion of a hard of hearing child. There were no individuals who would consider abortion of a hearing baby.

The future will bring even more advances in the ability to test for different genes for deafness. An important consideration in the future directions of genetics and the deaf community is to ensure that decisions about the availability of genetic testing be made by members of the deaf and hard of hearing community as well as people in the medical and health fields. The deaf and hard of hearing community should be involved and encourage the government to set enlightened policies. The more the members of the deaf community learns about genetics, the more power they have as individuals. They can then become empowered to make informed decisions about their future and the future of their children.

The medical community does not view deafness in the same way as the deaf community does. They view it as a disease. It is the responsibility of the deaf community to educate the medical community about deafness as a cultural condition and as a way of life. Members of the deaf community have a right to life, but all the stakeholders need to work together in cooperation with people in medical and research fields to make better decisions about how the government may choose to act with this new information so that the ethical use of genetics technology takes precedence. The more information deaf and hard of hearing people have as individuals about genetics, the better decisions they can make.

Questions and Answers

Question

Gallaudet is viewed as the leader within the deaf community. I understand that you all are doing research on genetic research and that you are leading that. I am wondering what sort of ethical principles you are using to conduct your research and what is your position on the genetic research that you are doing. I understand that you cannot predict what is going to be happening in the coming years; however, I am wondering where you are going with it. We obviously are concerned about what is going to happen in the future. I appreciate what you shared with us today. However, I would like to hear your position.

Answer

Any technology has implications and can be used in a positive or harmful way. The same is true with genetics. We focus on protecting human rights and the dignity of people. We cannot allow genetic technology to control our decisions. We certainly want to protect not only the rights of the deaf community, but the rights of all humans as well.

As a geneticist myself and working with the deaf community for almost the past twenty years, I know that individually many deaf people are very curious to know why they are deaf and to have information about themselves. As we said, this information can be very empowering for people. And as a geneticist I believe that individuals should have choices. They should be able to make choices, and those choices should not be dictated to them by other people. They should be able to make informed choices, and that is why we encourage people to learn as much about themselves in terms of the cause of their deafness and the implications for their children as possible. One very good thing about having a genetics center at Gallaudet for so long is that it has enabled us to initiate discussions with hundreds of deaf students about ethics, where this technology is leading us, and how they can become informed and knowledgeable, both about themselves personally and about the potential impact of this technology. We encourage deaf people to become more involved.

Question

I am from France, from Paris. There has been a considerable amount of research throughout the country into the whole area of deafness and genetics. The government of France has made links with those of the United States to carry out complementary research. But I am asking you, is it likely that there can be work between countries? I know that deaf people in France are very apprehensive about the research. We are very afraid the deaf community will disappear. Is this something that we can prevent? Is it something that working together with those of you in the United States we can work to contradict? I mean this is very new. This is new information for me in France. Are you sharing this information with other countries, particularly us in France?

Answer

It is important for all of us, regardless of what country we are in, to continue that research [on ethical implications]. We would be happy to share our studies with countries on an international level. In fact, the original studies of the attitudes of the deaf community toward genetic testing were done in Europe. Sharing this information is part of what Deaf Way II is all about. The National Association of the Deaf here in the United States has expressed interest in developing a position statement on this issue of genetics technology. Such a document could be the basis for discussion of this issue at the international level, and so that is a great point.

Question

I am from Britain. I have three questions. I was very interested in your presentation. I found it fascinating. But I have some anxieties. You were referring to hearing parents having given birth to deaf children and perhaps wanting to know whether their second child was going to be deaf. And they might then have an abortion. Is genetics that accurate that it can predict that? My second question: you put up a diagram of hearing parents who eventually gave birth to deaf children, and you identified connexin 26 as a factor. How many hearing people are actual carriers of connexin 26? Do we know? And third, what information do we have about connexin 26? I would like to know a lot more.

Answer

In the United States about one in thirty hearing people are carriers of the connexin 26 gene. In Spain, the number of hearing carriers is slightly higher than this. There is also a particular change in the connexin 26 gene that is very common in the Jewish population. About one in twenty-five people of Ashkenazi Jewish descent is a carrier of connexin 26. Prenatal testing for connexin 26 is currently possible and is offered in a few laboratories in the United States and Europe. We do not yet know the level of interest in prenatal diagnosis among hearing couples who have already had one child born deaf from connexin 26. It is possible that hearing parents who have experienced having a deaf child have a much more positive attitude than those parents who have never experienced that. That is to say, their interest in prenatal diagnosis of connexin 26 deafness may not be as high as it would be in hearing parents who have never had a deaf child.

WISDOM: Wireless Information Services for Deaf People on the Move

GUNNAR HELLSTRÖM

Wireless multimedia developments offer great opportunities for better accessibility to communication and information for deaf users. A European project called WISDOM is developing mobile terminals and services specifically aimed at deaf people's needs. Figure 1 shows a WISDOM terminal.

The terminal has enhanced mobile videophone functionality. It implements the total conversation concept, providing video, text, and voice communication, and aims to improve personal communication. It provides simultaneous real-time communication in the following media:

- ❖ Video, enabling fluent signed conversations or lipreading-supported voice communication.
- ❖ Character-by-character text communication, for fallback to text for single words or for performing the whole conversation in text.
- ❖ Speech, to complete the opportunities for all.

Figure 2 shows a typical total conversation user interface with video and text. The 3G mobile services make this important functionality possible, and the WISDOM project makes it happen.

The communication environment is composed of a set of services that are important to deaf users:

- ❖ Real-time conversation in sign language, lipreading, writing, and speech.
- ❖ Video relay service, forming a convenient link between sign language users and voice telephone users by translating between sign language and spoken language.
- ❖ Distant interpreter service, offering interpreting between sign language and speech for small meetings.
- ❖ Interworking with text telephones in the fixed telephone network.
- ❖ Internet access for the Web and e-mail.

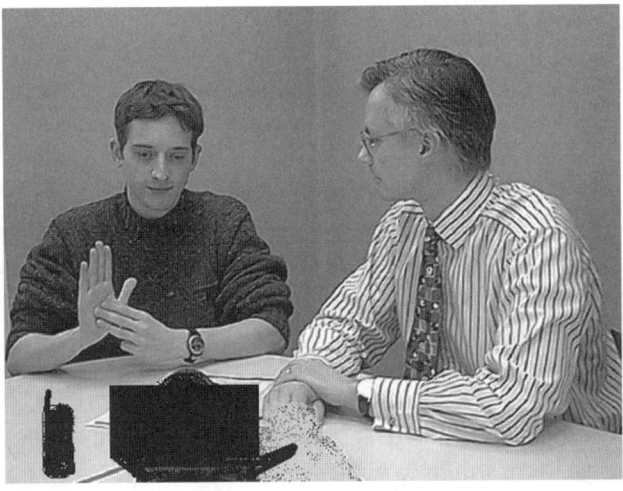

FIGURE 1: A WISDOM terminal

❖ Video information services where sign-language-based information can be retrieved.
❖ Sign language recognition to be researched, developed, and tried for control of the video information services.

With this package of services available from a handy terminal, it is expected that deaf people will have improved access to information and communication anywhere. It will be a big step toward equal opportunities for communication.

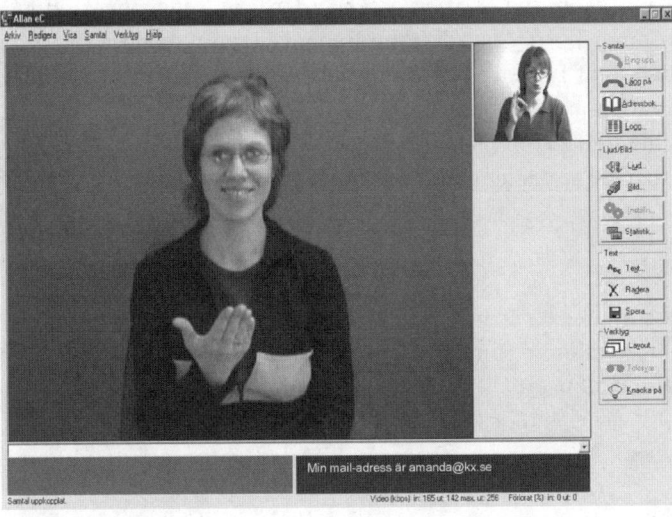

FIGURE 2: A total conversation user interface

The terminal will come in different shapes in the project. Specifically developed dedicated mobile terminals will be tried, as well as general-purpose, powerful small computers with built-in cameras, equipped with IP-based Total Conversation software.

Challenges include the following:

- to achieve sufficient video quality for signing through the 3G mobile network;
- to have enough processing power for good compression of video; and
- to make the right compromise in size, weight, power, and battery duration.

The project is partly funded by the European Commission within the Information Society Technologies (IST) program, number IST-2000-27512. Ten organizations from the United Kingdom, Sweden, Germany, and Spain, with strong deaf involvement, cooperate as a consortium to implement the WISDOM vision for its field trials during year 2003.

WISDOM aims to demonstrate models for deaf communication in future mobile and wireless networks.

Standards

One important goal of WISDOM is to contribute to standardization of telecommunications with features of value for deaf users. Standardization is an important way to make communication equipment of different types work well together. Some results of these activities are as follows:

- Validation of the quality requirements for video communication for sign language and lipreading; ITU-T H series supplement 1 states, for example, that twenty pictures or more per second are needed for good sign language communication.
- Contribution to the creation of a standard for total conversation in 3G networks, in 3GPP TS 26.235 IP multimedia, default codecs.
- Validation of gateway principles between mobile IP multimedia text communication and text telephony, as described in ITU-T H.248.2. This made it possible to have text telephone conversations between 3G mobile terminals and regular text telephones in the telephone network.

Conclusion

WISDOM was a forerunner in wireless sign language communication for deaf users and demonstrated the importance of providing wireless sign language communication services for deaf people. The first 3G networks are at the threshold of being usable for signing. By using wireless land area network connections, where available, for good quality and 3G for wider coverage, an important service can be created for deaf users.

References

International Telecommunications Union. 2000. Requirements on narrowband video communication for sign language and lipreading. ITU-T H-series Supplement 1, ITU-T. Geneva: Author.

International Telecommunications Union. 2000. Call discrimination, fax, text, and text telephony packages: ITU-T H.248.2. Geneva: Author.

3GPP. 2001. IP multimedia, default codecs: 3GPP TS 26.235. Retrieved from http://www.3gpp.org/ftp/Specs/html-info/26235.htm.

Telecommunications Access: An American Civil Right

KAREN PELTZ STRAUSS AND GREGORY HLIBOK

Telecommunications access in America has changed dramatically over the past decade. Much of this is due to new and innovative technologies, including e-mail, the Internet, and paging services, but much is also the result of new federal laws specifically designed to ensure telecommunications access for people with disabilities. Many, if not all, of these laws were secured with the understanding that telecommunications access is a civil right for all Americans, including Americans who are deaf and hard of hearing. As a vital link to jobs, education, news, entertainment, emergency services, and social activities, the ability to fully access our telecommunications technologies has become critical to the ability to lead an independent and productive life. We discuss the various laws that are making this possible.

Closed Captioning

Closed captioning provides visual text for the dialogue, sound effects, and background noise of a video program. A federal law—the Telecommunications Act of 1996—requires new television programs that are provided via broadcast, cable, satellite, and other distributors to be "fully" accessible through closed captioning. The law also requires video programming providers to "maximize" access to older television programs. The law covers television programs only—it does not cover home or educational videos, CD-ROMs, the Web, DVDs, or movies shown in theaters.

In 1997, the Federal Communications Commission (FCC)—the U.S. federal agency charged with overseeing telecommunications matters—issued a schedule to phase in captioned television. This schedule requires nearly all English-language programming shown on or after January 1998 to be captioned as of January 1, 2006. Of the programming shown before 1998, called "pre-rule programming," 75 percent must be captioned by 2008. Spanish-language programming is given additional time to achieve compliance: twelve years for newer programming first shown after January 1998 and fourteen years for programming first shown before that time.

Companies that are required to increase captioning are allowed to limit their captioning spending to 2 percent of their annual gross revenues. In addition, captioning is not required on programs which are shown between 2 a.m. and 6 a.m. local time, commercials less than five minutes long, public service announcements, and certain local programming, other than local news, that is not likely to be repeated. Video programming providers with revenues of less than $3 million per year also are not covered by the captioning rules, and any provider may request the FCC to exempt individual programs or networks if it can prove that supplying captions would cause it to experience an "undue burden."

Although there are some requirements in place to require real-time captioning for live news programs in large cities, for the most part the FCC's rules permit local stations to use news scripts provided on teleprompters, which are then converted into captioning text (which is also known as the electronic newsroom technique). This has been of concern to the deaf community, because teleprompter script does not capture late-breaking stories, field reports, or most weather or sports reports.

In the United States, the Television Circuitry Decoder Act of 1990 requires television sets with screens that are thirteen inches or larger to have closed caption decoders built into their circuitry. The law also requires that new television technologies support closed captioning. In July of 2000, the FCC adopted technical standards for the display of closed captioning on digital television (DTV) receivers. These standards, in effect as of July of 2002, could allow viewers to control the font, size, background colors, and foreground colors of captions. DTV receivers could also display multiple channels of captions for varying reading abilities.

Emergency Access

There are various legal protections to ensure that individuals who are deaf and hard of hearing have access to emergency information.

Telephone Access to Emergency Services

In the United States, public safety answering points (PSAPs) respond to telephone calls seeking emergency police, fire, and ambulance services. Most towns and cities offer direct voice telephone access to PSAPs through 9-1-1 dialing. Under Title II of the Americans with Disabilities Act (ADA), where 9-1-1 PSAP dialing is available, text telephone (TTY) users must be able to call that number to receive prompt emergency assistance. These callers do not need to go through relay services or a separate, longer telephone number.

Some communities have PSAPs that do not offer 9-1-1 dialing. Where a longer number is needed to access emergency services, PSAPs must still offer direct, TTY access to their services. In addition, not all individuals who use TTYs choose to call PSAPs directly. Some TTY users prefer to go through relay services for all their calls, even calls involving emergencies. If a relay center receives an emergency call, it must immediately and automatically transfer that call to the appropriate PSAP.

In addition to the ADA's mandate for TTY access to PSAPs, the FCC requires digital wireless systems to be able to handle enhanced 9-1-1 TTY calls. Several years ago, the FCC addressed this matter in a proceeding that required the wireless industry to provide enhanced 9-1-1 service, a service that enables PSAPs to ascertain the number and location of a caller when an emergency call is made over a wireless service. Specifically, the FCC directed the wireless industry to develop technical solutions to enable TTY transmissions to be carried over various wireless technologies (e.g., CDMA, TDMA, and GSM) so that these transmissions could reach the PSAPs. A consumer-industry forum set up for this purpose succeeded in developing compatibility solutions after several years of intensive efforts.

Television Access to Emergency Information

FCC rules require all audio emergency information presented on television to be visually accessible to people who are deaf or hard of hearing. The FCC defines emergency information as information that is televised to further the protection of life, health, safety, or property in dangerous situations such as floods, tornadoes, earthquakes, explosions, and criminal activity. This information must be provided visually and must include critical details regarding the emergency itself and how to respond, including information about shelters, evacuation routes, and school closings.

The FCC's emergency rules cover broadcasters, cable operators, satellite television services, and other video programming distributors. Closed captioning is the preferred method, but other methods are acceptable as well. These include open captioning, crawls, or scrolls that appear on the screen. Unlike the closed captioning rules discussed previously, there are *no exemptions* to the requirement that emergency information be made accessible to deaf viewers.

Telecommunications Relay Service

Telecommunications relay services enable people with hearing and speech disabilities to communicate by telephone with people who may or may not have such disabilities. Under Title IV of the Americans with Disabilities Act, all telephone companies have been required to provide relay services throughout the United States, free of charge, since July 1993.

There are now several types of relay services in the United States. Text-to-voice relay, required under FCC law, uses operators, called communications assistants (CAs), to relay conversations between individuals who use TTYs or computer modems and voice telephones. Speech-to-speech services, also mandated, use specially trained individuals to relay calls by or to individuals with difficult-to-understand speech. Spanish-language relay services, which relay calls between users of these services in Spanish, are required for interstate telephone services only but may also be provided within states that determine they have a need for these services.

Another type of relay service, video relay services, uses sign language interpreters and video equipment to interpret calls between American Sign Language (ASL) users and other individuals. Video relay services are not required by federal law; however, companies that provide this service may be reimbursed through the interstate relay fund. Internet protocol relay is yet another type of relay service that is authorized, though not mandated. Internet relay allows individuals to use their computers or portable devices to send relay text over the Internet. Finally, captioned telephone relay services can allow individuals to both hear (with their residual hearing) and read the message of the other party to the call.

FCC rules require relay services to be "functionally equivalent" to voice telephone services. This means that companies providing these services must meet minimum standards of relay quality, including service twenty-four hours a day, seven days a week; an appropriate speed of answer; a typing speed of at least sixty words per minute; the provision of skilled CAs; and access to emergency services.

The FCC allows the fifty states and the U.S. territories to provide relay services on behalf of telephone companies. To be permitted to provide relay services, a state must meet all of the FCC's minimum standards and provide relay service both within its state and to any other location in America. In addition to state relay programs, there are a few American long-distance telephone companies that compete with one another to provide long-distance relay service. Relay services provided within states are mostly funded by adding a few cents each month to the bills of all the telephone users within those states. Funding for relay calls between the states is provided through a fee that interstate telephone companies must pay, based on their revenues.

The FCC requires all telephone (wireline and wireless) companies nationwide to provide three-digit, 7-1-1 dialing to access all relay services. As noted previously, most states have their own relay service. As a consequence, in the past, it was very difficult for relay users who traveled to know what number to use when they wanted to call relay services in any given state. 7-1-1 access eliminates this problem for travelers and makes TRS access more convenient, fast, and uncomplicated. Some states have also reported that hearing people have used relay services more since 7-1-1 went into effect. Individuals are more likely to return calls to TTY users if they have an easy-to-remember number to dial.

Hearing Aid Compatibility

Wireline Telephones

The Hearing Aid Compatibility Act of 1988 has required all wireline telephones sold in the United States to be hearing aid compatible (HAC) since August of 1989. Under this act, phones must build compatibility into the phone itself; an add-on device or external accessory is not enough to meet the requirements of the act. Under FCC rules, HAC phones must emit magnetic impulses that are picked up by hearing aids with telecoils. The telecoil allows the hearing aid user to eliminate background and feedback noise so that he or she can hear more clearly. FCC rules also require workplaces, hotels, hospitals, prisons, and other institutions to install HAC phones. These latter rules are intended to ensure that certain phones sold before August of 1989 are also compatible with hearing aids. In addition, FCC rules have required all wireline telephones to have volume control since January 2000.

Wireless Telephones

When the U.S. Congress passed the HAC Act, it decided to temporarily exclude wireless telephones from the HAC requirement. Although analog wireless phones are generally HAC anyway, many digital phones are not accessible to hearing aid users because of the interference that occurs when such phones interact with hearing aids. Hearing aid users are concerned about the lack of access to digital phones because (1) digital wireless service is gradually replacing analog service and (2) digital service and handsets offer superior service quality, additional features, and more attractive pricing than do analog systems.

The HAC Act directed the FCC to periodically review the wireless exemption and to eliminate the exemption if the following conditions were met: (1) eliminating the exemption is in the public interest; (2) the exemption would have "an adverse effect" on individuals with hearing disabilities; (3) wireless compliance with the HAC requirement is technologically feasible; and (4) compliance would not hurt the successful marketing of wireless telephones.[1]

Section 255

Section 255 of the Communications Act, enacted by Congress in the Telecommunications Act of 1996, requires telecommunications manufacturers and service providers to make their equipment and services accessible to people with disabilities where readily achievable. Where it is not readily achievable to do so, manufacturers and providers must make these products and services compatible with specialized equipment (e.g., TTYs, artificial larynxes) that is commonly used by persons with disabilities, if doing so is readily achievable. To comply with Section 255, companies must consider the access needs of people with disabilities in the design, development, and manufacture of their products. Section 255 covers virtually any and all types of telecommunications equipment: telephones, fax machines, answering machines, and so forth. In addition, it covers all basic and "adjunct-to-basic" telephone services, such as call waiting, call forwarding, and caller ID. Section 255 also requires access to voice mail and interactive telephone menus. Finally, a separate section of the Communications Act, Section 251, prohibits telephone providers from installing network features, functions, or capabilities that do not comply with the Section 255 guidelines. In 1998, the FCC issued rules to implement Section 255. At the same time, the FCC began a proceeding to examine the extent to which IP telephony (telephone calls made over the Internet) and personal computers used for telecommunications are also covered under Section 255. This proceeding remains open at this time.

Some manufacturers and providers have begun to implement Section 255 by developing offices of accessibility and incorporating accessible design into some of their products and services. Others have done little to implement the law. Consumers wishing to file complaints about telecommunications services and products that are not accessible may do so with the Consumer and Governmental Affairs Bureau of the FCC.

Section 508

Section 508 of the Rehabilitation Act requires each U.S. agency to procure, use, and maintain electronic and information technology (E&IT) that is accessible to

---

1. In August 2003, after the Deaf Way II Conference but before the completion of this essay, the FCC issued rules requiring certain wireless phones to be compatible with hearing aids.

(1) federal employees with disabilities and (2) individuals with disabilities outside the federal government who need government information, unless doing so would impose an undue burden on the agency. Examples of E&IT include telecommunications equipment, computers (hardware and software), Web-based applications (including governmental Internet sites), information kiosks, videotapes, and office equipment such as copiers and fax machines. Section 508 is overseen by a federal agency called the Architectural and Transportation Barriers Compliance Board, also called the Access Board, which issued guidelines governing Section 508 compliance in June 2001. Federal agencies must now use the Access Board's guidelines to revise their own policies for procuring and using E&IT.

Consumers hope and expect that because the federal government purchases E&IT in very large quantities, major manufacturers of E&IT will now need to develop more accessible products. It is also hoped that the availability of more accessible equipment will improve employment opportunities for federal employees and make it easier for the general public to get access to governmental information.

Conclusion

Prior to the telecommunications access movement of the 1990s, Americans who were deaf and hard of hearing were typically denied access to telecommunications technologies. The successes gained over the past decade have begun to level the playing field with respect to the provision of telecommunications services. However, significant changes in the way that people all over the world communicate and obtain information continue to take place. Greater reliance on new types of technologies—computer technologies, the Internet, and broadband gateways—are raising new concerns about accessibility by individuals who are deaf and hard of hearing. Because these newer technologies are generally considered "information" rather than "telecommunications" technologies, they may not be covered under any of the federal laws that already exist. Efforts must be taken to protect and maintain access, as our nation joins others in moving to these and other advanced technologies.

Additional information about each of the federal laws discussed here is available at the Web site of the FCC's Disabilities Rights Office of the Consumer and Governmental Affairs Bureau: www.fcc.gov/cgb/dro.

Accessible Educational Media: Research, Development, and Standards

LARRY GOLDBERG, MADELEINE ROTHBERG, AND MARY WATKINS

The CPB/WGBH National Center for Accessible Media (NCAM; http://ncam.wgbh.org) is a research and development facility dedicated to the issues of media technology for people with disabilities in their homes, schools, workplaces, and communities. It is part of the Media Access Group at Boston public broadcaster WGBH. In addition to NCAM, the Media Access Group at WGBH consists of the Caption Center, established in 1972 as the first television captioning agency, and the Descriptive Video Service, established in 1990 as the first agency to make television and videos accessible to people who are blind or have low vision.

NCAM's mission is to expand access to present and future media; to explore how existing access technologies may benefit other populations; to represent its constituents in industry, policy, and legislative circles; and to provide access to educational and media technologies for special needs students.

NCAM is also pioneering the use of accessible multimedia, both on the Web and in the classroom, through projects that educate software and hardware developers, empower students and teachers, design new media access devices and procedures, and in general help assure that everyone can reap the benefits of electronic and educational media.

This essay provides an overview of several NCAM projects relating to education, including curriculum development, distance learning, and accessible multimedia, and includes information about the Media Access Generator (MAGpie), NCAM's freely available software for adding access features to digital multimedia.

Cornerstones: Building Blocks of Literacy

Cornerstones is a technology-infused approach to literacy development for early elementary children who are deaf or hard of hearing. Academic experts in literacy and deafness, along with teachers of deaf students, helped us develop an instructional approach that is demanding, engaging, research-based, and flexible for use with children who have a range of backgrounds, communication needs, and skills.

We are concerned with three key areas of literacy:

1. identification of words in print,
2. in-depth knowledge of words, and
3. story comprehension.

An essential element of Cornerstones is a story taken from PBS's literacy series *Between the Lions*, complemented by versions of the story in American Sign Language (ASL) and other visual-spatial systems for communicating with deaf children, such as Signing Exact English and cued speech. Other materials include a hypertext version of the story, an electronic storybook where children can click on a word to see a picture, example, or other meaning; clip art of target words; and supplementary games and activities. A teacher's guide includes a day-by-day sequence of rigorous learning objectives and lessons, with recommended instructional practices.

The Cornerstones Project developed a sample teaching unit for teachers to try out in their classrooms. We refined this sample unit; the resulting prototype Cornerstones unit is now available at ncam.wgbh.org/cornerstones. Cornerstones was featured in *Reading Online*, a journal of K–12 practice and research published by the International Reading Association (www.readingonline.org). Project staff conducted field tests and a pilot evaluation in 2000. A more rigorous evaluation took place in 2002 and 2003.

Funding for the Cornerstones project is provided by the U.S. Department of Education's Office of Special Education Programs.

Research on Edited Captions

The project is evaluating effects of edited captions—captions with a slower presentation rate and modified language—on comprehension. For many deaf children, reading is a frustrating experience, and reading captions is challenging. The goal of edited captions is to help children who are not fluent readers have greater success reading captions and understanding a program. If the research results support our hypothesis, this would argue for a second stream of captions on selected children's television programs, in addition to the original near-verbatim captions. Media with edited captions could be a new source of age-appropriate materials that match children's reading abilities.

The project is a collaboration between NCAM and researchers at Ohio State University.

The research questions are as follows:

1. Is there a difference in children's comprehension scores between the near-verbatim and edited videos?
2. Is there an effect due to the type of assessment used?
3. What are the children's preferences and attitudes with respect to the captioned programs in the study and to captioned media in general?

The study is using *Arthur*, an Emmy-award winning and extremely popular children's program on public television. Under a separate agreement with the U.S. Department of Education, all existing episodes of *Arthur* have two sets of captions, near-verbatim and edited.

The project is developing a set of videotapes for the study, half with edited captions and half with original, near-verbatim captions. We will set up after-school *Arthur* Clubs at up to eight New England schools, involving a total of thrity-eight children. Participating children will be between seven and eleven years old and read at a 2.0 reading level or higher.

During each club session, children will watch an *Arthur* program with either edited or near-verbatim captions, and an examiner will assess each child on his or her comprehension of the story. There will be two types of assessments—one known as QAR, question-answer relationships, and a retell format—to reduce the possibility of the assessment influencing comprehension scores. Approximately three-quarters of the students will be part of a group design, and the remaining students will be part of a single-subject design. Both the caption condition—edited and near-verbatim—and the assessment—QAR and retell—will be randomized. The project will also gather qualitative information and preferences about children's attitudes toward captioned media.

Funding for the Research on Edited Captions project is provided by the U.S. Department of Education's Office of Special Education Programs.

Access to PIVoT

NCAM is engaged in a collaboration with the Massachusetts Institute of Technology's Center for Advanced Educational Services (http://www.ceci.mit.edu/projects/pivot/) to make an online interactive physics course accessible to students with disabilities. Known as Access to PIVoT (Physics Interactive Video Tutor), this project is testing, implementing, documenting, and promoting the development of multimedia access solutions to make distance learning accessible to blind, low-vision, deaf, and hard of hearing students.

The Access to PIVoT project is built around MIT Professor Walter Lewin's popular introductory physics class. Web-based components include a complete digitized library of Professor Lewin's physics lectures as well as dozens of help sessions, interactive demonstrations and simulations, quizzes, and a full online textbook. Using the questions provided in an extensive FAQ list, students can choose second- and third-level follow-up questions, invoking appropriately linked video responses by the professor. Students will be able to get even more detailed information by typing in questions and receiving responses from an online teaching assistant.

The goals of the project are to enable science-focused high school and college students who are blind, visually impaired, deaf, or hard of hearing to participate in an innovative and challenging Web-based introductory physics curriculum; enable the MIT Center for Advanced Educational Services to institutionalize the technical capabilities developed through this project to apply access solutions to a range of future educational products; and provide developers, publishers, and distributors of distance-learning and educational multimedia with recommended practices and an applied demonstration of access-design principles for network-delivered multimedia.

Project activities include identifying the needs of deaf and blind students in the design of the user interface, navigation systems, and presentation of video, text, illustrations, graphs and tables; researching and evaluating the practical use of current and emerging solutions to provide access for blind or deaf students; developing and implementing a training and production plan to apply solutions to PIVoT; developing a set of recommended practices for design and implementation of access solutions in network-delivered educational multimedia; disseminating recommended practices; and publicizing project results.

Building upon NCAM's ongoing research into Web-based multimedia accessibility, the PIVoT project has developed a method for students to create captions and audio descriptions for the video tutorials on the Web site using MAGpie (NCAM's Media Access Generator tool). Testing and evaluation with disabled and nondisabled students and professionals is helping to gauge the usefulness of these accessibility enhancements. Please visit the PIVoT Web site at NCAM (http://ncam.wgbh.org/webaccess/pivot/index.html) for more information.

Funding for Access to PIVoT is provided by the National Science Foundation and by the Mitsubishi Electric America Foundation.

Specifications for Accessible Learning Technologies: The SALT Partnership

The Specifications for Accessible Learning Technologies (SALT) Partnership is a four-year initiative, which began in December 2000, focused on developing and promoting open access specifications and effective models that will enable people with disabilities to have equal access to the growing wealth of online learning resources.

NCAM is working closely with the IMS Global Learning Consortium, a worldwide coalition of more than 250 member organizations developing technical specifications for online learning. In early 2001, NCAM and IMS established an industry-led Accessibility Working Group to identify the features needed to make online learning accessible and to specify the resources and technologies needed to implement solutions. The IMS Accessibility Working Group is engaging leading companies involved in product development and institutions implementing distributed learning environments.

The IMS Accessibility Working Group has issued an initial draft of a set of accessibility guidelines targeted at the online distributed learning community, which are available from the IMS Web site (www.imsglobal.org). The group is concurrently working to add accessibility extensions to the IMS Learner Information Profile (LIP) specification and to the IMS Meta-data specification. The proposed additions will make it possible for learning systems to select and adapt content to ensure accessibility for learners with disabilities. Several industry partners have committed to serve as early adopters of specifications. With NCAM's help, technology providers will work with publishers to enable and implement access features within platforms, applications, and content.

Specifications will involve and serve organizations developing learning resources, learning systems, and the entire community of public and private online distributed learning companies. Results will impact the accessibility of online resources in every conceivable learning environment, including K–12, vocational and postsecondary education, the government and the military, and faculty development and workplace training.

Funding for the SALT Partnership is provided by the Learning Anytime Anywhere Partnerships program of the Fund for the Improvement of Postsecondary Education (FIPSE), Office of Postsecondary Education, U.S. Department of Education.

MAGpie

Developers of Web- and CD-ROM-based multimedia need an authoring application for making their materials accessible to people with sensory disabilities. The Media Access Generator (MAGpie), NCAM's digital captioning application, allows authors to add captions and audio descriptions to multimedia in two formats used by several popular players. MAGpie 2.0 is a Java-based tool, so it works nearly identically on both the PC (Windows 9x, 2000, NT, and Millennium Edition) and Macintosh (initially OS X, but subsequent versions will support earlier Macintosh operating systems). With more and more online distance-learning Web sites taking advantage of multimedia, MAGpie could have a significant impact on the amount of multimedia that is accessible to deaf, hard of hearing, blind, and visually impaired users.

Funding for MAGpie 2.0 is provided by the Mitsubishi Electric America Foundation; the National Institute on Disability and Rehabilitation Research (NIDRR), U.S. Department of Education; and the Trace Research and Development Center at the University of Wisconsin. MAGpie may be downloaded at no charge from ncam.wgbh.org/webaccess/magpie.

Further Information

NCAM's Access to Rich Media project (ncam.wgbh.org/richmedia) is an excellent resource for anyone interested in learning more about MAGpie and accessible multimedia. Visitors to this site will find a listing of applications used to create various types of multimedia, tutorials on creating captioned and described movies, and information on current research to help developers understand and deal with accessibility issues. Tutorials on adding captions and audio descriptions to multimedia, and making other forms of rich media accessible, may be found here, as well. Finally, users may download MAGpie or view many examples of accessible multimedia, many of which were created with MAGpie.

Funding for the Rich Media Accessibility resource center is provided by the National Institute on Disability and Rehabilitation Research (NIDRR; www.ed.gov/offices/OSERS/NIDRR), U.S. Department of Education.

PART TWELVE

Youth

Climbing the Seven Summits: A Deaf Woman's Dream

HEIDI ZIMMER

This conference is a celebration much like taking on the challenge of the seven summits. The "summits" refer to the highest peak in each of the seven continents. My goal is to climb all seven. I have completed three.

When I was young, my family lived in an old house that was built between 1915 and 1919 in Tempe, Arizona, next to a church on one side and the Arizona State University on the other, all on the same block. The house is no longer there. But when I was two years old, my mother let me out of the house one day to play in the yard. Later on, my mother could not find me because I wandered off. She went into complete panic, as any parent would. Well, I was up on the roof of the house. Of course, I nearly gave her a heart attack. She immediately called my father, who was over at the church, but he was afraid of heights. They noticed a student from the university walking by, and they asked for his assistance. He brought me down off the roof. I think that might have been the moment when I first became inspired to climb mountains.

There is also a famous book and film called *Heidi* about this a young girl who very much adored her grandfather, who lived in the mountains of Switzerland. Well, I was named Heidi, and that certainly was a perfect match to my lifestyle. It gave me additional inspiration in my life. I have been in Switzerland and actually seen the mountains described in this classic novel. The quote from that book that always inspires me is, "I will climb the mountain someday."

I have been involved in a variety of sports activities, including volleyball and track and field teams, during my junior high school, high school, and university years. I was fortunate to be selected on the U.S. team for the World Deaf Games in 1969 and 1973. I won third place in high jump in Yugoslavia in 1969. Such experiences of competition have continued to daily challenge and inspire me, physically and mentally.

One of my role models was a former teacher of mine, Dr. Lawrence Newman, who taught mathematics at the high school level at the California School for the Deaf—Riverside. He was also a former president of the National Association of the Deaf. He has always kept on saying to me, "Do it! You can do it!" He talked to me a great deal about the success a Deaf person can achieve and shared a number of stories and biographies of successful Deaf people as examples from the book *Deaf Heritage:*

A Narrative History of Deaf America, authored by Jack Gannon. At first I did not necessarily give it the kind of attention or interest that I should have, but after Newman repeatedly showed examples of successful Deaf leaders, my attention and interest eventually grew. At first, I did not necessarily want to be a leader myself, but he often challenged me to think differently.

My decision to climb the seven highest world mountains did not happen overnight. However, when I decided to take it on, I knew I had to consider it as a personal challenge, and I will always be very grateful for Dr. Newman for inspiring me to keep on challenging myself when I was young. It also was important to take on one mountain at a time and to realize that each climbing experience was of great value for the next climb.

I have read books on hiking and climbing. The one book that gives me the most inspiration is *Seven Summits*, written by Dick Bass, Frank Wells, and Rick Ridgeway (1988). The book is about their quest to reach the highest peaks on all seven continents. The book mentions that there were seventy-five international climbers who had reached the highest peaks. I often would go through this book to consider the different expeditions I would take and what would be the next one I would do. Now, Bass was a very wealthy man who owned a company and a ski resort, and he had done a number of climbs personally. At the time the book was written, Bass, during his fifties, was the oldest man to ever stand on top of the Everest summit.

Since then, Sherman Bull, a sixty-four-year-old guy from the state of Connecticut, became the oldest climber to reach the summit of Mount Everest. The oldest woman ever to reach the summit of Mount Everest was Yasuko Nambo, a forty-seven-year-old Japanese businesswoman, who unfortunately died on the mountain during the disaster of May 10, 1996. When I looked at the roster of various people who had climbed the various peaks, I noticed that no Deaf or disabled individuals had ever reached any one of the seven summits. So, at fifty years old, I took the challenge upon myself to be the first Deaf person and oldest woman to ever climb *all* seven summits.

Let me tell you about my actual climbing experience while on the Denali expedition in Alaska (North America). *Denali* actually is a term in a Native American language to denote height, meaning "the high one." Professional climbers and I like to refer to this mountain range by its native name, Denali, although it was later named Mt. McKinley after one of our former U.S. presidents. We needed to take a thirty-minute flight in a small plane from the airport at the foothills into a base camp higher up the mountains. We had to depart quickly so the plane could return and bring additional climbers before the weather got bad. There was a ranger's station there that looked like the shape of a hangar, where the radio controller could communicate with the airport at the foothills. We could not always land when we wanted to because of the weather, so some of us had to wait until the weather conditions improved before the entire expedition team could be transported to the base camp.

We had horrible weather, and so the guide decided that we had to do this expedition in twenty-five days. There were six people. Our equipment was weight-limited in accordance to each individual's weight and strength. We had to be strong enough to carry whatever we needed with us. Each of us had about a sixty-five- to seventy-five-pound pack, and there was a twenty-five- to thirty-pound sled to pull. We also had a rope that connected the climbers at thirty-foot intervals.

Our field rope has to be set up to keep three people together in each team as we started the climb. You may wonder why there was such a distance from one climber to the next. This is because often we encounter crevices. The crevices could vary from only a hundred to more than a thousand feet deep and are very dangerous, and so we wanted to keep a fair amount of distance from one climber to the next for safety reasons.

Our first task was to haul food and equipment from the base camp to another campsite on higher ground. Now, it would be impossible to bring all our food and equipment from one base camp up to the higher campsite in one day, because there were lots of things to bring. We had to identify certain food and equipment we would not immediately need, bring them up to the higher campsite, bury them in snow, and mark the site with flags so that we would know exactly where they were for later use. Then we had to return to the lower base camp and pick up the remaining food and equipment to bring to the higher campsite on the next day.

After the second trip to the higher campsite, we needed to set up a "kitchen." With the high altitude and the frozen temperature, it would take a great deal of time to melt ice into enough water to fill two bottles for each of six climbers. We needed to take the time to do that and make sure we were hydrated and had enough to eat and drink throughout the day. Again, we had to plan ahead, basically take what we had buried, brought it to the surface, and prepared the meal. Then we had to shovel a small hole for the tents, so that they could be somewhat buried to avoid collapsing or blowing away under strong winds, which ranged from fifty to eighty mph overnight. It was exhausting to bring your pack and all the equipment, do some cooking and shoveling, and then finally get the tent set up. It was quite a long series of events. Finally at the end of second day, we were able to have some rest. Before I went to bed, I always made a journal entry of our experiences.

We actually stayed at the higher campsite for two days to acclimate to the increased altitude before we started to do the strenuous climbing exercise. Now, higher up the angle of the slope would be at forty-five degrees or steeper, and so it was going to be quite a difficult day of climbing. Thus it was important to give our bodies the opportunity to adjust before we would be ready to move on to the next site higher up. Once our team arrived at a given site, the first person to arrive would not take off the rope until the last member of the team arrived. The process was repeated from one site to the next site higher up.

We then set up camp. Each of our tents was small, about three feet high. It turned out we had to stay in our tents for four days because of extreme weather and winds. The first day, I was overjoyed to get the rest I needed after several days of difficult climbing. On the second day, I immediately became terribly restless from being cooped up in the small tent. Communication was limited, because no one knew sign language. Also, I had run out of books to read. There were no TTY calls to make. I became crazier on subsequent days, and by the fourth day, I was basically out of my mind. We were trapped in these tents. We could roll over but we could not even stand up. Every hour we needed to take turns going out and digging the snow off our tents so that they would not collapse under the weight of accumulated snow. This was the last campsite before we actually took on the summit.

We certainly had quite the celebration when we finally reached the summit on June 13, 1991, at 5 p.m. It was sad for me in some ways that the people who could hear could call down and let their friends and family know they had reached the summit. I wish I had some video technology so that I could do the same and inform my friends and colleagues through the Internet that I, too, had reached the summit. If any of you are particularly gifted with technology, let me know if you could come up a way for me to spread the word from the top.

Anyway, it required lots of hard work and eighteen days to go from the base camp to the summit, but we were able to enjoy the view from the top for only five minutes! This is because we needed to quickly get back down to the last campsite before night when strong winds would arrive again. Many people asked how I felt about that climb, because I was able to stay on the top for only five minutes. My response was that my achievement gave me immense pleasure. I felt victorious. I was the first deaf woman to reach the Denali summit. I overcame many personal, emotional, and physical challenges along the way, which meant that nothing could stop me from accomplishing anything I wanted to do in life.

Next, I am going to briefly describe my second accomplishment with the Mt. Elbrus expedition in Russia (Europe), near the Black Sea area. Elbrus is a Slavic term for "white mountain." To get to the base camp, we needed to ride in a tram up and over rocky surface with some snow to a higher level on the mountain, then we got on a ski lift with our backpacks to yet another higher level, and then we got on a snow vehicle to bring us up to a certain higher point, at which we then had to go on foot a long way up the gentle slope to the base camp.

Now, this was very different from Denali, where we had to carry so much equipment and do all the hard work in setting up campsites in bitter cold climate. Instead, we had to spend a great deal of time hiking and climbing from point A to point B in a relatively mild climate. At the base camp, there was an oval-shaped hut the size of a small cabin along with bunk beds for us to sleep in. Again, we had to acclimate, staying for two days at the hut before we could move onto the summit on the third day, and then arrive back at the hut again on the fourth day.

On the third day, August 15, 1992, we woke up at 2 a.m. and actually left by 3:00 a.m. It was a beautiful trek because there was a full moon, and we could actually see our paths and the contours by the light of the moon. It was certainly an exhilarating experience. Some of us arrived at the summit before others did, and we were able to stay on the top for about an hour to enjoy the 360-degree view.

The third peak I climbed was at Mt. Kilimanjaro in Tanzania (Africa). Kilimanjaro means "great mountain" in the Tanzanian language. The mountain is unique in that its vegetation zones change with the increase in elevation after a few hours of walking along the climbing route. It starts out in a jungle-like forest, then becomes moorland, then alpine desert, and then an ice cap on the way to the Uhuru peak. *Uhuru*, in Tanzanian, means "freedom." Kilimanjaro is not in any mountain range, and it is known as the highest, single, isolated peak in the world. There is also a crater on one side of the top of the mountain.

Climbing the Seven Summits

We took the Marangu route to reach the Kilimanjaro summit, namely the Uhuru peak, on September 22, 1994. There were only three of us that went together. I went up the mountain with a porter and a guide. Neither spoke English. Neither had ever met a deaf person before, but we got along very well quickly. We were able to communicate through gestures to get our points across.

We got up at midnight. Again, luckily, there was a full moon, and we could enjoy the views all the way to the top. We had a great 360-degree view and could also view the crater formations there.

Certainly my goal is to climb all seven summits. I have tentatively set the dates for the four remaining summits: Carstensz Pyramid in Irian Jaya (Oceania) in September–October 2002, Mt. Vinson at about six hundred miles from the South Pole (Antarctica) in December 2002, Mt. Aconcagua in Argentine (South America) in February 2003, and Mt. Everest in Nepal (Asia) in March–May 2004.

This is not an easy task, because it requires a great deal of resources and funding. Let me give you the estimated cost for each of the remaining four expeditions to the summits: Carstensz Pyramid, $10,000; Mt. Vinson, $26,000; Mt. Aconcagua, $4,000; and Mt. Everest, $65,000.

You may wonder why Mt. Everest is so expensive compared with the others. There are several reasons. There is a $10,000 fee to enter the Everest Mountain Park (compared to about a $20 fee to enter most national parks here). There is a fee to pay for a climbing permit. Fees need to be paid to porters for carrying supplies and equipment to a base camp, up and down the mountain slope, and from the base camp back to the foothills over a period of three months. We need to pay rent for oxygen masks. We need to pay fees for guides, and we need to pay for accommodations, too.

Now, people could save money on the Mt. Everest expedition by independently arranging a group of up to seven climbers, but the earliest reservation you can make for this independent group is eight years from now. It is a long wait, and so you have to weigh the advantages and disadvantages of immediate opportunity at a very high cost versus waiting patiently for eight years for an expedition at a significantly lower cost.

It is critical that I get support from interested sponsors for me to achieve the goal of reaching the remaining four summits. I am still searching hard for potential sponsors. Fund-raising is probably the most difficult challenge for any climber, not just me, unless the climber is wealthy.

I have gone through a lot of self-sacrifice to achieve my climbing goals. Some people considered me to be a martyr, but I do not agree with that view, because I am a lover of adventure. I love to take challenges.

I encourage all of you to follow your hearts. Follow your dreams. Do not let anybody discourage you from trying and tell you to give up. Grab every opportunity you can. Never quit on yourself. Do not be afraid to take risks. You will make mistakes, but keep on going because you will learn and grow. Stay committed to yourselves and to your dreams.

What Makes a Good Deaf Leadership Camp in Germany, Thailand, and the United States?

DAN BRUBAKER, BEVERLY BUCHANAN, STEFAN GOLDSCHMIDT, AND SIMEON HART

DAN: We have four presenters here today, and let us introduce ourselves briefly. I am Dan Brubaker, and I have worked with Deaf youth over many years. My presentation is related to the American Youth Leadership Camp (YLC).

STEFAN: I am Stefan Goldschmidt, and I have been responsible for the German Youth Camp (Jugendcamp in German) over the past five years, and it is still running strong.

BEVERLY: Hello, my name is Beverly Buchanan. I am going to talk about Thai YLC. I currently work at Gallaudet University with the Campus Life as a program manager.

SIMEON: My name is Simeon Hart from England. I have worked with Beverly as her assistant at the Thai YLC. In England, I work as a training and development officer specializing in research into Deaf children in mainstream education.

DAN: Each of us will take turns back and forth several times, giving short presentations on different topics relative to our three youth camps, but we also include discussion on the following three questions: First, why are youth camps important? Second, what do the programs include in each of our camps? Third, how are the camps established, planned, and operated?

SIMEON: Why have we established a youth camp in Thailand? There young Deaf children do not have any exposure to Deaf adults and do not have self-confidence to achieve high goals. By having Thai YLC, we were able to share our experiences and skills. There were Deaf adults running the camp, and we included leadership activities and other activities so that they could feel good about themselves and become leaders in the future.

STEFAN: In Germany, historically the schools for Deaf students were predominantly oral, and thus Deaf students had limited opportunities to learn the sign language used by Deaf adults. Unsurprisingly, for many years Deaf people did not have a whole lot of pride in being Deaf. It was not until 1985, when German Sign Language was recognized as a language in its own right, that pride increased. By 1993, an increasing number of Deaf people learned to become proud of their own sign language and Deaf culture. I remember coming to Gallaudet University and asking Deaf students about their experiences growing up, and many of them talked about wonderful experiences as campers at the YLC. I realized then that that was something very important there. Such exposure gave me a strong encouragement to pursue the idea of having Jugendcamp. When I got back to Germany, I was fortunate to learn that someone else in Germany had been a camper at the American YLC in 1995. The two of us wanted to establish a camp in Germany, where Deaf staff members would be excellent role models to the younger generation of Deaf leaders. We could teach them a lot about Deaf culture, Deaf identity, and the Deaf community, which they did not learn at schools. These are the primary reasons for establishing Jugendcamp in Germany.

BEVERLY: In Thailand, I used to work as a volunteer teacher of Deaf students. After one year, I really became interested with their culture and tried to understand the culture as much as I could. After two years there, I realized that there was something missing, and that was youth leadership training. I talked with several friends about it, and I then contacted Simeon, who worked in the Philippines, to help us. We worked with four local Deaf adults to set up the Thai YLC. It started as a small program for graduating seniors at a school for Deaf students and provided them basic training to face challenges in the real world.

DAN: The American YLC was established in 1969 under the auspices of the National Associate for the Deaf (NAD), and this will be our thirty-fourth summer. In 1962, Junior NAD was established for high school students, and there were leadership activities held during the school year. However, the members of the NAD realized there was not enough training for the youth, and so a camp was set up for the first time in 1969. The American YLC program was not something that was created without any trial and error. We have learned what did not work well and then made some changes in the program. We have constantly fine-tuned the program every year to keep up with changing times. For example, we added the survival program in 1977. The length of the camp has varied between three and four weeks.

STEFAN: In Germany, the Jugendcamp was established in 1997. That was five years ago. I found my American experience along with my German background valuable in selecting activities for the camp. The other person who was an American YLC camper brought some ideas, or blueprints, from the American YLC, but we had to look at appropriateness of some activities in light of German Deaf culture and made some modifications to the program accordingly. In Germany, there are sixteen different states, and their schools have different schedules for their summer vacations. Thus, we realized it would be undesirable to have a one-month-long camp, because the longest overlapping summer break for most of the schools in these states is only two weeks. Thus, we planned on a two-week camp.

BEVERLY: In America, Deaf students at schools for Deaf students have a relatively strong educational foundation, and a good number of them have been exposed to a number of Deaf teachers, staff, or adults; thus a one-month-long youth leadership camp may be appropriate. However, in Thailand in general, Deaf students only study to eighth grade. Some of them continue to twelfth grade, but most of them get vocational training instead. We found it best to create a one-week camp at that time, focusing on light training, lots of hands-on experience, and team-building activities to enhance their self-esteem. Also, keep in mind that March is their summer month, and it is even hotter in April. We decided to have the camp in March for one week before they go home to work on farms with their families. We did receive money and were able to fund a retreat at various places including one at a resort with good food and some recreational activities as well. We hope to see it extended to two or three weeks in the future.

DAN: I remember I was asked by Stefan and his colleague Tomas to attend the planning meeting of Jugendcamp in 1997. They showed me the planned agenda and schedule for their first youth camp, with some doubts on its completeness. When I looked at what they had I indicated to them that their program was wonderful. We had this trial-and-error process over many years and then passed the framework along to Stefan and Tomas. They had adapted the program very well to mesh with German culture and customs. They nevertheless did make additional refinements each year to strengthen the program. The important thing is you have to remain flexible at all times and stand ready to make changes or refinements where appropriate.

SIMEON: There is one important thing I would like to mention. I went to Germany to work with Stefan last year and also went to Thailand twice to work with Beverly. Except for the first year when VSO covered my airfare to Thailand, in the remaining years I had to pay my own way and most other expenses to volunteer my time in the youth camps. Generally youth camps in Thailand and Germany, and America as well, work within limited budgets. We are doing this from our heart and not for money. They would provide us with room and board but for little or no pay. We may also get a small "thank you" gift, too. Basically, we volunteered our time because we wanted to.

DAN: Let us now look at the program activities. Although the different camps have specific activities unique to their country and culture, all of our basic programs include a good number of common elements. For the American YLC, the schedule of program activities for campers would include something like this: (1) Get up around 6:30 a.m. and do some physical exercise so that the campers would be wide awake for the day. (2) Watch lectures or participate in different workshops on public speaking, leadership, and self-esteem, among others. (3) Participate in team-building activities that are hands on and fun filled, rather than watch lectures that would put them to sleep. (4) Participate in a literacy program, including writing daily newsletters. (5) Compete in Camp Bowl, where they answered questions to develop their knowledge of a wide variety of topics. (6) Participate in a survival program. We would have them imagine that their plane made an emergency landing in an isolated place, and they were stranded and needed to learn how to survive on their own and how to cook with limited equipment or supplies. The campers' responses to this activity vary. Some of the campers found this experience rewarding, but others found it to be frustrating.

STEFAN: Now, remember Dan mentioned earlier that he thought our two-week program was wonderful. Actually, our program took some ideas and characteristics from the four-week YLC program. We incorporated the Camp Bowl, for example, but we changed some activities or English terms to better fit the German culture and language. There also is a new word that we have come up with: *Rübeau*. The letters of the word *Rübeau* are coined as follows. "RÜ" is from *rückblick*, which means "looking back," "BE" from *bekanntgabe*, which means "announcement," and "AU" from *aussicht*, which means "looking forward." The new activity called *Rübeau* is something that we do in the youth camp every evening. As it turned out, *Rübeau* is a very important activity in which the kids are encouraged to express themselves freely to the staff and to express their ideas, opinions, or concerns on any matter. The staff then considers the children's thoughts before the following evening, when they presented their explanations for their support or lack of support. Sometimes students get very frustrated, but we need to be able to allow them to uncork and vent their frustrations and give them an avenue to express themselves freely. The campers quickly realize from the *Rübeau* activity that we are listening to them and that their ideas or concerns can lead to something. This give-and-take process enhanced their self-esteem and confidence in expressing themselves freely rather than keeping their own concerns or anger to themselves. They all love this particular activity, and we found this to be a key part of our program.

SIMEON: In Thailand, at first Beverly worked alone for three years. She realized that to have a successful YLC, there was a need for additional individuals to increase the students' exposure to Deaf adults and role models. So Beverly asked three people, including me, to join her. The young kids saw our work in action and were impressed by our cooperative work. They also saw the importance of working together and realized that they could do the same thing and work together with their young peers. Based on an earlier evaluation, we agreed that a three-day camp was not long enough and extended it to five days. Each of us was responsible for planning activities for one day. One person was responsible for Monday, the next person was responsible for Tuesday, and so on. We showed the young kids the same cooperative process, even with different staff as role models. There are times when we as staff members got upset or disgruntled, but we would keep this to ourselves, take our problems outside, and resolve them among ourselves outside of the presence of the campers. We wanted to project positive images of working together, either as leaders or as support staff during each day. That is, we would never argue or get mad at each other publicly. Last year we had a new staff member from Cambodia who grew up in America, and we all worked together very well and projected positive images to the campers. This year Thai Deaf adults are now doing the planning and running the camp on their own, and we are thrilled about it. However, they indicated to us that they still would like for us to come in to support them because of our rich experience and information to share on culture, leadership, and other relevant things. At the Deaflympics in Rome, Italy, last year, Beverly and I met with Stefan, and he introduced us to a number of Deaf kids from Germany. They became fascinated with Deaf adults from other countries and the different sign languages we used. Stefan did the interpreting as we communicated to them. They learned that we have jobs at home and that we also are leaders with strong interest in running youth camps. Such informal conversation with the kids is an effective way to instill pride and confidence in them. They would start thinking, "Yes, I can become future leaders like them." So, it is important that a youth camp gives the kids the opportunity to see Deaf adults work cooperatively and to expose them to several Deaf role models.

DAN: Stefan explained about that particular *Rübeau* activity that they found so helpful in Germany, but we do not have its counterpart with the American YLC because we do not find that activity as being relevant in our American Deaf culture.

Conversely, some of the activities that work well for us in America may not work well in Germany or other countries. The program has to be relevant to the country's culture. For example, the physical exercise portion, and the expectation or demand that kids follow a rigid schedule or else suffer some consequences, work well with American and German campers but not with the Thai campers. Thus, you will need to make those necessary adaptations so that the program is appropriate to the country and culture.

STEFAN: At Jugendcamp, we had the campers on the first day ask the staff, "Are you Deaf?" Yes, we answered. They were astounded to find out that the entire staff was Deaf. They also were amazed to learn that our invited guest presenters were Deaf, too. We could see that they got a broader picture in their minds about the capabilities of Deaf adults than ever before and had significantly raised their expectations to greater heights for their future. They began to feel good about themselves.

BEVERLY: Guest presenters or volunteers can serve as excellent role models. The first year I was in Thailand as a teacher, there were seniors who had just graduated high school and they were going into the world of work. They never even thought of going to a college or university. During my several years there, I encouraged the school kids to set high goals for themselves and to attend college and work toward a bachelor's degree, a master's degree, or even a doctoral degree. After I left, I could see a good number of them attending colleges, which is great. Unquestionably, appropriate role models can serve as a strong motivator for young kids.

DAN: The American YLC program has several workshops on leadership skills. Generally they cover things such as communication skills, diplomacy (interacting with people in a pleasant way), feedback and listening skills, how to run meetings smoothly, parliamentary procedure (which is uniquely applicable to American culture), public speaking (most students were afraid to get on stage), self-esteem and assertiveness skills, Deaf culture and Deaf history (something that a lot of the campers did not know), positive and negative attitude/thinking (refrain from the negatives and focus on the positives), self-starting (not becoming dependent on others to get things started), brainstorming (the power of the group is stronger than the power of one individual), teamwork, networking (working together effectively), event planning, problem solving, time management, and volunteerism (importance of contributing time for others in the community and working from the heart rather than for pay). In addition, we teach political and advocacy skills (understanding the laws, knowing their rights, knowing how to push for changes) to advanced campers. For example, the campers would not know what to do about a noncaptioned program on television, so we would discuss several strategies or options to consider. We also teach them how to work with interpreters effectively in our advocacy efforts. We also discuss the importance of networking and working with other disability organizations for a common cause. Many times Deaf people think of themselves as not being a part of the bigger disability community, but there are power and strength in those numbers and so we have to teach people to work together in our advocacy efforts on access issues. The political skills workshop is one of the more advanced workshops, something we normally do not teach the kids right away or else they will be overwhelmed. They needed to progressively learn basic leadership skills first before they could be ready for the political skills workshop.

STEFAN: The political skills workshops Dan just described are appropriate for American YLC because their Deaf community has been advocating for captioning, interpreting, and other telecommunications access issues with other disability organizations. In Germany, we did not cover them in Jugendcamp. We had to first look at and assess the needs of German Deaf campers and determine what they lacked. We learned that schools do not teach Deaf culture, Deaf history, and relevant Deaf issues before we decided on certain areas to cover during the youth camp. The three primary areas we covered were communication and what effective communication involves; Deaf culture and what it means; and Deaf history. Then from these three primary areas, we would go into the development of selected leadership skills that Dan covered earlier such as public speaking, self-esteem and assertiveness, and positive and negative thinking, among others. Every effort has been made by staff to keep on pulling the kids toward higher skill levels. We may cover some political skills topics in the future, but that has to happen after the kids first develop high self-esteem and self-confidence.

BEVERLY: In Thailand, Simeon and I asked the schools for help in establishing these camps. We also worked with them to schedule camp activities. We would have staff come in for a weekend of planning before the camp starts on Monday morning. During the first year, we had our camp at a beach home belonging to one of the foundation's members, who generously allowed us to use it. The second year we had it at a school near the beach. It has been a challenge getting the needed materials for the kids to work with and take home. A minimal amount of time was needed to train the staff because we recruited the experts from other countries with some previous experience, who gladly volunteered, and they worked well with local staff. The campers were thirty graduating seniors from high school where I worked, and we had the school principal contact twenty-two other schools in Thailand and have each school send two students, one boy and one girl. Thus, we had a pretty good mix. We received some funding through the school from foundations, private donations, and some meals and other necessities from the local military bases and companies. Things worked out pretty well.

STEFAN: In Germany, we have Deaf staff, and the staff must be professionally trained in fields such as supervision, Deaf education, and counseling so that the parents could trust us with confidence. We want to make sure that they perceive that their children are being cared for professionally. We wanted to find a good place outside of the city and civilization. Jugendcamp is situated at a site at fourteen hundred meters above sea level, right in the mountain range. It is practically impossible for the campers to go any place near the city. This is what we wanted because it encouraged the campers to mix with each other, become close knit, and work together as a unit. The staff brought their own technology and equipment to camp for offices and workshops. To fund the camp, the German Deaf Association obtained grants and funds from the government. The government funds roughly half of the camp expenses, with the other half coming from tuition paid by the students and their families.

DAN: The NAD has a full-time staff person who is responsible for the overall planning and operation of the American YLC. The schedule is kept somewhat similar, with several refinements every year. Our survival program is something that cannot be taken lightly. It requires lots of planning and taking care of details for the staff to become ready to handle emergency situations and to ensure the safety of campers. We have about fifteen to twenty staff and sixty-four campers. Unlike Germany and Thailand, we do not get government support in America. The majority of expenses for running the camp are essentially paid for by the campers themselves, at the current tuition rate of $950 per camper for a four-week session. If families cannot afford the tuition, some of them can get support from state Deaf associations, charity organizations, private donors, and others. In our case we were able to keep our overall camp costs down because the staff members are mostly volunteering their time. The staff arrives early for one week of training. In Germany, they had professional staff, but in America, we have a small number of Deaf adult staff in administrative roles. We use college students who seek summer jobs and gain work experience for a lot of the staffing. Because our campers are between fourteen and eighteen and college students are about twenty or twenty-two years old, we need to train college students on appropriate roles and boundaries as staff so they avoid getting involved in inappropriate relationships with the campers.

SIMEON: In our Thai YLC, Beverly and I were fortunate to have one hearing teacher work with us as a staff member who did a lot of translating for us. We could use sign language, but neither of us could write in Thai. That particular teacher could write in both English and Thai. Whenever we communicated in sign language on a topic shown in written English, the hearing teacher was able to write its equivalent in Thai on the board for the benefit of campers. They saw that there was very good cooperation between the Deaf staff and the hearing teacher, which was a great example.

BEVERLY: Thanks for pointing this out, Simeon. Like we said earlier, we had four staff from outside the country working with four local staff during the first three years of camp, which was sort of a training period for the local staff. During the fourth year, and for the first time, the local staff members were conducting the Thai YLC on their own. We got goose bumps when we say that the local staff members became creative and added new things to the camp, including having the campers wearing colored bandanas as a way to identify different groups or teams of campers. It is really wonderful to see their camp program growing. I hope that this experience will apply to other countries in the future.

STEFAN: It was great to see local staff eventually take responsibility in running the YLC, like Beverly just described. In Germany, although we do recruit only professional staff, we make sure that there is at least a mixture of returning and new staff to run the camp in any given year, to maintain the integrity and continuity of the two-week program. We know an entire group of new staff cannot run the program effectively, because there are so many intangibles and small details that cannot possibly be fully covered on paper. The important principle is to have a mixture of returning and new staff each year so that new staff can learn and get some sense about the spirit and overall goals for the program to ensure continuity and stability of the program in years to come. We also have former campers who grew up to become some of our professional staff, which is great.

A National Organization of Deaf-Blind Youths

LINDA ERIKSSON, EVA JANSSON, AND EMIL BEIJERSTEN

LINDA: My name is Linda Eriksson. I have two other presenters with me, and the three of us discuss the national organization Deaf-Blind Youth (DBU) in Sweden. I was the President of DBU for eight years, but last April I resigned.

EVA: My name is Eva Jansson. I have Usher syndrome, and I am a former student at Gallaudet University.

EMIL: My name is Emil Beijersten, and I also have Usher syndrome. At the moment, I am the new president of DBU.

LINDA: The three of us want to share our experiences about how to create and run a national organization of young deaf-blind individuals. Our DBU was established in 1994 and is affiliated with FSDB, the Swedish National Association of Deaf-Blind People.

EVA: DBU is probably the only national organization of deaf-blind youth in the world with its own board and its own governmental support, aside from some smaller or local groups in other countries. Only people who are between seven and thirty years old and are deaf-blind, that is, have both visual and hearing impairments, can get full membership with voting rights.

EMIL: We have about seventy-five members in DBU. That means about half of the known number of deaf-blind youths in Sweden. It has taken lots of time and work to find and contact all these youths. FSDB started this work ten years ago, in 1991, and then FSDB invited young deaf-blind individuals to a meeting. About five youths attended this meeting. That meeting was the starting point of the youth work, later on known as DBU.

LINDA: In 1992, FSDB founded a youth council that consisted of three young deaf-blind members. I was one of them. This council went on to plan and arrange meetings and activities for young deaf-blind individuals between the ages of eighteen to thirty years. Also, in 1992, FSDB started a three-year project, called the School Project, and employed a project leader. This project worked to find and contact deaf-blind children and youths who were school aged, that is, seven to eighteen years old. The project leader tried to get in touch with all five deaf schools, with classes of hearing impaired students, and also with mainstream schools where there might be integrated deaf-blind individuals. Then the leader arranged summer camps to let the deaf-blind children and youths meet and socialize with each other.

EVA: An important result of the project was that every deaf school in Sweden got one person responsible to give support to the deaf-blind individuals, their parents, and their teachers.

EMIL: When this project approached the end, the youth council inside FSDB created DBU, and the new established board of DBU took over the responsibility of running the business. Also, a coordinator was employed by the FSDB, mainly to take care of administration, financial matters, and different things, working as a consultant or coordinator together with the board of DBU.

LINDA: There are five members of the board of DBU. One is the president and the four others are representatives. The five members of the board are elected to one-year terms, but they also have the opportunity to stay on the board if they want and if they are reelected. The people on the board work on a voluntary basis. They take turns for arranging different kind of activities, such as camps, conferences, meetings, and other work.

EVA: The purpose of the DBU is to make life better for deaf-blind children and youths, by breaking isolation, creating deaf-blind identity, getting together to meet other people within the same situation, encouraging each other, learning to overcome obstacles, and spreading information about deaf-blindness.

EMIL: To achieve these aims, DBU works in two ways. It advocates and provides information about deaf-blind children's and youths' rights and interests in the community, acts as a pressure group to influence authorities and politicians to give deaf-blind children and youth better service, and visits schools and the like to give speeches and information about the experiences of a young deaf-blind individuals. Then, of course, we work in cooperation with other youth organizations, deaf youth organizations, and hard of hearing and partially sighted organizations.

LINDA: The other area that DBU works within is member activities, which means seeking out the deaf-blind children and youth as early in life as possible to give them older role models and arrange different activities for them, for example, summer camps. Last week, we had a summer camp for fifteen children and youths in Sweden who are deaf-blind. We also arrange horse-riding camps, conference weekends, and theme seminars, where the deaf-blind children and youth are allowed to try and discuss new and unknown things, which they might not think they could manage, for example, horse riding, tandem bicycling, slalom, diving, bowling, tactile sign language, deaf-blind culture, independent living, and university studies.

EVA: DBU has organized and taken part in annual youth conferences and summer camps together with other Nordic countries, that is, Denmark, Finland, and Norway, since 1991 or 1992. Last July, the fourth Nordic camp took place in Sweden and was arranged by four members of DBU.

EMIL: Also DBU has been represented in European seminars of young deaf-blind individuals in 1995 and 1997. Several times DBU has tried to arrange another European seminar, too, but there have been some financial problems, and so it has not happened yet.

AUDIENCE: My name is Frank, and I am here from Maryland, and I know that there are deaf-blind camps in other countries. I am curious about how long these camps last and whether they are one-day camps, three-day camps, or week-long camps? Do campers stay in facilities such as cabins in the woods or sleep in tents? How many years has this been going on?

LINDA: We started arranging the camps in 1992. That was part of the school project, and so in 1992, we started the camps. We have had summer camp every year since then. They usually last for one week, but sometimes we have arranged two camps. Sometimes we have had a lot of deaf-blind young people who want to attend the camps, and so we then have arranged two camps in one summer. However, for example, this year we had the camp for one week, and we only had one camp. It is a camp-like place, but we stayed in cabins. Sometimes we sleep outside for one or two nights in tents. We have done different activities, and some of those activities included staying overnight in a tent.

AUDIENCE: How you do advertise these camps to the deaf-blind community? I think it is important to get the information out to people in other countries such as here in America, because there may be people who would be interested in coming from far away to attend these camps. Perhaps you can even extend the time of the camp beyond one week because I know that we have an organization, a national organization of the deaf-blind community. We have several camps, and we have lots of information here. We could do some networking and provide some information to your organization in your country.

LINDA: Yes. Maybe we could establish some kind of exchange program for the youth so that deaf-blind youth from different countries get the opportunity to meet each other. I know that there are many countries that do not have youth association for deaf-blind people, so I would like you all to go back to your own countries and to create them.

AUDIENCE: My name is Marcia Martinez. I am from New York, and I am a teacher. I work at the Helen Keller National Center for deaf-blind students. I am the coordinator of our SSP program. Here in America, there are a few states that have support service provider (SSP) programs. Some of them are paid positions. Some of the SSPs work as paid individuals. Others are volunteers. How are you handling the situation of getting SSPs? What are you all doing about that in your organization in your camps?

LINDA: In Sweden, the system is a bit different from the United States. In the DBU, we usually have about five leaders on our camps, and the ones who are the leaders on the camp are deaf-blind. However, some of the deaf-blind children or youth need their own SSPs or interpreters, so they bring those people with them. They have the SSPs or the interpreters provided by the province where they live. In Sweden, the government pays the salary to the interpreters and to the SSPs.

AUDIENCE: My name is Alice Haggemeyer. I worked for the Washington, D.C., public library system for many years, and I retired about ten years ago. I retired because I wanted to get more involved with international library awareness programs for deaf and deaf-blind individuals and deaf communities around the world. Last year, I went to the International Federation of Librarians, an international conference that happened to be here in America, in Boston. At that conference, I asked librarians if they provide any services for individuals who are deaf; of course, many of them replied that they did not. However, they did provide services for individuals who have other disabilities. The librarians have expressed concerns and wanted to do something about this, and so we have been working through the World Federation of the Deaf (WFD) to set up a network of libraries on an international level to better serve deaf and deaf-blind individuals. I do have some information about this, a pamphlet, so if you are interested in working on this effort, please take a pamphlet and send me your e-mail address. My e-mail address is on this pamphlet, and I believe it is information we can get disseminated through the library system that will be of benefit to all of you. Have you or your organization done any advocacy on behalf of people who are deaf-blind to ensure their access the public library system?

LINDA: Your question is a bit difficult to answer, but in Sweden, we have one library that is responsible for giving out books in Braille. However, not all the deaf-blind individuals do read Braille, of course, and so they have a limited service that is good only for the deaf-blind individuals who use Braille. This library also takes responsibility for all the deaf-blind individuals, no matter what type of reading they do (ordinary text or Braille). If I would like to have some information on a certain topic, then I would try to send that information to this specific library and have it translated into Braille or appropriate textual form. It is true that generally the public libraries do not have any service for blind or deaf-blind individuals in Sweden. We have not worked on that area yet.

AUDIENCE: I have talked to a few librarians in Sweden who have said that they are interested in doing something about this. Because other countries are interested in this as well, I have decided to get involved on the international level. Just a few months ago in America, President Bush allotted $500 million for the public libraries to improve literacy. Because of that support, I am able to get involved on an international level. Bill Gates and his wife have given quite a bit of money to the public library systems worldwide. I highly recommend that you tap into those resources. If you are interested, you can get more information about that through the World Wide Web.

AUDIENCE: My name is Barry Sega. I live here in the D.C. area. I have been involved with a lot of recreational activities, including camping. I am wondering about your camp in Sweden. Do you have a director who runs the camp or some sort of administrative structure to the camps that you are doing, such as an activities director or someone who is responsible for outdoor activities?

EMIL: Actually, we have different camps, and we would go to different places for camps. We have a summer camp, which has one person in charge to run and direct that week. That person divides the tasks with others so he or she can have overall responsibility for the different things going on. During the summer camp, we have five leaders working together. We planned all those activities during the week. As we said before, we also have a coordinator or a consultant working for DBU, and he or she works together with the five leaders during the camp week. During the spring and fall, we have a meeting with the president of the DBU, who takes care of the practical things. During those meetings, we take turns in assuming responsibility for what is going to happen during those meetings. It is a heavy responsibility, but we work together well.

AUDIENCE: I am here from Germany. I have two questions. In Germany, we are doing quite a bit of work with deaf-blind individuals. However, we do not have any

SSPs. We only have interpreters, and the interpreters are usually volunteers because there are not any funds available. In the German Association of the Deaf, there is a volunteer section within the association for working with deaf-blind individuals specifically and usually individuals with Usher syndrome. In Berlin, we do have a small group of five people who have Usher syndrome and who really are not in "youth" category. We are working together to better the lives of deaf-blind people. Historically, we had two groups, one for people with Usher syndrome and one was for people who are deaf-blind for other reasons. This past April was the first time that we all got together. The Usher syndrome individuals have been much more progressive in their efforts of getting together and working together. There is one man who is younger. He is twenty-one, and he is in a college now. However, he has had a lot of frustrations there. He is having a difficult time because he is losing his peripheral vision, and he is not getting the support that he needs. In your group in Sweden, do you all work together, all deaf-blind individuals together, or do you have a separate group for people who have Usher syndrome? My second question is this: how are you finding funding to support SSPs and to pay for that support? Also, in Germany, the deaf-blind community has been more aligned with the blind population rather than the deaf community. Is that the same trend you see in Sweden?

EVA: We have the group of deaf-blind there all together. We do not have a special group for Usher syndrome. We all have an organization together, hearing impaired, visual impaired, deaf-blind. We have a lot of members. The second question was about governmental support for interpreting service and SSPs. It is the government who pays for the SSPs for us in Sweden.

LINDA: Deaf-blind individuals are a separate group from blind individuals and deaf individuals. In our association, all deaf-blind people are grouped together, no matter what language they use (sign language or spoken Swedish). We are all integrated in our organization. Of course, we work closely together with both the blind association and with the deaf association depending on the question or issue.

The Past, Present, and Future of Deaf Youth in Russia

VLADIMIR V. KOTENEV

Let me introduce the past, present, and future of Deaf youth organizations in the Russian federation.

Nonprofit organizations for deaf youth play major roles in the creation and development of Deaf youth culture and help protect rights and interests of Russian youth with hearing losses. They have difficult enough periods in personal and professional development. Their youth is a time of uncertainty about their status and role, a time of unstable feelings, lack of confidence, and stress.

Ivan K. Arnold founded the first school for Deaf-mute people in Moscow, Russia, in 1912. This school celebrated its ninetieth anniversary in October 2002. Archives mentioned that in this new society of the school all Deaf people were united, and young people were among them.

Tsar Nikolay II Romanov resigned from his throne in March 1917 before the October Revolution. His throne was inherited by his blood brother Prince Michael, but he refused to be a Russian tsar because of the political crisis. Later, Russia was seized by Bolsheviks (future communists). The Bolsheviks plundered and nationalized all properties. Prince Michael's residential palace in St. Petersburg was captured by Bolsheviks and transferred to their properties. Later, they contributed this palace to the St. Petersburg Deaf Organization. At this time, the St. Petersburg Deaf Organization organized activities and support for youth with hearing loss, and they became Bolshevik supporters.

According to story of the well-known Russian deaf woman, Agrippina Kalugina (Iampolskiya), many deaf people, especially youth, lived in the Zamoskvorechy area (in the heart of Moscow). The Deaf club was located on Ulansky Lane. Later, a second Deaf club was established on Kaluzhsky Street. It was more spacious and convenient than the first club on Ulansky Lane. Agrippina Kalugina mentioned that there were many empty classic buildings after the Bolsheviks' revolution. Members made a stage and washed all the rooms. The club occupied the second floor, and on the third floor made a hostel. In this club, members began to work constantly, to send reports and conversations on political themes, and to arrange assemblies related to Bolshevik activities.

In autumn of 1920, the Komsomol league and the Deaf youth became members of the Youth Communist League. They spent all hours together in the organization after work and at their club on Kaluzhsky Street in Moscow.

The members of the Youth Komsomol League (YKL) effectively arranged and organized their activity, support, and cooperation. Twice per week they wrote political letters. Also, they studied the history of their party and its policies. Certainly, each member of the YKL attentively kept up on news and events in the world and in the Soviet country. They did not miss or pass any news around the world.

Members of the YKL tried to help the country. Deaf young people, with the senior communists, provided community services every Saturday, such as cutting trees; preparing firewood for hospitals, schools, and children's houses; helping senior citizens, and so forth.

According to Agrippina Kalugina, "We loved our club. It always shone by cleanliness: members of the YKL cleaned, washed a floor, and windows. We were very young—almost boys and girls. Serious large business always mixed with pranks, folks, and jokes. Certainly, we had art, sport, romance, feelings, and love too."

One of the Deaf Komsomol leaders, P. A. Savelev, was the secretary of the Regional Communist Party for the Deaf. He criticized deaf youth activity and told them: "It is time for you to straighten young wings and to take off from walls of the club. You must represent as a member of deaf youth society for Communist activities. At the same time, assembly have decided to ask the Moscow Committee of the YCL to hire one of them in order participate in Communist activities, and to serve for youth needs."

Later, the Bureau of the Moscow Komsomol Committee approved Agrippina Kalugina for a staff position serving deaf community. She arranged and organized a new Komsomol group of Deaf students. Komsomol development and exposure among the Deaf population were not easy. Most deaf people were not educated. She frequently provided Komsomol propaganda and educated deaf youth. Komsomol development started to rise in the cities where Deaf society expanded, lived, and worked.

Agrippina mentioned that Komsomols accepted only the best Deaf young people. They usually joined an upper level in the Komsomol organization after a pioneers' membership. Pioneer is a lower and young level of the Communist Party. Deaf young people were in pioneer organizations. The laws of the young pioneers of the former Soviet Union were as follows:

> The pioneer is devoted to a native country and Communism.
> The pioneer prepares to become member of the YKL.
> The pioneer aligns themselves with the heroes of struggle and work.
> Also prepares to become the defense counsel of a native country.
> The pioneer perseveres in school, work, and sport.
> The pioneer is an honorable and correct comrade, always safely questing for the truth.
> The pioneer is comrade and leader of Octobrians.
> The pioneer is a friend to the pioneers and children around world.

The Communist Party ran the pioneer organization, and the party supervised, organized, and showed "care" for the young. Komsomols were created at each special school where deaf and hard of hearing children were trained. They took part in the activity, as well as hearing youth.

In the thirty years after the revolution, the pioneers and members of the YKL, both Deaf and hearing, actually had no independence or freedom of speech in the Soviet republics. They idolized Stalin. The All-Russian Society of the Deaf-Mutes joined with the whole country in supporting the Communist ideology.

Eventually, USSR President Mikhail Gorbachev began to restructure and reform the system. All the people joined in the process to democratize their society. The Komsomol League of the Deaf and Hard of Hearing discontinued activity between 1985–1991.

In 1997–2001, a young leader, Dmitry Rebrov, and I put forward our idea of establishing a new youth organization in Moscow, Russia. At the end of September 1999, the Moscow Public Organization of the Deaf called a general meeting of Deaf and hard of hearing young leaders, which elected Sofia Shmelkova as chairperson.

We officially registered the Regional Youth Public Organization of the Deaf (RYPOD) in February 2000. Unfortunately, Mrs. Shmelkova focused only on youth parties. The members of council were dissatisfied by unilateral character of activity of youth organization. On April 21, 2000, elections were held for a president of the Deaf youth organization. They selected me. The general program and plan for 2001 were successful; sessions of the council of the RYPOD were regularly held. We organized youth trips to Scotland, Nizhny Novgorod, Yaroslavl, St. Petersburg, and so forth. In 2000, Ruslan Kulikov and I gave a presentation regarding our leadership at the National Association of Deaf Conference in Norfolk, Virginia. The plans and measures were productive, and we worked with unbelievable enthusiasm. We empowered our generation and gave an opportunity to new Deaf youth leaders to take care of youth activities and leadership. Then, everything changed and Russian youth leadership split. There is a lack of support from governments and organizations.

Probably, the Society of the Deaf should coordinate the isolated efforts of Deaf youth. Youth organizations are not always capable of independently finding their place. To define their function and role, it is necessary to create a system of state and public support and subsidize prospective youth movements.

In general, any normal democratic country should have three directions in youth policy: state, public, and political. Let me mention a state youth policy in modern Russia. The state youth policy's elements are departments, committees, and others, which are under governmental control.

The function of state regulation of youth policy is assigned to the State Committee of Youth. A core part is the federal program "Youth of Russia." One of the directions is the civil, spiritual–moral, and patriotic education of youth. The committee should work on social and economic problems of the young people generally. Many regions have created several centers for social-psychological help for youth. Their mission is to help drug-addicted and criminal youth, who have serious trouble or come from places of deprivation.

In January 1995, part of the first Civil Code of Russian Federation fixed practically all norms related to nonprofit organizations (clauses 116–123, paragraph 5, and chapter 4). In 1995, the State Duma (representative body) accepted five basic federal laws determining the legal status of nonprofit organizations. In particular, on June 28, 1995, it accepted and approved a federal law regarding state support for youth and children's associations.

The Russian legislation is supposed to support all youth organizations in various forms. But Russian Deaf youth are separated from the government's support, general nonprofit organizations for the youth, and hearing youth society. This legislation is not functional for young people with hearing loss at the present time. Modern Russian Deaf youth are abandoned. At the present time, Russian Deaf youth have been struggling with silent discrimination and inactive modern laws. They still do not have clear goals in their future for leadership and development.

Vital Self-Determination of Deaf Youth in Russia in Conditions of Social Instability

DMITRY REBROV

The dynamically varying social conditions require developing the qualities of initiative and independence in our youth. The changing cultural-historical inheritance puts new fundamental problems before education. If in the past, the basic task of school was to transfer the cultural experience as a system of knowledge to the youth and to have them form a scientific picture of the world, nowadays the new function of education is to be "a genetic matrix" society, subject of transformation society, and a generation of the new forms of public life.

Youth is a difficult period in development. It is characterized as a time of status and role uncertainty, as the period of stress and instability of social values of the young man. The main task of individual development during youth is the self-determination and formation of identity.

The psychological content of this period as a whole is defined by a situation of multiple choices. It is an important feature in the process of self-determination in an unstable situation and a crisis of habitual norms and values. Thus, potential difficulties of youthful self-determination follow, first of all, from the fact of destabilization of social life.

Aggravation of crisis processes in the economy and the increase of social intensity create negative processes in all layers of a society, but especially in the environment of youth. Social trouble shows up in changes in social and related communications, vagrancy of children, criminal offenses, drunkenness, and drug addiction. Group forms of criminal activity in the youth environment increase. The change of the political form of authority has resulted in destruction. The new system of preventive maintenance in our society has not yet arisen.

This social instability is shown in three interconnected levels: society as a whole, social groups, and the individual level. The individual psychological level, factors that influence the vital self-determination of youth, and the civil state of health of this social group should be investigated.

As a result of a break in economic and sociopolitical devices, the formation of a new and essentially different public structure, and a new system of requirements for the youth community, a break in generations was formed. Research shows that psychological groups of youth do not have the psychological readiness to live and to work in new conditions and the moral stability to preserve themselves from deformation and degradation in conditions of social instability. Lack of essential exposure, full knowledge, practical skills, and pragmatic thinking make youth uncompetitive in the job market, and from this the economic, social, and political status falls. Youth are dependent, not self-assured, and socially inactive. In the youthful environment, feelings of aggression, irritation, and uncertainty about tomorrow increase.

At the same time, youth have psychological potential: aspirations to knowledge and harmony with the environment, creativity, and self-knowledge. All this objectively creates the necessity of action on the part of societies and the state to promote the preservation, reproduction, and development of culture for connections between generations and also the creation of conditions for free development of the person and society. These functions should include the following:

1. society can devote resources to youth;
2. youth can and should give to society; and
3. various communities should figure out how to mobilize and to use youth as a resource for the creation of new developments in social and economical life.

These factors influence the socialization and formation of self-consciousness of Deaf people.

V. S. Sobkin stated that "the character of teenage experiences of the child with an acoustical defect is complicated by his experience of the defect as a social defect." L. S. Vygotsky, the well-known psychologist, wrote "Blindness or the deafness is normal, instead of an unhealthy condition for the blind or mute child, and the specified defect is felt by him only secondarily, as reflected on him as the result of his social experience."

The expansion of the social environment for seniors with hearing loss frequently is connected to fixing the defect in an aggressive environment: "About every fourth senior is strongly frustrated about hearing loss" (Sobkin).

The child's identity grows out of identification with a significant other person. The feeling of belonging to a subculture or community increases the self-esteem of an individual. There is accelerated development of norms of behavior, characteristic for the members of Deaf society, using RSL (Russian Sign Language) or another effective communication in the subculture of the Deaf community. Thus, not only for hard of hearing people but also for Deaf people, self-determination in culture assumes formation of individual qualities, including the following:

- ❖ the need to construct behavior and activity on the basis of available cultural norms;
- ❖ conviction of the value of perceived displays of culture for the person, for self-development;
- ❖ the ability to realize his place in cultural space and the features of cultural behavior, so he can fine-tune his interpersonal interactions;
- ❖ the ability to gauge cultural activity and correct his interactions with an environment; and

❖ the need to selectively perceive validity of the environmental and make conscious choices about certain cultural values.

We shall not overlook the fact that Deaf people are under pressure from the dominant culture to seize incompatible norms and values. Therefore, the processes of self-determination are important.

For a survival of a young man, the formation of his spiritual world is decisive. The function of formation of the spiritual world in many respects is allocated to the system of education. The role of the spiritual factor sharply grows in crisis and extreme situations. In these conditions, more often people with spiritual beliefs survive.

Young people with hearing loss need organizations or outreach communities to support their search for identity, education, and opportunity.

The absence of information, opportunity, and support has resulted in serious deformations in psychological and social aspects of the young generation to master education, work, and life. The basic condition of self-determination is essential to develop moral principles and to be guided by them in action and goals.

Global crisis, which has captured all spheres of life of the modern Russian society, represents real threats to the self-determination and educational system of Deaf youth. Many forms of the self-determination and survival are broken. In the Communist era, these were carried out through education and career development under the government's control.

Disturbing symptoms of the fall of a culture are the occurrence and strengthening of negative tendencies, such as criminal behavior, increase of conflicts, and aggression. Deaf people are strongly focused on material assets to survive, and they ignore participation in Deaf society.

Researchers consider the teenage years as a period of stress caused by emotional turmoil, role conflicts, vague status, and unstable social values. The individuals at this stage have psychological discomfort, caused by factors including low self-esteem.

Deaf teachers and psychologists mention that Deaf youth have difficulty forming moral-ethical representations and concepts, overestimating particular qualities of particular people, and in preventing their emotions from overwhelming their reasoning. These slow down the process of forming a Deaf youth society.

The school psychologists ascertain that many Deaf teenagers psychologically are not ready for independent life. School conditions and small social circles frequently have resulted in social dependency and selfishness, and some graduates are excessively trusting and believe that the help and care of others is obligatory. Therefore, let me emphasize that the development of moral life values is the central task of society, family, and education.

contributors

Isaac O. Agboola, United States
Rune Anda, Norway
Kathleen Arnos, United States
Cynthia Neese Bailes, United States
David Barber, United States
Robert Bayley, United States
Abbas Ali Behmanesh, Iran
Emil Beijersten, Sweden
Elizabeth Beldon, United States
Barbara Brauer, United States
Kelby Brick, United States
Nancy Bridenbaugh, United States
Bernard Brown, United States
Dan Brubaker, United States
Beverly Buchanan, United States
Thomas H. Bull, United States
Steven Chough, United States
John B. Christiansen, United States
Emilia Chukwuma, United States
Steven Collins, United States
Jeffrey E. Davis, United States
Clark Denmark, United Kingdom
Jane Dillehay, United States
Kristina Dobyns, United States
Raphael Domingo, Philippines
Jordan Eickman, United States
Lynne Eighinger, United States
Frances Elton, United Kingdom
Linda Eriksson, Sweden
Carol J. Erting, United States
Lynne C. Erting, United States
Meir Etedgi, Israel
Anthonia Ngozika Euzouwa, Nigeria
David Fowler, United Kingdom
Jan Fried, United States
Kostas Gargalis, Greece
Heather Gibson, Canada
Larry Goldberg, United States

Stefan Goldschmidt, Germany
Maria Tanya de Guzman, Philippines
Kika Hadjikakou, Cyprus
Simeon Hart, Philippines
Rachel M. Hartig, United States
Mark Heaton, United Kingdom
Gunnar Hellström, Sweden
Gregory Hlibok, United States
Rob Hoopes, United States
Eva Jansson, Sweden
Peoungpaka Janyawong, Thailand
Paul Johnston, United States
Nayantra Kanaye, South Africa
Liisa Kauppinen, Finland
Alok Kumar Kejriwal, India
Vladimir V. Kotenev, Russia
Vassily Kourbetis, Greece
Marlon Kuntze, United States
Paddy Ladd, United Kingdom
Linda Lambrecht, United States
Carole Lazorisak, United States
Irene W. Leigh, United States
Ceil Lucas, United States
Jim Macfadden, United States
Maricar Marquez, United States
Ricardo Vianna Martins, Brazil
Carla M. Mathers, United States
Yuri Maximenko, United States
Johanna Mesch, Sweden
Betty Miller, United States
Carly Munro, United Kingdom
Joseph J. Murray, United States
Wilma Newhoudt-Druchen, South Africa
Paul W. Ogden, United States
Raymond J. Oglethorpe, United States
Adebowale Ogunjirin, Nigeria
Gina A. Oliva, United States
Yukata Osugi, Japan

Sue E. Ouellette, United States
Gladis Perlin, Brazil
Cynthia Peters, United States
Karen Petronio, United States
Bert Pickell, United States
Cynthia J. Plue, United States
Paul Preston, United States
Dmitry Rebrov, Russia
Ruth Reed, United States
Madeleine Rothberg, United States
Julie Elaine Roy, Canada
Ilissa Rubinberg, United States
Robyn Sanford, United States
Krister Schönström, Sweden

Elena Silianova, Russia
Laurene Simms, United States
Deborah Sonnenstrahl, United States
Benjamin Soukup, United States
Kevin Stanley, Ireland
Karen Peltz Strauss, United States
Ronald Sutcliffe, United States
Sarah Taub, United States
Carlene Thumann-Prezioso, United States
Michel Turgeon, Canada
Mary Watkins, United States
Alex Wilhite, United States
Amy Wilson, United States
Heidi Zimmer, United States

Index

Page numbers in italics denote figures, photographs, or tables.

abortions, 354–55, 373
ADA (Americans with Disabilities Act), 201
Adamopoulou, A., 42
adolescents. *See* youth
adoption, 121–26
advocacy, political, 17–20, 203–4, 249
African Americans, 81–85, 200–1, 202
Agboola, Isaac, 73–77
AIDS/HIV service delivery, 178–80
Alker, D., 245
Allen, T.E., 81
Amami Islands, 27–28
American Deaf culture, 227–32, 248–49, 272–77
American Indian Sign Language, 234–38
American Samoa, 32–37
ANC (African National Congress), 17–20
Anda, Rune, 121–26
Andersson, Yerker, 7
Anzaluda, Gloria, 274
AOL (America Online), 361–62
Apter, Haim, 206, *207*, *209*
Araujo, M.U., 341
Arnos, Kathleen, 370–75
art exhibits, 251–63
Arthur program, 387–88
Asian Deaf culture: American Deaf culture comparison, 227–32; deaf education, 107–13; sign language and, 26–28; views of deafness/disabilities, 109, 123
ASK model, *316*, 316–21, *317*
ASL (American Sign Language): bilingualism and literacy, 87–95, 101–2, 114–17; in Deaf literature, 276; origins, 227–28, 236–37, 260; poetry, 278–83, 284–89; tactile ASL, 324–25, *325*, *329*; variation studies, 322–35, *323*, *326*, *327*, *329*, *331–32*, *334*
attitudes. *See* societal attitudes
automotive driving, 229

Baghchaban-Pirnazar, 194
Baghcheban, Samineh, 193–94
Bahan, Ben, 134–35, 136, 138, 139, 274, 276, 345
Baird, Chuck, 262–63
Bamberger, Moshe, 206
Barber, David, 66–72
Bass, Dick, 394

Bayley, Robert, 322–35
Behmanesh, Abbas Ali, 193–98
Beijersten, Emil, 405–9
Beldon, Elizabeth, 154–56
Berg, I., 181–83, 184
Berthier, Ferdinand, 245–46, 310
Between the Lions, 360, 387
bilingualism, 87–95, 100–6, 114–17
bioethics, 11–13
Bloch, David, 261
book sharing, 35, 89–91
Borderlands (Anzaluda), 274
Brauer, Barbara, 163–65
Brazil, 53, 336–39
Bridenbaugh, Nancy, 32–37
Bridges, Ruby, 85
Brown, Bernard, 66–72
Brown v. Board of Education, 81–82
Brubaker, Dan, 398–404
BSL (British Sign Language), 220–24, 241–44
Buchanan, Beverly, 398–404
Bull, Sherman, 394
Bull, Thomas, 152–54
Bullard, Douglas, 273
Burke, Jamie, 125

Canada, 100–6, 178–80
cancer awareness projects, 172–77
Cane (Toomer), 274
captioning, 360, 380–81, 387–88
Chang, W.B.C., 341
China, 122–23
Chough, Steven, 227–32
Christiansen, John, 363–69
Chukwuma, Emilia, 66
CID (Catholic Institute for the Deaf), 38–40
"Circle of Life", 285–89
civil rights, 81–86, 200–4, 340–41, 380–85
cochlear implants: about, 363–64, 364n1; Deaf community and, 351–55, 367–68; educational settings/services, 365–66, *366*; parental perspectives, 365–67; team availability, 130, 132
CODAs (Children of Deaf Adults), 152–59
Collins, Steven, 322–35
communication styles, 231

connexin 26 gene, 353, 371, 374–75
Cornerstones literacy project, 386–87
court interpreting, 340–43
"The Cowboy Story", 275
CSD (Communication Service for the Deaf, Inc.), 4, 6–8
Csikszentmihalyi, M., 306–7
cultural differences: about, 145; Asian vs. American, 227–32; Deaf vs. hearing, 157; in education, 229; United Kingdom vs. American, 248–49; views of deafness/disabilities, 55–56, 109, 123. *See also specific cultures*
Cummins, J., 101
Cyprus, 127–33

DANS (Deaf Adoption News Service), 125–26
Davis, H., 134
Davis, J.E., 235–36
Davis, Jeffrey, 233–40
DBU (Deaf-Blind Youth), 405–9
Deaf art. *See* Deaf View Image Art
Deaf-blind services, 48–51, 407–8. *See also* tactile sign language
Deaf-Blind Youth (DBU), 405–9
Deaf Cancer Wise, 172–77
Deaf clubs, 155, 219–20, 295, 299
Deaf community: changes over time, 219–20; on cochlear implants, 351–55, 367–68; Deaf sport and, 295–96, 299; development of, 24–25, 42–47, 205–12; old/young interaction, 230; partnerships in, 38–41; technology impact, 150, 155
Deaf cultural patterns, 247–48. *See also* cultural differences
Deaf education. *See* education
Deaf Empowerment Project, 42–47
A Deaf Family Diary, 276
Deafhood, 245–50
Deaf literature: on CODA families, 153; Deaf American literature, 272–77; Helen Keller biography, 267–71; poetry, 278–83, 284–89
Deaflympics, 295
Deafology 101, 273
Deaf pride, 230–31. *See also* Deafhood
Deaf sport: Deaflympics, 295; identity development and, 293–300; women in, 301–4; Zimmer's seven summits, 393–97. *See also* leisure activities
Deaf theater, 247
Deaf View Image Art, 251–63
de Guzman, Maria Tanya, 166–71, 215
Denmark, Clark, 219–26
de Shazer, Steve, 181–83, 183–84
developing countries: assistance to, 52–57, 61–63, 75–76; entrepreneurship, 64–65, 66–72, 73–77; human rights, 14–15; political advocacy, 17–20; technology in, 62, 231

Dillehay, Jane, 370–75
Dobyns, Kristina, 227–32
Domingo, Raphael, 213–16
DPN (Deaf President Now) protest, 201, 202
DPSA (Disabled People of South Africa), 17
Dupor, Susan, 259

education: accessibility issues, 81–86, 202; Asian Deaf perspectives, 107–13; bilingual/bicultural, 87–95, 100–6, 114–17; cochlear implant support services, 365–66, *366*; cultural differences, 229; higher education, 139; as human right, 28–31; interpreter training, 83, 221–22; in Iran, 193–95; mainstreaming/inclusion, 29–30, 203, 219, 308–9; Pacific Outreach Initiative, 32–37; parental perspectives, 138–39; pedagogical approaches, 87–88, 96–99; residential schools, 219; statistics, 14, 28–29; teacher training, 21–23, 229; tutor training, 222–24. *See also* literacy
educational media, 359–60, 386–90
Eguzouwa, Anthonia Ngozika, 301–4
Eickman, Jordan, 293–300
Eighinger, Lynne, 315–21
Elton, Frances, 219–26
emergency access, 381–82
employment: entrepreneurship, 64–65, 66–72, 73–77; in government, 203; investment capital and, 62–63; state-funded, 66–70, 189–92
England, 398–404
Ennis, Bill, 274–75, 276
entrepreneurship, 64–65, 66–72, 73–77
Eriksson, Linda, 405–9
Erting, Carol, 87–95
Erting, Lynne, 87–95
Estiller, Maritess Raquel, 215–16

families: adoption, 121–26; attitude toward disabilities, 109; CODAs, 152–59; coping strategies, 142–44; Deaf parents with teenage children, 145–51; financial support, 229; guidance programs, 127–33; intermarriages, 230. *See also* parents
Ferentinos, S., 42
fingerspelling, 231
Finland, 69
Fowler, David, 241–44
Fried, Jan, 32–37
friendship, 230
FSM (Federated States of Micronesia), 32–37

Gallaudet, Thomas, 236–37
Gallaudet University, 55, 201, 256, 373–74
Gargalis, Kostas, 42–47

Index

genetic science, 351–56, 370–75
Germany, 398–404, 408–9
Gibson, Heather, 100–6
Glickman, Ken, 273
Goff-Paris, D., 236
Goldberg, Larry, 386–90
Goldfield, M., 337
Goldschmidt, Stefan, 398–404
government funding/support, 66–70, 189–92, 229
Goya, 258
Greece, 42–47
Grosjean, F., 138

Hadjikakou, Kika, 127–33
Haggemeyer, Alice, 407–8
hair cell regeneration, 370
Hands across the Pacific, 32–37
Hart, Simeon, 398–404
Hartig, Rachel, 267–71
Haüy, Valentin, 269–70
health, 172–77, 178–80. *See also* mental health
hearing aid compatibility, 383–84
hearing aids, 53, 136
Heaton, Mark, 241–44
Helen Keller Home, 210, *210*
Hexter, Richard, 206
Hinkle, J., 185
Hlibok, Gregory, 380–85
Hoffmeister, R., 134–35, 136, 138, 139
Holcomb, T., 42
Holocaust, 261
Hoopes, Rob, 322–35
Human Genome Project, 370–71, 372
human rights, 10–16, 28–31, 81–86. *See also* civil rights
humor, 272–73
Humphries, T., 241

iconicity, 284–85
IDEA (Individuals with Disabilities Education Act), 201, 202, 203
identity development: in CODAs, 157; Deaf sport and, 293–300; nationality vs. deafness, 249; sign language and, 276, 336–39; in youth, 414–16
IM (instant messaging), 358
inclusion/mainstreaming, 29–30, 203, 219, 308–9
indigenous populations, 233–40. *See also* Native Americans
intermarriages, 230
Internet access, 357–58
interpreting: attitude component, 315, 317; court interpreting, 340–43; education/training, 83, 221–22; expectations of, 315–16, 317; in families, 150; model of cultural relationships, *316*, 316–21, *317*; pricing issues, 319–20

Iran, 193–98
Ireland, 38–41
Islay (Bullard), 273
Israel, 205–12

Jansson, Eva, 405–9
Janyawong, Peoungpaka, 21–25
Japan, 26–27
Jefferson, Thomas, 236
Johnston, Paul, 251–63

Kalugina, Agrippina, 410–11
Kanaye, Nayantra, 134–40
Kannapell, Barbara, 255
karma, 228–29, 230–31
Kauppinen, Liisa, 7, 10–16
Kejriwal, Alok, 64–65
Keller, Helen, 208, *209*, 267–71
Kemp, Mike, 21
King, Martin Luther, Jr., 356
KODA Camp program, 156–57. *See also* CODAs
Kotenev, Vladimir, 410–13
Kourbetis, Vassili, 42–47
Kraft, Elinor, 276
Kuntze, Marlon, 87–95

Ladd, P., 219, 245–50
Lambrecht, Linda, 32–37
Lane, Harlan, 134–35, 136, 138, 139, 352n1
Lazorisak, Carole, 315–21
legislation, 200–3, 380–85
Leigh, Irene, 363–69
leisure activities, 305–11. *See also* social life
Lentz, Ella Mae, 285–89
Liddell, S., 284
literacy: achievement levels, 81, 87–88, 139; bilingualism and, 87–95, 101–2, 114–17; online tools, 359–60, 386–87; parental perspectives, 138–39; shared reading, 35, 89–91; statistics, 109, 193. *See also* education
Lucas, Ceil, 322–35

Macfadden, Jim, 66–72
MAGpie, 390
mainstreaming/inclusion, 29–30, 203, 219, 308–9
Markides, A., 131
Marquez, Maricar, 48–51
Martha's Vineyard Sign Language, 234
Martinez, Marcia, 407
Martins, Ricardo Vianna, 336–39
Maslow, Abraham, 306
Mathers, Carla, 340–43
Maximenko, Yuri, 66–72
McClendon, Frankie, 82–83

media influences, 221
medical model of deafness, 136–37, 373
mental health, 163–65, 166–71, 181–86
Mesch, Johanna, 344–48
Miller, A., 342
Miller, Betty, 251–63
Miller, Mary Beth, 275
Moores, D.F., 134–35, 136
mountain climbing, 393–97
Munro, Carly, 172–77
Murray, Joseph, 351–56
My Third Eye, 273, 275

NAD (National Association of the Deaf), 5, 200, 202, 367
Nambo, Yasuko, 394
Native Americans, 83–85, 233–38
NCAM (National Center for Accessible Media), 360, 386–90
Neese Bailes, Cynthia, 87–95
Nepal, 30, 229
Newhoudt-Druchen, Wilma, 17–20, 204
Newman, Lawrence, 393–94
Nigeria, 61–62, 301–4
"Nitty", 274–75
Nolan, Kevin, 203–4
Une nuit rayonnante: Helen Keller (Pitrois), 267–71

Ogden, Paul, 141–44
Oglethorpe, Raymond, 357–62
Ogunjirin, Adebowale, 61–63
Oliva, Gina, 305–11
onomatopoeia, 241–44
oralism, 136–37, 137, 227, 245–48
Osugi, Yukata, 26–31
Ouellette, Sue, 181–86

Pacific Outreach Initiative (POI), 32–37
Padden, C., 241
Pahlavi, Farah, 194
parents: bilingual practices, 91–94; cochlear implants and, 365–67; coping strategies, 142–44; counseling, 129–32, 135; Deaf culture involvement, 137–38, 147; Deaf parents with teenage children, 145–51; diagnosis reaction, 134–35, 141–42, 364; on education, 138–39; guidance programs, 127–33; medical model impact, 136–37. *See also* families
Peller, J., 182–83
Perlin, Gladis, 96–99
Peters, Cynthia, 272–77
Petronio, Karen, 322–35
Philippines, 52–53, 166–71, *167*, 213–16
Pickell, Bert, 156–57
pinky extension study, *323*, 323–24, 328, *329*, 330
Pitrois, Marguerite, 268

Pitrois, Yvonne, 267–71
PIVoT, 388–89
"Planet Way over Yonder", 273
Plue, Cynthia, 107–13
poetry, 278–83, 284–89
Poetry in Motion, 276
POI (Pacific Outreach Initiative), 32–37
political advocacy, 17–20, 203–4, 249
Preston, Paul, 145–51

Quebec Deaf Aids Coalition, 178–80

rear window captioning, 360
Rebrov, Dmitry, 414–16
recreation. *See* leisure activities
Reed, Ruth, 322–35
Rehabilitation Act, 200, 384–85
relay services, 6, 382–83
religious beliefs, 109, 228–29, 230–31
Rennie, Debbie, 276
residential schools, 219
Ridgeway, Rick, 394
Rocky Mountain Deaf School, 30
Rothberg, Madeleine, 386–90
Roy, Julie Elaine, 178–80
Rubinberg, Lissa, 48–51
Russia, 189–92, 410–13, 414–16
Rutherford, S., 43
Ryan, Stephen, 273

Sales, Jose, 214
SALT Partnership, 389–90
Samii, Julia, 196
Sandford, Robyn, 278–83
Santos, Pedro, 213–14
scaffolding, 92–93
Schönstrom, Krister, 114–17
Scotland, 172–77
Scott, Hugh, 235
SDAD (South Dakota Association for the Deaf), 4
SEE (Signed Exact English), 34
Sega, Barry, 408
Seven Summits (Bass et. al), 393–94
shared reading, 35, 89–91
A Shining Night: Helen Keller (Pitrois), 267–71
sign languages: bilingualism and literacy, 87–95, 101–2, 114–17; changes over time, 220–21; Deaf culture and, 26–28, 248–49; fingerspelling, 231; iconicity in, 284–85; identity development and, 276, 336–39; in indigenous populations, 233–40; interpreter/tutor training, 83, 221–24; onomatopoeia in, 241–44; poetry, 278–83, 284–89; preoralist principles, 246; tactile, 324–25, *325*, *329*, 344–48, *345*; variation studies, 322–35, *323*, *326*, *327*, *329*, 331–32, 334

Silianova, Elena, 189–92
Silverman, R., 134
Simms, Laurene, 81–86
social life, 155, 219–20, 230, 305–11
social status, 230
societal attitudes: cultural differences, 55–56, 109, 123, 229; in education, 97–98; entrepreneurship and, 76–77; impact of, 3–4; mental health and, 169–70; volunteer projects and, 55
socioeconomic status, 203
Sonnenstrahl, Deborah, 251–63
Soukup, Benjamin, 3–9
South Africa, 17–20, 138–39
Spain, 375
Spradley, James, 296
Stokoe, William, 227–28
Strauss, Karen Peltz, 380–85
Sullivan, Anne, 268–69
Supalla, Sam, 276, 345
surdophrenia, 165
Sutcliffe, Ronald, 66–72
Sutton-Spence, R., 242, 244
Svarthom, Kristina, 114, 117
Sweden, 114–17, 138, 405–9

tactile sign language, 324–25, *325*, *329*, 344–48, *345*
Taub, Sarah, 242, 284–89
TDCA (Television Decoder Circuitry Act), 201–2
teacher training, 21–23, 229
Teaching Indians to be White, 83–84
technology: captioning, 360, 380–81, 387–88; communication impact, 150, 155; in developing countries, 62, 231; educational media, 359–60, 386–90; genetic science, 351–56, 370–75; hearing aids, 53, 136; home networks, 361; Internet access, 357–58; telecommunications access, 18, 201–2, 358–59, 380–85; wireless communications, 358–59, 376–79, *377*. *See also* cochlear implants
teenagers. *See* youth
telecommunications access, 18, 201–2, 358–59, 380–85
Telecommunications Act, 202, 380, 384
Television Circuitry Decoder Act, 381
Thailand, 21–25, *22*, 398–404
theater, 247, 268–69

Three Lights in the Darkness (Pitrois), 269–70
Thumann-Prezioso, Carlene, 87–95
Tibet, 229
Toomer, Jean, 274
Torres, M., 185
Trois lumières dans la nuit (Pitrois), 269–70
Turgeon, Michel, 178–80
tutor training, 222–24

UH (University of Hawai'i), 33
Ukraine, 66–70
United Kingdom, 219–26, 248–49, 293–300
United States ex rel. Negron v. New York, 341
UN (United Nations), 13, 15–16, 29

vaudeville theater, 268–69
Veditz, George, 233–34
Vehmas, Simo, 11–12
Vietnam, 21, 24
Villacin, Cecilia, 215
Vukotic, Dragoljub, 214

Walter, J., 182–83
Watkins, Mary, 386–90
WDL (World Deaf Leadership) project, 21–25
Wells, Frank, 394
WFD (World Federation of the Deaf), 7, 15
White, Barbara, 125
Wilhite, Alex, 251–63
Wilson, Amy, 52–57
wireless communications, 358–59, 376–79, *377*
WISDOM project, 376–79, *377*
Woll, B., 242, 244
women and sports, 301–4
Wood, S., 236
Woodward, James, 21, 23
Wright, C.A., 342

youth: about, 145–51; CODAs, 152–59; DBU (Deaf-Blind Youth), 405–9; identity development, 414–16; interaction with older Deaf people, 230; programs for, 8, 398–404; Russian organizations, 410–13

Zimmer, Heidi, 393–97

Silianova, Elena, 189–92
Silverman, R., 134
Simms, Laurene, 81–86
social life, 155, 219–20, 230, 305–11
social status, 230
societal attitudes: cultural differences, 55–56, 109, 123, 229; in education, 97–98; entrepreneurship and, 76–77; impact of, 3–4; mental health and, 169–70; volunteer projects and, 55
socioeconomic status, 203
Sonnenstrahl, Deborah, 251–63
Soukup, Benjamin, 3–9
South Africa, 17–20, 138–39
Spain, 375
Spradley, James, 296
Stokoe, William, 227–28
Strauss, Karen Peltz, 380–85
Sullivan, Anne, 268–69
Supalla, Sam, 276, 345
surdophrenia, 165
Sutcliffe, Ronald, 66–72
Sutton-Spence, R., 242, 244
Svarthom, Kristina, 114, 117
Sweden, 114–17, 138, 405–9

tactile sign language, 324–25, *325*, *329*, 344–48, *345*
Taub, Sarah, 242, 284–89
TDCA (Television Decoder Circuitry Act), 201–2
teacher training, 21–23, 229
Teaching Indians to be White, 83–84
technology: captioning, 360, 380–81, 387–88; communication impact, 150, 155; in developing countries, 62, 231; educational media, 359–60, 386–90; genetic science, 351–56, 370–75; hearing aids, 53, 136; home networks, 361; Internet access, 357–58; telecommunications access, 18, 201–2, 358–59, 380–85; wireless communications, 358–59, 376–79, *377*. See also cochlear implants
teenagers. *See* youth
telecommunications access, 18, 201–2, 358–59, 380–85
Telecommunications Act, 202, 380, 384
Television Circuitry Decoder Act, 381
Thailand, 21–25, *22*, 398–404
theater, 247, 268–69

Three Lights in the Darkness (Pitrois), 269–70
Thumann-Prezioso, Carlene, 87–95
Tibet, 229
Toomer, Jean, 274
Torres, M., 185
Trois lumières dans la nuit (Pitrois), 269–70
Turgeon, Michel, 178–80
tutor training, 222–24

UH (University of Hawai'i), 33
Ukraine, 66–70
United Kingdom, 219–26, 248–49, 293–300
United States ex rel. Negron v. New York, 341
UN (United Nations), 13, 15–16, 29

vaudeville theater, 268–69
Veditz, George, 233–34
Vehmas, Simo, 11–12
Vietnam, 21, 24
Villacin, Cecilia, 215
Vukotic, Dragoljub, 214

Walter, J., 182–83
Watkins, Mary, 386–90
WDL (World Deaf Leadership) project, 21–25
Wells, Frank, 394
WFD (World Federation of the Deaf), 7, 15
White, Barbara, 125
Wilhite, Alex, 251–63
Wilson, Amy, 52–57
wireless communications, 358–59, 376–79, *377*
WISDOM project, 376–79, *377*
Woll, B., 242, 244
women and sports, 301–4
Wood, S., 236
Woodward, James, 21, 23
Wright, C.A., 342

youth: about, 145–51; CODAs, 152–59; DBU (Deaf-Blind Youth), 405–9; identity development, 414–16; interaction with older Deaf people, 230; programs for, 8, 398–404; Russian organizations, 410–13

Zimmer, Heidi, 393–97

Flagler College Library
P.O. Box 1027
St. Augustine, FL 32085